W9-BUC-787

REVIEW COPY

Please submit two tear sheets of review.

U.S. list price: $98.00

With the compliments of
FUTURA PUBLISHING COMPANY, INC.
135 Bedford Road, PO Box 418,
Armonk, NY 10504-0418
Web Site: www.futuraco.com

Endocarditis

A Multidisciplinary Approach to Modern Treatment

edited by

Angelo A. Vlessis, M.D., Ph.D.

Albert Starr Academic Center, St. Vincent Hospital,
Portland, Oregon
Clinical Assistant Professor of Surgery
Oregon Health Sciences University
Portland, Oregon
Director of Cardiac Surgery, St. Charles Medical Center,
Bend, Oregon

Steven F. Bolling, M.D.

Professor of Cardiac Surgery, Section of Thoracic Surgery
University of Michigan Medical Center
Ann Arbor, Michigan

**Futura Publishing
Company, Inc.**
Armonk, N.Y.

Library of Congress Cataloging-in-Publication Data
Endocarditis : a multidisciplinary approach to modern treatment /
   edited by Angelo A. Vlessis, Steven F. Bolling.
         p.   cm.
   Includes bibliographical references and index.
   ISBN 0-87993-433-6 (alk. paper)
   1. Endocarditis.   2. Infective endocarditis.   I. Vlessis, Angelo
A.   II. Bolling, Steven.
   [DNLM: 1. Endocarditis.   WG 285 E569 1999]
   RC685.E5E545   1999
   616.1′1—dc21
   DNLM/DLC
   for Library of Congress   99-26873
                                                                                      CIP

Copyright 1999
Futura Publishing Company, Inc.

Published by
Futura Publishing Company, Inc.
135 Bedford Road
Armonk, NY 10504

LC#: 99-26873
ISBN#: 0-87993-433-6

Every effort has been made to ensure that the information in this book is
as up to date and as accurate as possible at the time of publication. However, due to the constant developments in medicine, the author, the editor,
or the publisher cannot accept any legal or any other responsibility for
any errors or omissions that may occur.

All rights reserved.
No part of this book may be translated or reproduced in any form without
written permission of the publisher.

Printed in the United States of America
This book is printed on acid-free paper.

Dedication

To all the physicians, surgeons and scientists
who have struggled to understand this devastating disease,
this book celebrates the culmination of their efforts.

Angelo A. Vlessis
Steven F. Bolling

Contributors

David H. Adams, M.D.
Assistant Professor of Surgery; Co-Director, Cardiac
Transplantation Division of Cardiac Surgery, Brigham and
Women's Hospital, Harvard Medical School, Boston,
Massachusetts

Lishan Aklog, M.D.
Assistant Professor of Surgery; Division of Cardiac Surgery,
Brigham and Women's Hospital, Harvard Medical School, Boston,
Massachusetts

Agustin Arbulu, M.D.
Clinical Professor of Surgery, Division of Cardiothoracic Surgery,
Wayne State University, Detroit, Michigan

Wendy S. Armstrong, M.D.
Fellow in Infectious Disease, Department of Internal Medicine,
Division of Infectious Disease, University of Michigan Medical
Center, Ann Arbor, Michigan

David S. Bach, M.D.
Assistant Professor of Medicine, Department of Internal Medicine,
Division of Cardiology, University of Michigan Medical Center,
Ann Arbor, Michigan

Suhas Bendre, M.D.
Fellow in Cardiac Surgery, Albert Starr Academic Center,
Providence St. Vincent Medical Center, Portland, Oregon

John Blizzard, M.D.
Staff Cardiothoracic Surgeon, Veterans Administration Hospital
and Medical Center, Portland, Oregon

Steven F. Bolling, M.D.
Professor of Cardiac Surgery, Section of Cardiac Surgery,
University of Michigan Medical Center, Ann Arbor, Michigan

Edward L. Bove, M.D.
Professor of Cardiac Surgery, Section of Cardiac Surgery, University of Michigan Medical Center, Ann Arbor, Michigan

Blasé A. Carabello, M.D.
Professor of Medicine, Charles Ezra Daniel Professor of Cardiology, Division of Cardiology and Gazes Cardiac Research Institute, Ralph H. Johnson Department of Veterans Affairs, Medical University of South Carolina, Charleston, South Carolina

Julia Dahl, M.D.
Fellow in Surgical Pathology, Department of Pathology, University of Washington Medical Center, Seattle, Washington

G. Michael Deeb, M.D.
Professor of Cardiac Surgery, Section of Cardiac Surgery, University of Michigan Medical Center, Ann Arbor, Michigan

N. Cary Engleberg, M.D.
Professor of Internal Medicine; Chief, Division of Infectious Diseases, University of Michigan Medical Center, Ann Arbor, Michigan

Steven Gellman, M.D.
Assistant Professor of Medicine, Division of Cardiology, Wayne State University, Detroit, Michigan, Chief of Cardiology, Detroit Receiving Hospital, Wayne State University, Detroit, Michigan

Reuben Gobezie, M.D.
Division of Cardiac Surgery, Brigham and Women's Hospital, Harvard Medical School, Boston, Massachusetts

Gary L. Grunkemeier, Ph.D.
Director, Medical Data Research Center, Providence St. Vincent Medical Center & Albert Starr Academic Center, Portland, Oregon

Donald Levine, M.D.
Professor of Medicine, Division of Infectious Diseases, Wayne State University, Detroit, Michigan, Chief of Infectious Diseases, Detroit Receiving Hospital, Wayne State University, Detroit, Michigan

Hui-Hua Li, M.D.
Postdoctoral Research Fellow, Providence St. Vincent Medical Center & Albert Starr Academic Center, Portland, Oregon

Bruce W. Lytle, M.D.
Surgeon, Department of Cardiothoracic Surgery, Cleveland Clinic Foundation, Cleveland, Ohio

Ralph S. Mosca, M.D.
Assistant Professor of Cardiac Surgery, Section of Thoracic Surgery, University of Michigan Medical Center, Ann Arbor, Michigan

Amy A. Pruitt, M.D.
Associate Professor of Neurology, Department of Neurology, University of Pennsylvania Medical Center, Philadelphia, Pennsylvania

Charles F. Schwartz, M.D.
Fellow in Cardiac Surgery, Section of Cardiac Surgery, University of Michigan Medical Center, Ann Arbor, Michigan

Michael Shea, M.D.
Professor of Internal Medicine, Department of Internal Medicine, Division of Cardiology, University of Michigan Medical Center, Ann Arbor, Michigan

Albert Starr, M.D.
Director, Heart Institute, Providence St. Vincent Hospital, Portland, Oregon, Director, Albert Starr Academic Center, Providence St. Vincent Hospital, Portland, Oregon, Professor of Surgery, Oregon Health Sciences University, Portland, Oregon

Larry W. Stephenson, M.D.
Ford-Webber Professor of Surgery, Chief, Division of Cardiothoracic Surgery, Wayne State University, Detroit, Michigan

David C. Stuesse, M.D.
Surgery Resident, Department of Surgery, Oregon Health Sciences University, Portland, Oregon

Donald D. Trunkey, M.D.
Professor of Surgery, Chairman, Department of Surgery, Oregon Health Sciences University, Portland, Oregon

Angelo A. Vlessis, M.D., Ph.D.
Director of Cardiac Surgery, St. Charles Hospital, Bend, Oregon, Principal Investigator, Albert Starr Academic Center, Providence St. Vincent Hospital, Portland, Oregon, Clinical Assistant Professor of Surgery, Oregon Health Sciences University, Portland, Oregon

Foreword

Our book on endocarditis differs significantly from past publications in that it reflects the explosive advancements in medical and surgical technology that have been made over the last few decades. Endocarditis was uniformly fatal less than 50 years ago. With the discovery of antibiotics, a few select individuals were able to survive. Over the last 40 years, the introduction of cardiopulmonary bypass, newer antibiotics, better blood culture techniques, echocardiography and valve replacement devices has fueled the decrease in mortality to between 10% and 15% at experienced centers. The patient's ability to survive this treacherous disease today is undoubtedly a culmination of technological advancement and an better understanding overall of the disease process by the treating physicians and surgeons.

With this in mind, this book focuses on the multidisciplinary aspects of the diagnosis, management and treatment of endocarditis which have evolved and continue to evolve at a rapid pace. In order to provide the best treatment to a patient with endocarditis, the clinician must be aware of these advancements and know how, and when, to implement them. Therefore, contemporary clinicians who encounter patients with endocarditis must have an understanding of: infectious disease, cardiopulmonary dysfunction from sepsis and valvular destruction, the application and interpretation of echocardiography, the use of inotropic and vasoactive drugs, surgical options to eradicate and treat valvular infection, clinical laboratory tests used to diagnosis and assess adequacy of treatment, and so on. The book contains up-to-date information on all of these topics prepared by recognized experts in each discipline. The clinician who absorbs this knowledge will be better suited to provide the advanced up-to-date care required to reliably guide the endocarditis patient toward a cure.

Angelo A. Vlessis, M.D., Ph.D.
Steven F. Bolling, M.D.

Preface

Progress in all fields is most rapid and develops the most beneficial consequences at the interface between disciplines. This is true not only where basic science and technology come together but also where the various disciplines in medicine rub up against one another for the benefit of the patient. In this book, this is clearly the case. History, physiology, infectious disease, radiology, cardiology, pathology, echocardiography and surgery, among other specialties, contribute to our understanding and treatment effectiveness of endocarditis in all of its ramifications.

My own involvement, in addition to encouraging the senior author, Dr. Angelo A. Vlessis, to undertake this project, has been to deal with the surgical technicalities of endocarditis since the dawn of open-heart surgery. In the beginning of this era, endocarditis was basically a medical disease. It was hoped that antibiotics would prevent the patient's demise, but replacing or repairing infected valves was not yet an option. With the emergence of open-heart surgery, it became possible to close punched-out holes in the leaflets of heart valves but it was not until artificial valves became available that surgical treatment began to make a reliably significant difference in the patient outcome. With valve replacement as a backup, more complex valve repairs could be performed. The ability to completely excise the area of infection and restore valvular function by means of an artificial valve with predictable success emerged in the early 1960s. At this point in time, the extent of infection became a more consequential risk factor in determining the ultimate result of combined medical and surgical treatment. Clinical and echocardiographic determination of the extent of infection became more and more relevant along with antibiotic sensitivity and hemodynamic deficit. The pathways towards modern treatment of endocarditis were thereby established with early surgical intervention available as a powerful new tool.

The advent of valve replacement bore with it an unwelcome form of endocarditis, namely prosthetic valve endocarditis. In the beginning, we thought prosthetic infection would be a severely limiting factor to the development and use of valve replacement devices, since many of our early valve replacement patients developed prosthetic endocarditis, frequently due to *Staphylococcus*. These infections were catastrophic, resulting in major dehiscence of the prosthetic valve or death from unrelenting sepsis. We subsequently realized that a large number of infected patients in our early series of prosthetic valve replacement were more of a local epidemiological problem than one intrinsic to the long-term success of valve replacement. Several preventive measures were established, but the problem remains incompletely solved, of course, since the implantation of a prosthesis lowers the threshold for infection in any location, including the heart.

A disease-oriented approach involving multiple disciplines is currently the favored method to evaluate and treat patients with endocarditis. Astute clinicians can acquire a more thorough understanding of the disease by examining the viewpoints of experts in the various disciplines that care for endocarditis patients. Clearly, the beneficiary of this multidisciplinary insight is the patient. The authors have provided us with just such an opportunity in this text.

Albert Starr, M.D.
Director, Heart Institute,
St. Vincent Hospital
Professor of Surgery
Oregon Health Sciences University
Portland, Oregon

Contents

Part IV: SPECIAL CONSIDERATIONS

I

Scientific Foundation

Chapter 1

Understanding the Cardiovascular Effects of Sepsis and the Medical Therapy of Acute Valvular Destruction in Endocarditis

Blasé A. Carabello, M.D.
Angelo A. Vlessis, M.D., Ph.D.
Donald D. Trunkey, M.D.

Introduction

Profound hemodynamic changes occur secondary to the valvular dysfunction associated with endocarditis. Superimposed on these changes are the hemodynamic alterations incited by the septic syndrome itself. The overlapping effects of septicemia and valvular dysfunction often complicate the clinical picture and make the decision to operate or to continue medical therapy more difficult. A sound clinical decision can be made more effectively when an appreciation for the alterations due to septicemia and those due to valvular destruction are understood.

The concept of the sepsis syndrome has undergone recent change.[1] Current concepts incorporate the fact that the inflammatory cascade can be initiated by conditions other than bacteremia, fungemia or viremia.[2,3] The nonmicrobial forms of the septic inflammatory response syndrome (SIRS) may be important in patients undergoing cardiopulmonary bypass,

From: Vlessis AA, Bolling S (eds): *Endocarditis: A Multidisciplinary Approach to Modern Treatment.* © Futura Publishing Co., Armonk, NY, 1999.

since cardiopulmonary bypass can initiate or contribute to the inflammatory cascade. These additional factors may amplify the bacteremia-induced cardiac dysfunction after surgical treatment of endocarditis.

This chapter describes the effects of septicemia on myocardial function and vascular resistance. The effects of acute valvular dysfunction induced by the infectious process are also described. These 2 issues are discussed throughout in a manner that provides a broader understanding of their interrelationship in clinical endocarditis.

Left Ventricular Dysfunction During Sepsis

Multiple studies have repeatedly demonstrated an increase in left ventricular compliance and a decrease in the Frank-Starling relationship during human septic shock.[4-9] These changes are effectively studied using measurements obtained from the combination of the pulmonary artery catheter and the radionucleotide scan. The pulmonary artery catheter allows the measurement of cardiac output by thermodilution technique, while the radionucleotide scan provides the ventricular ejection fraction. Stroke volume is calculated from the pulmonary artery catheter determination of cardiac output as cardiac output equals stroke volume times heart rate. Since stroke volume equals the ejection fraction (determined from radionucleotide scan), ventricular end diastolic and end systolic volumes can be calculated. These studies have provided significant insight into the functional changes of the heart during sepsis.

As early as 1951, myocardial dysfunction was suspected as a cause of septic shock.[10] In a series of publications from 1984 to present, Parker and colleagues[4-6,9] describe the alterations in myocardial function. Briefly, sepsis is associated with left ventricular dilation and increased end diastolic and end systolic volumes. Ventricular performance is depressed with a marked reduction in the ejection fraction. Stroke volume is maintained, however, by the increase in ventricular volumes, an effect similar to that seen in chronic heart failure. Cardiac output is enhanced by an increase in heart rate and aided by a decrease in systemic vascular resistance. When challenged with volume, septic patients have very little increase in left ventricular stroke work. In other words, enhanced preload is not accompanied by increased performance representing a downward shift or blunting of the Frank-Starling relationship.[4] Left ventricular volumes increase with little change in left ventricular end diastolic pressure indicating a marked increase in left ventricular compliance.

In terms of treatment, volume resuscitation becomes essential during sepsis. With normal functioning left-sided cardiac valves, as left ventricular compliance increases, adequate preload is critical to maintain the filling pressures necessary to sustain stroke volume. In endocarditis, when these changes are superimposed on mitral or aortic insufficiency, the situation becomes synergistically worse. Stroke volume is maintained by regurgitant volumes which do not contribute to forward flow and the cardiac output falls dramatically from the contribution of decreased cardiac performance and valvular dysfunction.

Right Ventricular Dysfunction During Sepsis

The right ventricle has significant functional differences as compared to the left ventricle. The right ventricle is a low-pressure chamber with a thinner, and more compliant, ventricular free wall. These morphological and functional differences reflect the markedly lower resistance of the pulmonary versus systemic vascular beds. Consequently, despite the right and left ventricular stroke volumes being obligatorily equal, the right ventricular stroke work is much lower than the left ventricular stroke work. With this in mind, sepsis is associated with a characteristic increase in pulmonary vascular resistance.[11–13] As a result, right ventricular stroke work increases in sepsis.[14] Right ventricular compliance also increases (as in the left ventricle) leading to increased right ventricular end diastolic volumes. Ejection fraction decreases, as overall stroke volume remains the same.[8,14–18] Therefore, although both the right and left ventricle demonstrate increased compliance during sepsis, the right ventricle must work against an increased pulmonary vascular resistance while the left ventricle works against a decreased systemic vascular resistance.

In endocarditis, valvular dysfunction places additional demands on the right ventricle. Mitral or aortic insufficiency will increase left atrial pressures and further increase pulmonary vascular resistance, thereby demanding further increases in right ventricular stroke work. Tricuspid regurgitation increases right ventricular end diastolic and systolic volume in addition to the volume changes associated with the increased right ventricular compliance incited by sepsis. Since the pressure-to-volume relationship is lower over a wider range in the right ventricle as compared to the left ventricle, massive right ventricular enlargement may often accompany the active phase of tricuspid endocarditis.[14]

Other factors related to sepsis may affect right ventricular function. Coagulation abnormalities and pulmonary microemboli may increase pulmonary vascular resistance, right ventricular pressure and right ventricular end diastolic pressure.[19,20] Diastolic dilatation of the right ventricle combined with confinement by the relatively rigid pericardium can cause the ventricular septum to encroach on the left ventricle, thereby reducing left ventricular stroke volume and decreasing cardiac output.[21,22]

Mechanisms of Myocardial Dysfunction During Sepsis

Early studies suggested that myocardial perfusion and oxygen delivery were impaired during sepsis and that the decreased perfusion and oxygen delivery led to the myocardial dysfunction observed in septic patients.[23] This premise was refuted by subsequent studies that found no correlation between coronary blood flow and myocardial oxygen consumption in septic patients studied with coronary sinus catheters. Further studies in 40 patients with septic shock confirmed the fact that coronary blood flow is not reduced in sepsis and that it is actually increased.[24] In addition, they found a net lactate extraction by the heart, which argues against tissue hypoxia.[25] Substrate studies demonstrate a decrease in the uptake of glycolytic substrates and a possible shift toward the use of amino acid fuels, particularly glutamate and glutamine, during sepsis.[26] Interestingly, sepsis is associated with an enormous potential for reactive oxygen generation from the total body white blood cell mass.[27] In a recent review, a hypothesis is set forth suggesting that increased rates of reactive oxygen metabolism by the heart and other organs (kidneys, lungs, liver) may account for the myocardial and multiorgan dysfunction as well as the metabolic shifts observed during sepsis.[28]

Other investigators describe a circulating myocardial depressant factor with a molecular weight of 500 kd to 5000 kd.[29] Serum from septic patients depresses the extent and velocity of contraction in cultured neonatal myocytes. The serum from the same patients after recovery from the septic episode had a limited effect on the contractile function of the cultured myocytes. Additionally, the extent of myocyte contractile inhibition correlated with the extent of decreased left ventricular ejection fraction observed in the septic patients.

Other factors that contribute to SIRS relate to excitation-contraction coupling. SIRS can induce a drop in ionized calcium that correlates with mortality.[30] Excitation-contraction coupling is also adversely affected by a drop in myocyte intracellular cyclic adenosine monophosphate levels[31] and decreased responsiveness to adrenergic stimulation.[32,33] The blunted myocardial response to catecholamines has been confirmed in septic humans.[34] Therefore, it appears there are multiple alterations in cardiac excitation-contraction coupling that contribute to the clinical myocardial dysfunction in sepsis.

Myocardial dysfunction is a consistent, yet reversible, finding in septic patients. Despite its identification over 40 years ago, the etiology remains an elusive topic of intense investigation.

Changes in Vascular Resistance During Sepsis

Sepsis induces a profound systemic vasodilation.[35,36] The vasodilatation is global, with increased blood flow to most organs. The resultant elevation in cardiac output and enhanced oxygen delivery remains a paradox since there is little increase in tissue oxygen extraction; the difference in systemic to venous oxygen saturation narrows.

The systemic vasodilatation associated with sepsis is protective in the sense that it reduces the afterload on the dysfunctional left ventricle. Mean arterial pressure is lower and the lower diastolic perfusion pressures may impair myocardial perfusion in the presence of coexisting coronary artery disease. In the presence of normal coronary arteries, however, no evidence of myocardial ischemia exists.[24,25] Pharmacological manipulations to increase the mean arterial pressure by increasing systemic vascular resistance should be employed with caution, as they will be associated with further left ventricular dilation and decreased stroke volume by the dysfunctional myocardium. Fortunately, systemic vasodilation is often the appropriate treatment for the mitral and aortic valvular insufficiency that may accompany endocarditis (see discussion below). As antibiotics control the active phase of the infection, one can expect the vasodilatory response to subside. As systemic vascular resistance increases, vasodilating drugs such as milrinone and nitroprusside may be added to palliate the valvular component of the disease process.

Interestingly, the mechanism of systemic vasodilation appears to involve increased nitric oxide generation from activated leukocytes.[37,38] Plasma nitrate levels, an end product of nitric oxide metabolism, are elevated several-fold in septic patients and correlate with the decrease in systemic vascular resistance.[39,40] Several clinical reports using inhibitors of nitric oxide synthetase in septic patients demonstrate an increase in systemic vascular resistance and possibly a detrimental effect on survival.[41] The fact that nitric oxide synthetase inhibitors do not improve survival in septic patients is not surprising, as any increase in systemic vascular resistance would increase left ventricular end systolic volume and place additional work demands on the dysfunctional myocardium.

Acute Mitral Regurgitation

In acute mitral regurgitation, a second pathway for left ventricular ejection suddenly develops as mitral incompetence allows a large portion of the

Normal

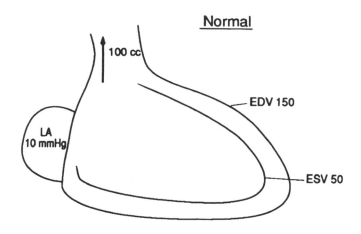

Acute MR

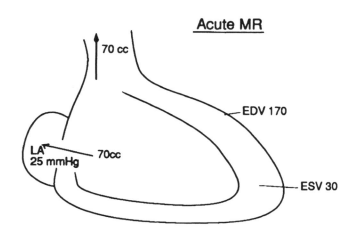

	Preload SL μ	Afterload ESS Kdyn/cm²	CF	EF	RF	FSV CC's
N	2.07	90	N	.67	.0	100
AMR	2.25	60	N	.82	.50	70

stroke volume to be regurgitated into the left atrium. The extra volume stored in the left atrium during systole increases filling of the left ventricle during diastole, making use of the Frank-Starling mechanism.[42] Thus, end diastolic volume increases, as does the work-generating capacity of the ventricle. The new pathway for ejection lowers the left ventricular imped-ance to emptying, and end systolic volume is reduced (Figure 1).[43] These changes in preload and afterload increase total stroke volume. However, 50% or more of the total stroke volume is regurgitated into the left atrium and is "wasted." Therefore, forward stroke volume decreases. At the same time, volume overload of the left atrium increases left atrial and pulmo-nary venous pressure leading to pulmonary congestion. These effects pro-duce the elements of congestive heart failure (reduced cardiac output and increased filling pressure) even though left ventricular muscle function is normal or even enhanced by activation of the sympathetic reflexes.

The presence of acute mitral regurgitation is suggested by the appear-ance of a new systolic murmur. Because acute mitral regurgitation results in a large atrial V wave, the systolic pressure gradient between the left ventricle and the left atrium rapidly equilibrates, reducing the gradient and shortening the murmur. The murmur may therefore be early systolic in nature rather than the usual holosystolic murmur of mitral regurgita-tion. The murmur may be obfuscated by the rales of pulmonary conges-tion. Unlike in chronic mitral regurgitation where left ventricular enlarge-ment is the rule, the heart is small in acute mitral regurgitation. Thus, the left ventricular apical impulse is not displaced. Reduced forward left ventricular stroke volume results in a brisk but reduced carotid upstroke with early closure of the aortic valve, sometimes causing wide splitting of S_2.

Medical therapy for acute mitral regurgitation is aimed at reducing aortic impedance and total vascular resistance. By doing so, more blood flows preferentially into the aorta (and therefore less flows into the left atrium) resulting in an increase in forward output together with a decrease in regurgitant volume. Specific therapy is chosen based on the amount of

◄───

Figure 1. Acute mitral regurgitation (AMR) is compared to normal (N) physiol-ogy. In acute mitral regurgitation, the volume overload increases preload (sarcom-ere length, SL) and end diastolic volume (EDV) increases. The regurgitant pathway unloads the left ventricle, decreases afterload (wall stress, ESS), and facilitates left ventricular ejection. Thus, end systolic volume (ESV) decreases while ejection fraction (EF) increases. Although total stroke volume increases, forward stroke volume (FSV) decreases because 50% (regurgitant fraction, RF, 0.05) of the total stroke volume is ejected into the left atrium (LA) thereby increasing left atrial pressure. Contractile function (CF) is normal. Taken from Carabello[43] with permis-sion.

regurgitation that has developed and the subsequent amount of hemodynamic compromise. In mild to moderate mitral regurgitation, there is likely to be no significant decrease in the forward output because output is maintained by use of the Frank-Starling mechanism alone; in such cases, therapy is often unnecessary. In more severe regurgitation that leads to pulmonary congestion but in which systemic blood pressure is adequate for vital organ perfusion, vasodilators and diuretics are the treatments of choice. Sodium nitroprusside is the most common agent used in acute therapy because of its potency and short half-life, which allow rapid dose titration. Nitroprusside accomplishes both arteriolar and veno dilatation, thereby simultaneously increasing forward output while decreasing left atrial pressure (Figure 2).[44] The drug is administered intravenously at a

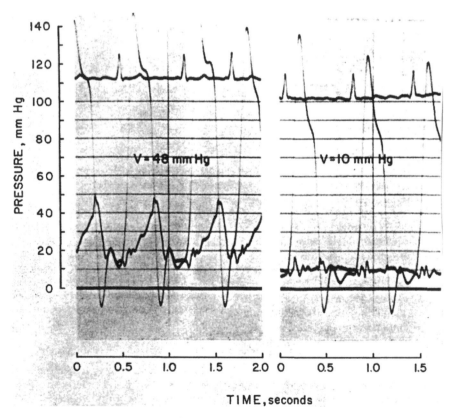

Figure 2. Simultaneous pulmonary capillary wedge pressure and left ventricular pressure tracings before (left) and after (right) sodium nitroprusside infusion. Following nitroprusside, the large V wave is reduced as is mean pulmonary capillary wedge pressure. Taken from Grossman[44] with permission.

beginning dose of 0.25 μg/kg/min and increased to the maximum dose tolerable without hypotension. Hypotension can be defined as a systolic pressure less than 90 mm Hg or a blood pressure at which renal perfusion—and therefore urinary output—falls instead of increases. In general, patients sick enough to require nitroprusside infusion also require hemodynamic monitoring with a Swan-Ganz catheter to guide therapy. By monitoring blood pressure, pulmonary capillary wedge pressure and forward output, the rate of drug infusion can be adjusted to provide the maximum benefit. Nitroprusside is continued until surgery is performed to correct the acute mitral regurgitation or until orally administrated vasodilators replace the intravenous infusion. Angiotension-converting enzyme inhibitors are the most commonly used oral agents because of their balanced arteriolar and venodilatation similar to that of nitroprusside. However, no controlled studies exist to compare angiotension-converting enzyme inhibitors to any other vasodilators. Therefore, calcium channel blockers that lack negative inotropic effects, such as amlodipine or isradipine, may also be effective. If these drugs are ineffective, hydralazine or minoxidil might also be employed. In patients in whom the mitral regurgitation is severe enough to produce hypotension, intra-aortic balloon counterpulsation is the treatment of choice. Counterpulsation reduces systolic afterload while increasing diastolic and mean blood pressure.[45] This therapy is contraindicated if there is coexistent aortic regurgitation.

In patients with acute mitral regurgitation due to endocarditis, antecedent left ventricular function is usually normal. Pressor agents may therefore have little beneficial effect in the hypotensive patient with acute severe mitral regurgitation. Pure beta agonist agents can only increase forward stroke volume by decreasing end systolic volume. However, in acute mitral regurgitation with normal left ventricular function, afterload reduction created by the regurgitant pathway allows for ejection to near-obliteration of the cavity, so end systolic volume is already reduced to the minimum. Pressor agents that cause vasoconstriction produce the unwanted effect of increasing afterload, thereby worsening the mitral regurgitation. When intra-aortic balloon counterpulsation is necessary to stabilize the patient, surgery should usually be performed once the stabilization has occurred.

Acute Aortic Regurgitation

Acute severe aortic regurgitation with even mild heart failure is usually a surgical emergency. Treated medically, mortality may be as high as 75% once heart failure becomes manifest.[46] Although no randomized trials between medical and surgical therapy have ever been performed (nor should they ever be performed), mortality in patients treated surgically appears to be one third that of patients treated medically.[47] However, there is generally a desire to send the patient to surgery with the best hemodynamic compensation that can be provided. While this approach is reasonable, medical therapy should be rapidly abandoned in favor of surgery if it is clear that hemodynamic improvement is not being effected.

The diagnosis of acute aortic regurgitation due to endocarditis is often elusive.[48] In chronic aortic regurgitation, a large stroke volume is discharged into the aorta during systole to compensate for that portion of the stroke volume which leaks back into the ventricle during diastole.[49] This high stroke volume creates most of the hyperdynamic physical signs of chronic aortic regurgitation (Corrigan's pulse, Duroziez's sign, etc.). However, in acute aortic regurgitation, eccentric hypertrophy has not had time to develop; thus, the high stroke volume, wide pulse pressure and the signs created by the 2 are absent. The only clues that severe aortic regurgitation might be present are the diastolic blowing murmur heard along the left sternal border and a soft first heart sound. The high left ventricular end diastolic pressure present in the uncompensated ventricle of acute aortic regurgitation produces rapid diastolic equilibration between the aortic and left ventricular pressure (Figure 3),[50] shortening the

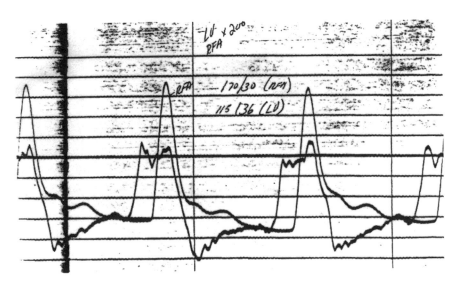

Figure 3. Simultaneous left ventricular and femoral artery pressure tracings for a patient with severe aortic regurgitation. In diastole, there is rapid early equilibration of the 2 pressures. Augmentation of femoral systolic pressure (Hill's sign) is also demonstrated. Taken from Carabello et al[50] with permission.

murmur of aortic regurgitation and making it seem unimpressive. This high diastolic pressure also causes mitral valve preclosure (before ventricular systole). Thus, when ventricular systole is initiated, the mitral valve is already closed and S_1 is soft. Because acute aortic insufficiency can be severe despite an unimpressive physical examination, echocardiography should be performed in all cases where aortic regurgitation is suspected. During echocardiography, the cause of acute aortic insufficiency can usually be demonstrated. Mitral valve preclosure can be confirmed and is an ominous sign, usually indicative of the need for surgery.[51]

The goal of medical therapy in acute aortic regurgitation is to decrease the regurgitant volume and to decrease left ventricular filling pressure. This is generally accomplished by the infusion of nitroprusside. However, if the patient has borderline systemic pressure, vasodilators may worsen hypotension. Pressor agents will cause peripheral vasoconstriction and may actually increase the amount of regurgitation. Intra-aortic balloon counterpulsation is not effective and is in fact contraindicated because it increases the amount of aortic regurgitation. In acute aortic regurgitation caused by infective endocarditis, there is always concern that urgent surgery prior to a sustained period of antibiotic administration will lead to reinfection of the new valve. Fortunately, studies indicate that the reinfection rate is low, 0% to 10%.[52] Therefore, surgery should not be delayed in unstable patients.

Tricuspid Regurgitation

Tricuspid regurgitation is usually recognizable by the presence of a holosystolic murmur heard along the left sternal border. Murmur intensity increases with inspiration. However, murmur augmentation may not occur if right ventricular function is compromised, because in that case inspiration cannot augment right ventricular stroke volume. Examination of the neck veins in tricuspid regurgitation demonstrates a large V wave. The right ventricle is enlarged and is detectable as a parasternal lift. The liver is enlarged and may be pulsatile.

The acute tricuspid regurgitation that occurs in endocarditis is usually well tolerated, as is the total removal of the valve.[53] Diuretics alone are usually sufficient to lower right atrial pressure and to treat the edema which may develop. Vasodilators have less of an effect on the pulmonary circulation than on the systemic circulation and thus are not usually effective in treating the disease. If acute tricuspid regurgitation is due to pulmonary hypertension, treating the cause of the pulmonary hypertension will reduce the amount of the tricuspid regurgitation. Therefore, if severe obstructive pulmonary disease is responsible, improvement in pulmonary function to improve oxygenation and decrease hypercarbia will diminish pulmonary vasoconstriction, helping to decrease the tricuspid regurgitation. If tricuspid regurgitation is secondary to the pulmonary hypertension that develops from left ventricular failure, intensification of the heart failure regimen is indicated. As diuretics and vasodilators lower the patient's left ventricular filling pressure, pulmonary artery pressure also diminishes, thus helping to improve right ventricular function and to restore tricuspid valve competence. If valvular disease such as mitral stenosis is responsible for pulmonary hypertension and subsequent tricuspid regurgitation, and surgery is not planned, balloon valvotomy will reduce pulmonary hypertension and help to reduce tricuspid regurgitation.[54]

Summary

The sepsis syndrome induces characteristic changes in myocardial and circulatory function during the active phase of endocarditis. These changes are often superimposed on the hemodynamic alterations resulting from valvular destruction. In order to fully understand the disease process in a given patient, one must separate the cardiovascular effects of sepsis from those of the valvular insufficiency. Only then can a reasonable and appropriate decision be made about the timing and mode of therapy. Sepsis incites an increase in left and right ventricular compliance and suppresses systolic function. This leads to increased end diastolic and systolic volumes and a reduced ejection fraction. Stroke volume is maintained and increases in cardiac output result from an increase in heart rate and a decrease in systemic vascular resistance. Knowledge of these septic-induced changes in cardiac function can facilitate the clinical decision-making process. For example, effective antibiotic treatment may control progression of infection within 24 to 48 hours and reverse the cardiovascular effects of sepsis. With improved cardiac performance, valvular insufficiency is more easily compensated for and the patient's overall hemodynamic condition may stabilize. In this instance, an emergent operation for valvular insufficiency in a patient with depressed cardiac function may be postponed to a semielective operation in a patient with improving cardiac function. Likewise, sound knowledge of the physiologic consequences of acute valvular dysfunction leads to earlier identification and initiation of appropriate medical therapy. This aids in the stabilization of the patient with infective endocarditis and can deliver him or her to the operating room in a more compensated condition or palliate him or her while sustained doses of antibiotics are administered.

References

1. Bone C. Sepsis, the sepsis syndrome, multi-organ failure: A plea for comparable definitions. *Ann Intern Med* 1991;114:332–341.
2. Rangel-Frausto SM, Pittet D, Costigan M, et al. The natural history of systemic inflammatory response syndrome. *JAMA* 1995;273:117–123.
3. Vincent JL, Bihari DJ, Suter PM. Prevalence of nosocomial infection in intensive care units in Europe. *JAMA* 1995;274:639–644.
4. Ognibene FD, Parker MM, Natanson C, et al. Depressed left ventricular performance: Response to volume infusion in patients with sepsis and septic shock. *Chest* 1988;93:903–910.
5. Parker MM, Shelhamer JH, Bacharach SL, et al. Profound but reversible myocardial depression in patients with septic shock. *Ann Intern Med* 1984;100:483–490.
6. Parker MM, Suffredini AF, Natanson C, et al. Responses of left ventricular function in survivors and nonsurvivors of septic shock. *J Crit Care* 1989;4:19–25.
7. Jardin F, Brun-Ney D, Auvert B, et al. Sepsis-related cardiogenic shock. *Crit Care Med* 1990;18:1055–1060.
8. Kimchi A, Ellrodt AG, Berman BS, et al. Right ventricular performance in septic shock: A combined radionucleotide and hemodynamic study. *J Am Coll Cardiol* 1984;4:945–951.
9. Parker MM, Ognibene FP, Parrillo JE. Peak systolic pressure/end-systolic volume ratio, a load-independent measure of ventricular function, is reversibly decreased in human septic shock. *Crit Care Med* 1994;22:1955–1959.
10. Waisbren BA. Bacteremia due to gram-negative bacilli other than *Salmonella*. *Arch Intern Med* 1951;88:467–488.
11. Clowes GHA, Farrington GH, Zuschneid W, et al. Circulating factors in the etiology of pulmonary insufficiency and right heart failure accompanying severe sepsis. *Ann Surg* 1970;171:663–678.
12. Vito L, Dennis RC, Weisel RD, et al. Sepsis presenting as acute respiratory insufficiency. *Surg Gynecol Obstet* 1974;138:896–900.
13. Sibbald WJ, Paterson NAM, Holliday RL, et al. Pulmonary hypertension in sepsis: Measurement by the pulmonary artery diastolic-pulmonary wedge pressure gradient and the influence of passive and active factors. *Chest* 1978;73:583–591.
14. Hoffman MJ, Greenfield LJ, Sugerman HJ, et al. Unsuspected right ventricular dysfunction in shock and sepsis. *Ann Surg* 1983;198:307–317.
15. Dhainaut JF, Lanore JJ, de Gournay JM, et al. Right ventricular dysfunction in patients with septic shock. *Intensive Care Med* 1988;14:488–491.
16. Schneider AJ, Teule GJJ, Groeneveld ABJ, et al. Biventricular performance during volume loading in patients with early septic shock, with emphasis on the right ventricle. *Am Heart J* 1988;116:103–112.
17. Vincent JL, Reuse C, Frank N, et al. Right ventricular dysfunction in septic shock. *Acta Anaesthesiol Scand* 1989;33:34–38.
18. Redl G, Germann P, Plattner H, et al. Right ventricular function in early septic shock states. *Intensive Care Med* 1993;19:3–7.
19. Sturm JA, Lewis FR, Trentz O, et al. Cardiopulmonary parameters and prognosis after severe multiple trauma. *J Trauma* 1979;19:305–318.

20. Blaisdell FW. Pathophysiology of the respiratory distress syndrome. *Arch Surg* 1974;108:44–49.
21. Glantz SA, Misbach GA, Moores WY, et al. The pericardium substantially affects the left ventricular diastolic pressure-volume relationship in the dog. *Circ Res* 1978;42:433–441.
22. Maughan WL, Shoukas AA, Sagawa K, et al. Instantaneous pressure-volume relationship of the canine right ventricle. *Circ Res* 1979;44:309–315.
23. Hinshaw LB, Archer LT, Spitzer JJ, et al. Effects of coronary hypotension and endotoxin on myocardial performance. *Am J Physiol* 1974;227:1051–1057.
24. Dhainaut JF, Huyghebaert MF, Monsallier JF, et al. Coronary hemodynamics and myocardial metabolism of lactate, free fatty acids, glucose and ketones in patients with septic shock. *Circulation* 1987;75:533–541.
25. Cunnion RE, Schaer GL, Parker MM, et al. The coronary circulation in human septic shock. *Circulation* 1986;73:637–644.
26. Hotchkiss RS, Song SK, Neill JJ, et al. Sepsis does not impair tricarboxylic acid cycle in the heart. *Am J Physiol* 1991;260:C50–C57.
27. Vlessis AA, Bartos D, Muller P, et al. Role of reactive O_2 in phagocyte-induced hypermetabolism and pulmonary injury. *J Appl Physiol* 1995;78:112–116.
28. Vlessis AA, Goldman RK, Trunkey DD. New concepts in the pathophysiology of oxygen metabolism during sepsis. *Br J Surg* 1995;82:870–876.
29. Parrillo JE, Burch C, Shelhamer JH, et al. A circulating myocardial depressant substance in humans with septic shock. *J Clin Invest* 1985;76:1539–1553.
30. Woo P, Carpenter MA, Trunkey DD. Ionized calcium: The effect of septic shock in the human. *J Surg Res* 1979;26:605–610.
31. Carmona RA, Tsao T, Dae M, et al. Myocardial dysfunction in septic shock. *Arch Surg* 1985;120:30–35.
32. Shepard RE, McDonough KH, Burns AH. Mechanism of cardiac dysfunction in hearts from endotoxin treated rats. *Circ Shock* 1986;19:371–384.
33. Reithmann C, Hallstrom S, Pilz G, et al. Desensitization of rat cardiomyocyte adenyl cyclase stimulation by plasma of noradrenaline-treated patients with septic shock. *Circ Shock* 1993;41:48–59.
34. Silverman HJ, Penaranda R, Orens JB, et al. Impaired beta adrenergic receptor stimulation of cyclic adenosine monophosphate in human septic shock: Association with myocardial hyporesponsiveness to catecholamines. *Crit Care Med* 1993;21:31–39.
35. Ognibene FP. Hemodynamic support during sepsis. *Clin Chest Med* 1996;17(2):279–287.
36. Hotchkiss RS, Karl IE. Reevaluation of the role of cellular hypoxia and bioenergetic failure in sepsis. *JAMA* 1992;267:1503–1510.
37. Wagner D, Young V, Tannenbaum S. Mammalian nitrate biosynthesis: Incorporation of $^{15}NH_3$ into nitrate is enhanced by endotoxin treatment. *Proc Natl Acad Sci USA* 1983;80:4518–4521.
38. Payen D, Bernard C, Belouif S. Nitric oxide in sepsis. *Clin Chest Med* 1996;17(2):333–350.
39. Ochoa J, Udekwu A, Billiar T, et al. Nitrogen oxide levels in patients after trauma and during sepsis. *Ann Surg* 1991;214:621–626.
40. Petros A, Lamb G, Leone A, et al. Effects of a nitric oxide synthase inhibitor in humans with septic shock. *Cardiovasc Res* 1994;28:34–39.
41. Preiser J, Lejeune P, Roman A, et al. Methylene blue administration in septic shock: A clinical trial. *Crit Care Med* 1995;23:259–264.

42. Urschel CW,Covell JWS, Sonnenblick EH, et al. Myocardial mechanics in aortic and mitral valvular regurgitation: The concept of instantaneous impedance as a determinant of the performance of the intact heart. *J Clin Invest* 1968;47: 867–883.
43. Carabello BA. Mitral regurgitation, part 1: Basic pathophysiologic principles. *Modern Concepts Cardiovasc Dis* 1988;57:53–58.
44. Grossman W. Profiles in valvular heart disease. In Grossman W, Baim DS (eds.) *Cardiac Catheterization, Angiography, and Intervention*, 5th ed. Baltimore, MD. Williams & Wilkins, 1996. pp 735–756.
45. Horstkotte D, Schulte HD, Niehues R, et al. Diagnostic and therapeutic considerations in acute, severe mitral regurgitation: Experience in 42 consecutive patients entering the intensive care unit with pulmonary edema. *J Heart Valve Dis* 1993;2:512–522.
46. Croft CH, Woodward W, Elliott A, et al. Analysis of surgical versus medical therapy in active complicated native valve infective endocarditis. *Am J Cardiol* 1983;51:1650–1655.
47. Cohn LH, Birjiniuk V. Therapy of acute aortic regurgitation. *Cardiol Clin* 1991; 9:339–352.
48. Mann T, McLaurin L, Grossman W, et al. Assessing the hemodynamic severity of acute aortic regurgitation due to infective endocarditis. *N Engl J Med* 1975; 293:108–113.
49. Carabello BA. Aortic regurgitation: Hemodynamic determinants of prognosis. In Cohn LH (ed.) *Aortic Regurgitation*. New York, NY. Marcel Dekker, 1986. pp 87–106.
50. Carabello BA, Ballard WL, Gazes PC. In Sahn SA, Heffner JE (eds.) *Cardiology Pearls*. Philadelphia, PA. Hanley & Belfus, 1994. pp 45–46.
51. Sareli P, Klein HO, Schamroth CL, et al. Contribution of echocardiography and immediate surgery to the management of severe aortic regurgitation from active infective endocarditis. *Am J Cardiol* 1986;57:413–418.
52. Agnihotri AK, McGiffin DC, Galbraith AJ, et al. The prevalence of infective endocarditis after aortic valve replacement. *J Thorac Cardiovasc Surg* 1995;110: 1708–1720.
53. Arbulu A, Thoms NW, Wilson RF. Valvulectomy without prosthetic replacement: A lifesaving operation for tricuspid *Pseudomonas* endocarditis. *J Thorac Cardiovasc Surg* 1972;64:103–107.
54. Skudicky D, Essop MR, Sareli P. Efficacy of mitral balloon valvotomy in reducing the severity of associated tricuspid valve regurgitation. *Am J Cardiol* 1994; 73:209–211.

Chapter 2

Pathological and Clinical Laboratory Diagnosis Of Infective Endocarditis

Julia Dahl, M.D.
Angelo A. Vlessis, M.D., Ph.D.

Introduction

Historically, the diagnosis of infective endocarditis has been difficult to secure. The role of the clinical laboratory is to provide objective evidence of endovascular infection by documenting continuous bacteremia. Infecting organisms are identified and antimicrobial therapy is guided by antibiotic sensitivities. Associated hematologic and immunologic manifestations are easily documented; however, these measurements currently have little impact on diagnosis and treatment.

The roles of the clinical laboratory and pathologist continue to evolve with the disease process. Antimicrobial resistance, demographic alterations and emerging pathogens in immune compromised patients require modifications and expansion of culture techniques. Technological advancements such as continuous monitoring blood culture systems, immunologic assays and polymerase chain reaction continually refine the laboratory's role. Managed care and cost containment measures are superimposed on these changes and may lead to decreased on-site testing and outpatient management of endocarditis. The result is an evolution in the criteria used to establish the diagnosis of endocarditis and a constant re-evaluation of these criteria as newer technologies are applied.[1-3]

From: Vlessis AA, Bolling S (eds): *Endocarditis: A Multidisciplinary Approach to Modern Treatment.* © Futura Publishing Co., Armonk, NY, 1999.

Most recently, the Duke criteria have demonstrated improved diagnostic value compared to previous criteria, both in reaching the diagnosis of "definitive endocarditis" and in excluding patients from the diagnosis.[4–6] A definitive diagnosis of endocarditis requires culture or histological examination of surgical and/or autopsy specimens. In the absence of tissue for evaluation, the diagnosis hinges on blood culture results as well as echocardiographic and clinical findings which collectively imply endocardial infection. Identifying the etiologic organism directs the choice and duration of antimicrobial therapy and may obviate the need for further diagnostic testing. Antimicrobial sensitivity testing is essential in the age of resistant microorganisms and helps predict therapeutic outcome. Methods of monitoring the effectiveness of therapy have traversed times of controversy and emerged with an emphasis on methods that assist in the early detection of inadequate therapy, complications, or recurrence.

Mortality and morbidity for patients with endocarditis remain significant despite recent improvements in both diagnosis and treatment. While blood cultures are currently the "gold standard" for microorganism identification, molecular techniques of microorganism identification are being developed rapidly and promise a means of earlier diagnosis and possibly a new gold standard. Antimicrobial sensitivity testing remains critical. Advances in antibiotic pharmacokinetic understanding may eventually allow the translation of serum bactericidal activity to antibiotic activity within foci of endovascular infection and allow a more accurate therapeutic outcome estimation. Currently, response to therapy is evaluated by nonspecific measures of inflammation. These may be replaced by specific serum component measurements which differentiate inflammation from continuing infection. Continued advancements in laboratory techniques should effect a more rapid and accurate diagnosis of endocarditis, leading to an earlier institution of effective treatment, thus further decreasing the morbidity and mortality.

Clinical laboratory physicians are instrumental in the development, evaluation and implementation of new methodologies while also remaining a valuable resource to clinical practitioners. Consultation of laboratory physicians may become more commonplace as laboratory techniques and their interpretation continue to be increasingly complex.

Pathological Criteria for Definitive Infective Endocarditis: Tissue Culture, Gross and Histological Examination

A definitive diagnosis of endocarditis is attained by demonstrating microorganisms by culture or histology in a valvular vegetation or intracardiac abscess, or by demonstrating histopathological features of active endocarditis within a vegetation or intracardiac abscess.[1-3] Material for examination is obtained during open heart surgery or peripheral embolectomy, via percutaneous endocardial biopsy, or at autopsy.

Tissue Culture

Tissue culture is warranted if blood cultures have not recovered the infecting microorganism or if results are pending at the time of surgery or autopsy. Cultures may be performed on excised valves, prosthetic valve material or abscess/fistulae material. Communication with the pathologist and/or the microbiology laboratory prior to the operation is strongly recommended as knowledge of the pertinent clinical history and the suspected infectious organism may influence tissue handling and culture technique. A pathologist should supervise proper specimen evaluation and handling whenever possible.

Requirements for submitting tissue for culture and histological examination vary among institutions. Generally, all excised valvular vegetation or abscess material should be placed in sterile containers. It is unnecessary to add media or sterile saline to the tissue unless transport to the laboratory requires longer than 1 hour. [7-9] Viable organisms present on the surface of the vegetations and within microabscesses are protected from dessication. At some institutions, all tissue may be directed to surgical pathology. The pathologist or assistant will oversee culture prior to continuing with the gross and histological examination. Indicate clearly on the surgical pathology requisition "rule out endocarditis" and "submit for culture." The clinical history should be written directly on the surgical pathology requisition, especially if specific or uncommon organisms are suspected.

At other institutions, it may be necessary to submit tissue to the microbiology laboratory separately from tissue submitted to surgical pathology. If so, place equal portions of the tissue material into sterile containers. Placing both tissue samples in sterile containers may provide an additional tissue source for culture in the event of mishandling or mislabeling. If separate tissue is submitted for culture, indicate on the surgical pathology specimen "rule out endocarditis" and "separate tissue submitted for culture." This will avert duplication of resources.

In the microbiology laboratory, the initial processing of tissue samples begins with touch preparation smears for Gram's stain examination. The remaining tissue is homogenized before culture. Tissue homogenization by grinding may destroy hyphal elements and reduce the recovery of some fungal organisms.[7,8,10] Therefore, it is essential that any suspicion of fungal endocarditis be conveyed to the microbiology laboratory. Homogenized tissue is then inoculated for aerobic and anaerobic culture. Most causative organisms are recovered using enrichment broth, blood agar, chocolate agar, anaerobic agar, MacConkey agar and eosin-methylene blue (EMB) agar.[7–11] Unused tissue should be stored at 4°C for several weeks in the event repeated cultures are required.[7–10] Quantitative tissue cultures are superfluous. Endocardium is normally sterile, therefore all organisms recovered from endovascular surfaces imply infection, even in immune compromised hosts. Culture requirements for unusual microorganisms are discussed in the section headed Culture-negative Endocarditis, below.

Postmortem tissue can be submitted for bacteriologic examination when infection is suspected as cause of death. In this case, the utility of tissue culture may be in differentiating community-acquired from nosocomial infections. Resident microflora overgrowth limits the usefulness of postmortem cultures to cadavers maintained at room temperature for less than 4 hours or at 4°C beyond 24 hours.[7,9,10] Normally, there is no resident microflora of the heart and valves. Pericardium or vessel disruption during surgery may interfere with the accepted "sterility" of this area. Necropsy tissues acceptable for bacteriological evaluation are processed as routine tissue cultures.[7–10] If blood or previous tissue culture has recovered a causative organism, postmortem examination is limited to the histological findings.

Routine culture of excised tissue at valve replacement surgery is not warranted in the absence of a history of infective endocarditis. Giladi and colleagues cultured excised valve material and valve identification tags of newly inserted prosthetic valves in 224 patients undergoing valve replacement and demonstrated a 12% culture positivity rate.[12] The spectrum of recovered organisms was similar to that seen in native valve endocarditis. No patient had evidence of preoperative infection, postoperative prosthetic valve endocarditis, or another infection with the same organism that had been isolated from the valve tissue. Additionally, the histological examination did not show features of endocarditis. Therefore, routine valve tissue or valve identification tag cultures have no clinical utility in the absence of a prior history of endocarditis.[12]

Gross Valvular Tissue Examination

Most valvular tissue received at our institution receives only gross examination. Histological evaluation is performed upon request or if there is a grossly apparent vegetation. Again, communicating the clinical history is essential to proper specimen handling.

Grossly, vegetations are the hallmark of endocarditis. Vegetations are collections of platelets, fibrin, microorganisms, exopolysaccharides and necrotic debris produced by the microorganism and inflammatory cells. Vegetations may occur on any endocardial surface including native valve leaflets, ventricular endocardium, mural thrombi, atrial endocardium (MacCallum's patch) and the intimal surface of the great vessels.[13,14] Prosthetic material (e.g. the sewing ring, valve leaflets and vascular patches) may also develop vegetations. Infective lesions are impacted by blood flow patterns and correspond to sites of turbulent or high velocity flow.[13,14] Atrioventricular valve vegetations usually occur on the atrial surface of the valves, while involvement of the ventricular surface predominates on the semilunar valves.[14,15] Vegetations more typically occur along valve closure lines and may spread to adjacent valve cusps, forming "kissing" lesions (Figure 1).[14] Congenital abnormalities (i.e., bicuspid aortic valve and ventricular septal defect), rheumatic and degenerative valve disease all predispose to infective endocarditis via alterations in blood flow patterns.[13,16] These features should be noted in both the operative and surgical pathology reports.

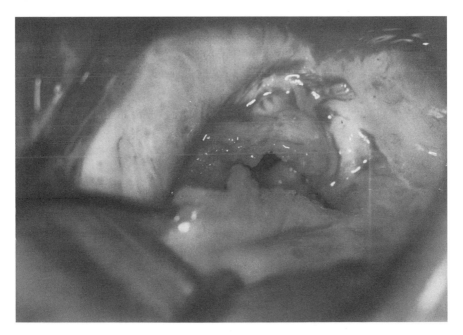

Figure 1. Mitral valve endocarditis intraoperative view involving both the anterior and posterior leaflets, a "kissing" lesion. Reproduced with permission: Antunes, MJ. *Mitral Valve Repair*. Starnberg, Germany, Verlag RS Schulz, 1989. p 49. (See color appendix.)

The appearance of vegetations and the supporting valve will vary with the infecting organism, the presence or absence of pre-existing valvular disease and the virulence of infection. Active vegetations of acute and subacute bacterial endocarditis can be quite colorful (pink, red, yellow, green) with loss of color to a dull gray or tan during healing.[13,14] More virulent bacterial organisms, such as *Staphylococcus aureus*, *Hemophilus influenzae*, gram-negative aerobic microbes and some anaerobes as well as fungi tend to form larger vegetations (Figures 1 and 2) that may embolize distally or occlude

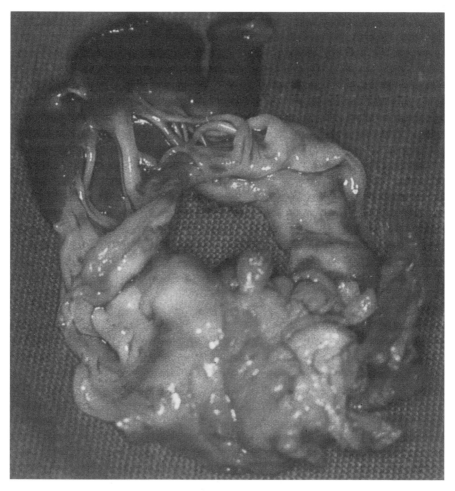

Figure 2. Fungal mitral valve endocarditis with extensive destruction of the anterior leaflet. Note the large size. Reproduced with permission: Antunes MJ. *Mitral Valve Repair*. Starnberg, Germany, Verlag RS Schulz, 1989. p 49. (See color appendix.)

blood vessels and valvular orifices. Subacute endocarditis can have subtle gross findings with areas of the valve containing small vegetations alternating with various stages of healing. Contracted areas of fibrosis may be seen as healing progresses. In some cases, ulceration may be the only evidence of endocarditis. A "worm-eaten" appearance is characteristic of subacute bacterial endocarditis involving the mitral valve with a pre-existing stenotic lesion.[14] Valve perforation may be seen; however, not all perforations result from endocarditis as normal valves can have small perforations.[17] Both acute and subacute endocarditis can extend to involve adjacent structures, such as chordae tendineae (Figure 3) and papillary muscles, or form myocardial abscesses, mycotic aneurysms, septal perforations and even purulent or fibrinous pericarditis.[13,14,16]

Grossly, prosthetic valve lesions vary with valve type and tend to be more extensive than native valve lesions. Prosthetic valvular material obtained at operation may contain large vegetations confluent with the valve ring surface. Pathological changes of porcine prostheses are primarily on the inflow surface which may show crumbling vegetations, fraying

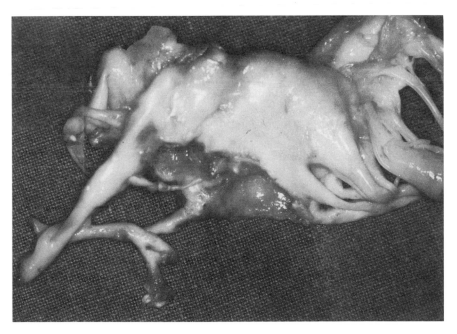

Figure 3. Ruptured chordae tendineae of mitral valve endocarditis. This patient had been operated on for extensive infective endocarditis of the aortic valve and mitral valve vegetations were found incidentally. Reproduced with permission: Antunes MJ. *Mitral Valve Repair.* Starnberg, Germany, Verlag RS Schulz, 1989. p 51. (See color appendix.)

or perforation.[13] With tissue valves, vegetations may initiate on the valve cusps but frequently extend to involve the sewing ring, adjacent connective tissue and myocardium.[13,14] Annular abscesses occur in both mechanical and tissue prosthetic valve endocarditis with sewing ring involvement.

Valve Tissue Histological Examination

Histological examination of suspected infective endocarditis vegetations can rule out other disease processes which may mimic infective endocarditis.[11,14] These include:

- Nonbacterial thrombogenic endocardial lesions (the proposed precursor lesions to infective endocarditis)
- Postsurgical valvular changes (suture, foreign body granulomatous inflammation, thrombus)
- Autoimmune disease associated changes (rheumatic valvulitis, Libman-Sacks endocarditis of systemic lupus erythematosus, polyarteritis nodosa and Behçet's disease vasculitic changes, antiphospholipid syndrome associated vasculitic and thrombotic changes)
- Neoplasm associated endocarditis (atrial myxoma, marantic endocarditis associated with adenocarcinoma, valvular involvement with lymphoma, rhabdomyosarcoma or carcinoid).

Differentiation of these abnormalities from infective endocarditis can be made only by histological examination.

An appreciation of the normal valvular histology is essential in order to identify the architectural disruptions characteristic of both active and healing phases of endocarditis. The normal semilunar valve has a distinct 3-layer histological structure with endothelium continuous over the arterial, atrial and ventricular surfaces. The ventricular endothelium directly overlies the ventricularis, which is composed of numerous, thickened elastic fibers. The ventricularis extends to the free edge of the semilunar cusp. The spongiosa is subjacent to the ventricularis and occupies the central position in the thickness of the cusp, but does not extend to the free edge of the valve cusp. The spongiosa contains fibroblasts and poorly differentiated mesenchymal cells scattered amongst loosely woven collagen fibrils within a proteoglycan matrix. The major structural component of the cusp is the fibrosa. The fibrosa blends into the collagen of the valvular ring in the region of the commissures and extends to the free edge of the cusp. Densely packed collagen bundles separate fine elastic fibers and form the structural matrix of the fibrosa.

Atrioventricular valves differ significantly from semilunar valves with the presence of the annulus and chordae tendineae. The annulus forms a circumferential ring of collagen and elastic fibers with extensions into the ventricle and the atrium. The collagen bundles of the annulus are continuous with the valve leaflets, forming the central fibrosa, which continues on into the chordae tendineae and spreads into a network that covers the tip of the papillary muscles. The dense elastic fiber network of the ventricularis, which in turn is covered by the ventricular endothelium, abuts the ventricular aspect of the fibrosa. The spongiosa overlies the atrial aspect of the fibrosa, again containing abundant proteoglycans, which is then covered by the atrial auricularis layer for the proximal two-thirds of the leaflet. The auricularis layer contains elastic fibers and smooth muscle cells. The atrial endothelium completes the layers. The endothelium of the atrial surface may appear plump, with irregular nuclei. The layers of the valves and their respective components can be seen vaguely with hematoxylin and eosin preparations, but are highlighted with trichrome and elastic stain preparations (Figure 4).

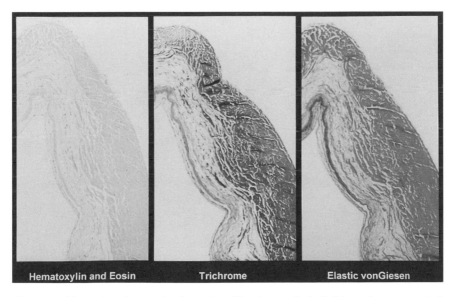

| Hematoxylin and Eosin | Trichrome | Elastic vonGiesen |

Figure 4. Normal atrioventricular valve. The thin endothelial layer is represented with the occasional hyperchromatic oblong nucleus covering the valve surface. The endothelium is commonly abraded during process and may not be seen on routine examination. The layering of valve material is vaguely discernible with hematoxylin and eosin stain. Trichrome stain highlights collagen bundles with a deep blue hue. The fibrosa contains densely packed collagen bundles. Elastic von Giesen delineates the elastic fibers of the ventricularis with silver, resulting in a black appearance. (See color appendix.)

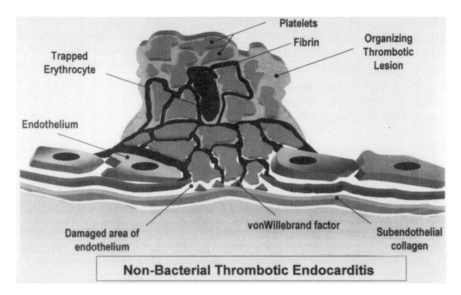

Figure 5. Nonbacterial thrombotic endocarditis begins with a damaged endothelium. Platelets, fibrin and trapped erythrocytes aggregate over the area of injury. Infection results in an endocarditis vegetation.

Infective vegetations may be formed on a pre-existing area of damaged endothelium or by interaction of microorganisms with an intact endothelium. Endothelial surface disruption exposes the thrombogenic subendothelial valve collagen, leading to platelet and fibrin deposition and subsequent formation of a nonbacterial thrombotic endocardial lesion (NBTE) (Figure 5).[13–15] NBTE may lyse and resolve or persist. Persistent NBTE may embolize, organize or calcify. When bacteria colonize an NBTE lesion, an infective vegetation is formed. Microorganisms in the vegetation multiply within the platelet-fibrin environment. Portions of the vegetation are shed into the blood once the vegetation reaches a critical size. Microorganisms deep inside the vegetation persevere with reduced metabolic activity and are not released into the circulation. Invasion into the valve fibrosa results in microabscess formation, containing microorganisms that subsist in a markedly reduced metabolic state. In approximately 30% of endocarditis cases, no pre-existing cardiac abnormality (including NBTE) can be identified and other pathogenic mechanisms must be considered.[13,14,18] Several microorganisms, among them *Staphylococcus aureus*, some streptococci, *Salmonella*, *Rickettsia*, *Borrelia* and *Candida*, are capable of infecting intact endothelial cells. Endothelial infection may occur via interaction of specific glycoproteins (*S. aureus*, viridans streptococci) or by endothelial phagocytosis.[14,18] In fact, endothelial cells may also harbor metabolically latent organisms.[18] The microorganisms eventually damage the endothelial cells, exposing subendothelial collagen, which promotes platelet aggregation and fibrin polymerization resulting in vegetation formation on the valvular surface. The vegetation provides a portal of entry to the valve connective tissue. Vegetations formed by endothelial infection also have a metabolically biphasic microorganism population.

Histologically, a vegetation is an amorphous platelet and fibrin mass in which abundant microorganisms and inflammatory cells are enmeshed (Figures 6–9). The remaining histological features show some variability dependent on the organism, the predisposing conditions, the valve(s) involved and the virulence of the disease process.

Acute endocarditis has a characteristic uniform appearance owing to the rapidly destructive process. Fibrin and platelet aggregates in untreated patients contain a predominance of neutrophils and bacteria which may be large enough to view with hematoxylin and eosin stained tissue (Figure 10). Elastin and collagen disruption by inflammatory cells and microorga-

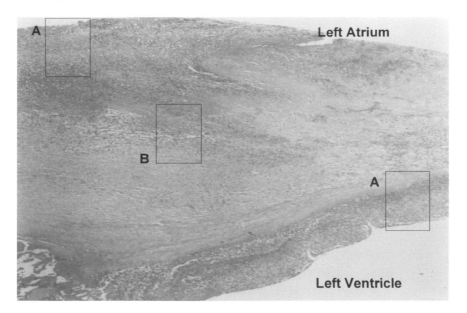

Figure 6. Infective endocarditis vegetation. A gradient of inflammatory cells present in the vegetation is apparent, with fewer inflammatory cells over the atrial and ventricular surfaces (A) and numerous inflammatory cells at the vegetation and supporting connective tissue junction (B). The vegetation is composed primarily of fibrin, platelets, inflammatory cells and microorganisms. (See color appendix.)

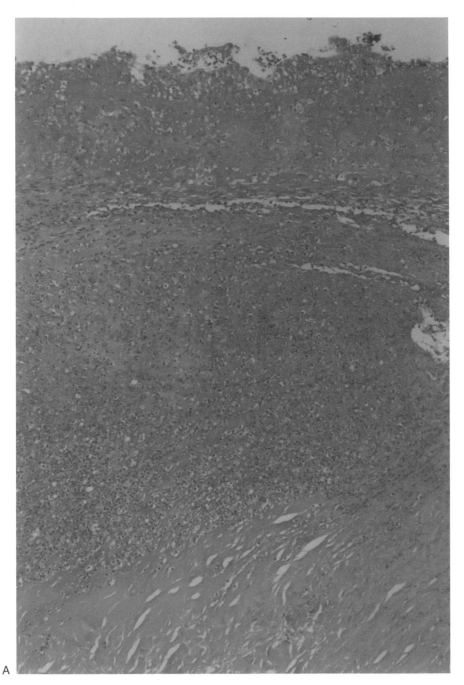

A

Figure 7. Higher magnification corresponding to Figure 6, area delimited in (A). Note the paucity of inflammatory cells within the dense eosinophilic fibrin matrix at the vegetation surface. (See color appendix.)

Figure 7. *(continued)* (B) The inflammatory cells are seen in dense collections within the valve tissue. (See color appendix.)

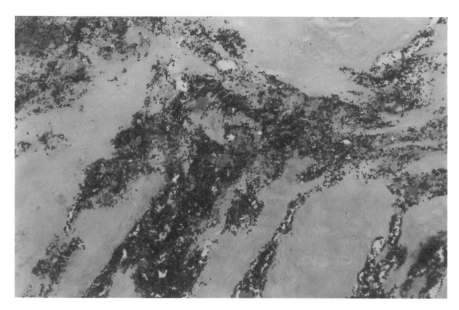

Figure 8. Tissue Gram's stain highlights the dense collections of cocci deep within the vegetation. The area depicted corresponds to Figure 6, area delimited in (B). (See color appendix.)

nisms can be fulminant and can quickly lead to valve destruction (Figures 10–13). Thrombus organization, fibroblast infiltration and neovascularization–all forms of repair–are conspicuously absent. Without repair, the propensity toward valve leaflet and chordae tendineae rupture is striking. The rapidly forming, large, friable vegetations of acute endocarditis frequently extend into the surrounding tissue and have a tendency toward embolization. Associated myocardial lesions are the rule rather than the exception and occur in 88% to 100% of cases.[13,14] Although the myocardium may show only edema, the most commonly encountered lesions are myocarditis with neutrophils and areas of suppuration.[13] Vegetation embolization to the coronary vessels may result in myocardial infarction with its consequent histological appearance.

Subacute endocarditis results in destruction and replacement of the valve parenchyma by varying stages of infection and healing respectively. As a result, the microscopic appearance varies from field to field. Scattered vegetations on and below the surface will be present. In contrast to the large collections of microorganisms seen in acute endocarditis, infecting organisms may be present only focally. Thrombus with organizing collections of fibrin and inflammatory cells may be appreciated. The inflammatory reaction consists predominantly of lymphocytes with histiocytes and multinucleated giant cells containing ingested bacteria. Neutrophils are

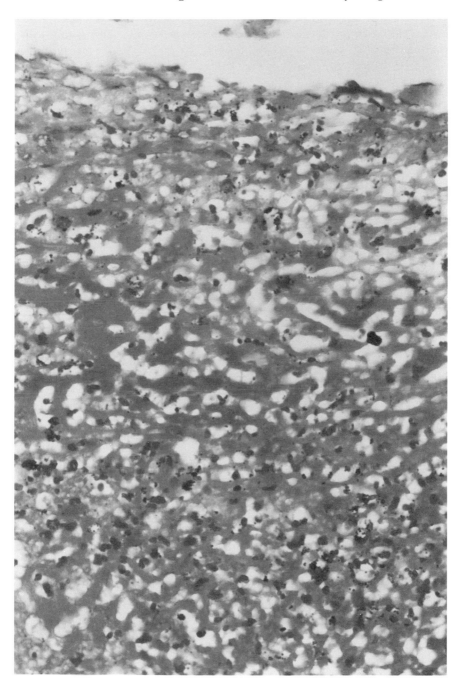

Figure 9. Exosaccharide polymers produced by some bacteria along with fibrin polymers create a seal over the vegetation (a "biofilm") which may inhibit the diffusion of antimicrobial drugs into the deeper layers within the vegetation. (See color appendix.)

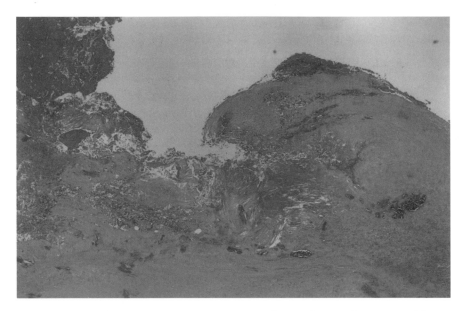

Figure 10. Virulent microorganisms may produce colonies that are visible on routine hematoxylin and eosin microscopic preparations. The organism in this case was *Staphylococcus aureus*. (See color appendix.)

not the dominant inflammatory cell and are limited to areas of extension. Abscess formation may be evident with dense collections of microorganisms walled off by fibrin and fibroblasts and few inflammatory cells in the surrounding tissue. Areas of resolving infection, marked by a decrease in the quantity of microorganisms, fibrosis, granulation tissue with neovascularization and the deposition and even calcification of collagen and elastic fibers, will be juxtaposed with the areas of active infection. The myocardium may reveal distinguishing features with larger debridement and postmortem examinations. Adjacent myocardium may show diffuse or localized collections of lymphocytes, monocytes and neutrophils often in a perivascular distribution. Necrosis, with muscle fiber degeneration and various stages of fibrosis and healing, may also be present. Vasculitic changes, such as arteriolitis or media or adventitia necrosis, are occasionally seen. The endothelium can appear reactive with hyperchromatic nuclei surrounded by abundant cytoplasm.

Histological examination of prosthetic valvular material obtained at surgery is limited to the biological material of the valve, the supporting myocardium and fibrous tissue. Marked fibrin deposition and disintegration of supporting collagen is seen. Macrophages and neutrophils prevail.

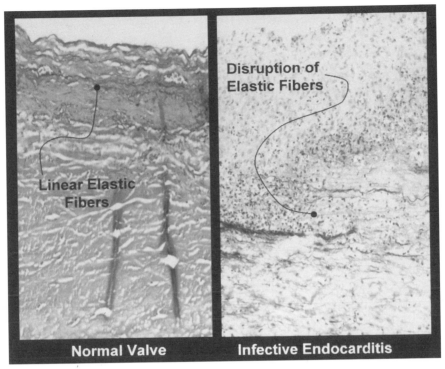

Figure 11. Normal and infected aortic valve with intact and disrupted elastic layers, respectively, stained with elastic von Giesen. Neutrophils are evident in the background of the infected specimen. (See color appendix.)

When fungal organisms are present, granuloma formation may be a prominent feature.

Unfortunately, microorganisms, bacteria, fungi and intracellular parasites are not likely to be evident with routine hematoxylin and eosin stains. Various staining techniques can highlight the microorganism's cell wall and reveal its presence. Tissue Gram's stains (bacteria) are fairly insensitive while periodic-acid Schiff and Grocott's/Gomori's methenamine silver (fungal elements) stains results are more rewarding.[7,14] Immunofluorescent and immunohistochemical stains for some microorganisms have limited use with paraffin-embedded tissue.[19,20] Additional histological and immunologic methods are available to detect less commonly encountered microorganisms (see discussion below).

Electron microscopy may be indicated in some culture-negative cases, to demonstrate organisms which are difficult or impossible to culture. A

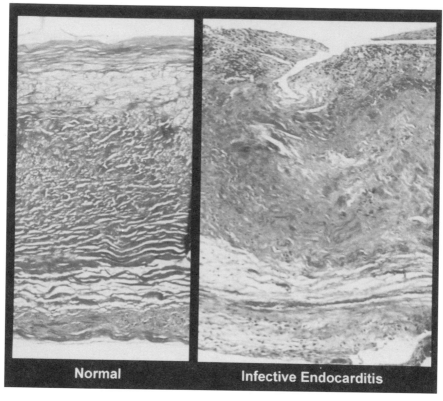

Figure 12. Normal and infected aortic valve stained with trichrome, highlighting the collagen bundles of the fibrosa blue. The fulminant inflammatory process destroys the fibrillar organization and integrity of the valve. (See color appendix.)

small portion of the valve material should be placed in 2.5% glutaraldehyde solution or 4% paraformaldehyde with 2.5% glutaraldehyde for electron microscopic processing. Differential features of these organisms are detailed below.

Clinical Criteria for Definitive Infective Endocarditis: Blood Culture and Related Methods

Clinical suspicion of the causative microorganisms can be made on the basis of the overall presentation (nocosomial versus community acquisition, patient population, comorbid disease states, exposure and risk factors) and the virulence of infection. Definitive treatment, however, relies

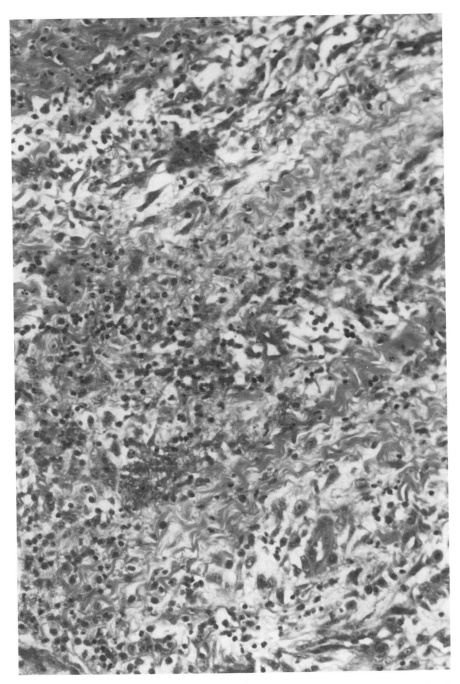

Figure 13. Trichrome stain of infected aortic valve. Neutrophils, extravasated red blood cells and edema separate the fibrosa collagen bundles. (Magnification 400X.) (See color appendix.)

on culture, organism identification and antimicrobial susceptibility testing.

Blood culture defines bacteremia and remains the most sensitive method of recovering and partially identifying many microbial pathogens.[21,22] No independent gold standard test exists to evaluate the blood culture. As such, several distortions in the analysis of the sensitivity and specificity are present and result in an artificial increase in the value of both parameters. New molecular methods with multiple primers are currently under investigation which may directly identify bacterial DNA from blood cultures.[22] A recent review by Weinstein, however, states that despite published reports of molecular methods to detect both culturable and nonculturable microorganisms implicated in endocarditis, none of these methods have yet received FDA approval for use on blood culture material nor are they widely available.[23] Thus, while it is unlikely that molecular methods will completely replace culture, they may lead to a more definitive assessment of the sensitivity and specificity of blood culture methods. Immunological methods may help establish causative organisms in culture-negative endocarditis. Many of these methods are available within reference laboratories, while others remain limited to the research facilities that have developed them.[24,25] Blood culture remains the mainstay of diagnosis.

Of all blood cultures performed, only 8% to 11% of blood cultures recover potentially pathogenic microorganisms.[8,21,26,27] A minimum of 1% to 3% of all blood cultures are contaminants.[26,27] This implies that at least one third and up to one half of all positive blood cultures represent contaminant, not pathogenic, microorganisms. Our institution considers each positive culture bottle to be a true positive and continues to isolate the organism and perform antimicrobial sensitivity testing even when the isolate is a commonly encountered contaminant. Our false positive rate varies between 2% and 3% with the majority of cultures performed on a continuous monitoring blood culture system (unpublished data). The blood culture test result depends on timing, sample number, blood draw and handling technique, blood volume sampled, media growth characteristics, culture growth detection system and the clinicians' interpretation.[7,8,10,21,23,27]

Much advancement has been made since the introduction of the blood culture. The most recent advancements include the continuous monitoring blood culture systems, refinement of rapid methods of organism identification and growth media alterations that improve recovery of fastidious microorganisms and possibly counteract the effects of antimicrobials in the blood culture sample.[23] Keep in mind that no single medium or blood culture system is capable of detecting all microorganisms. Most commercially marketed blood culture media, however, perform quite well.[23,28]

Table 1 provides an overview of currently available blood culture systems.[8,29]

Endocarditis can be caused by a wide variety of microorganisms (Tables 2 and 3). Viridans streptococci, staphylococci, nonenterococcal group D streptococci, enterococci and aerobic gram-negative bacilli account for more than 95% of native valve endocarditis.[7,15,30] A recent 10 year review of cases at our institution corroborates these findings (Table 4).[31]

The organisms most commonly encountered are generally simple to culture. Among patients with tissue culture-proven endocarditis who do not receive antibiotics prior to blood culture, 97% are positive for the causative microorganism.[32] The vegetations of untreated infective endocarditis constantly discharge bacteria into the circulation and produce a continuous bacteremia. In patients with endocarditis, the likelihood that a subsequent culture would be positive after an initial positive result was 95% to 100%. With bacteremia from other causes, the likelihood that a subsequent culture would be positive after the first positive culture was 75% to 80%.[21]

The standard blood culture procedures of each institution will vary. For optimal utilization of blood cultures and pathogen recovery, it is essential that the clinician be fully aware of the type of blood culture system used for standard cultures and the ancillary methods available for culture.[23,26,33] Knowledge of blood culture systems may impact the number of culture sets drawn, as well as specific requests for ancillary cultivation methods, nonroutine subculture and prolonged incubation times. The expected reporting and interval times between cultivation, identification and antimicrobial sensitivities are determined by laboratory staffing, the system used and the identification and antimicrobial sensitivity methods used. An understanding of these factors may circumvent clinician frustration with unexpected "delays" in reporting.

An exhaustive review of blood culturing systems is beyond the scope of this text. Reviews by Aronson,[21] Weinstein[23] and Wilson[27] are suggested for those interested in a complete treatment of the topic.[33] The significant aspects and developments will be reviewed briefly.

Blood Culture Acquisition, Processing and Evaluation

Blood obtained from arterial and venous sources is culture positive at similar rates.[8,10,23] Peripheral venipuncture is the method of choice. Increased contamination rates have been reported when blood for culture is obtained from intravenous catheters.[7–9, 21, 23, 27,33] The American College of Physicians guidelines recommend that blood for culture not be obtained

Table 1
Selected Specifications of the Currently Available Blood Culture Systems

System/Bottle	Broth Volume (mL)	Inoculum Volume (mL)	Blood: Broth Ratio	Continuous Agitation?	Routine Subculture	Method of Detection	Monitor Interval	Antibiotic Binding or Enhanced Media Available
Manual	30–40	3–5	1:8–1:10	No	Blind and Terminal	Visible detection	Q day	No
Septichek (BDDIS*)	30	3–5	1:6–1:10	No	Blind q day	Visible detection of colonies on immersion/paddle	Q day	No
Isolator/Lysis Centrifuge (Wampole Laboratories)	N/A	10 mL	N/A	N/A	No	Visible colonies on agar plate	Q day	Enhanced for fungal recovery
BACTEC 460 (*Becton Dickinson Diagnostic Instrument Systems)								
6B, 7D, 8B, 13A	30	5	1:6	Yes	Not required	Radiometric $^{14}CO_2$	BID first 2 days, then q day	Yes, Media 16B and 17D
BACTEC 660, 730 or 860 (Becton Dickinson Diagnostic Instrument Systems)								
6A, 7A, 8A, 16A, 16B, 17A, 17D Plus 26, Plus 27	30	5	1:5	Yes	Not required	Infrared spectrophotometry	BID first 2 days, then q day	See Plus 26 and Plus 27
Plus 26, Plus 27	25	10	1:2.5	Yes	Not required	Infrared spectrophotometry	BID first 2 days, then q day	Contains resins and glass beads
Ped Plus	20	4	1:5	Yes	Not required	Infrared spectrophotometry	BID first 2 days, then q day	No
HBV—Fungal Medium	25	10	1:2.5	Yes	Not routine	Infrared spectrophotometry	Q day × 7 days	No

BacT/Alert (Organon Teknika Corporation)							
Aerobic	40	10	1:4	Yes	Not required	Colorimetric	Q 10 to 24 min	Yes
Anaerobic	40	10	1:4	Yes	Not required	Colorimetric	Q 10 to 24 min	Yes
PediBacT	20	4	1:5	Yes	Not required	Colorimetric	Q 10 to 24 min	Yes
BACTEC 9120/9240 (Becton Dickinson Diagnostic Instrument Systems)							
Standard aerobic/F	40	5	1:8	Yes	Not required	Fluorimetric	Q 10 min	Yes
Standard anaerobic/F	40	5	1:8		Not required	Fluorimetric		BACTEC resin
Plus aerobic/F	25	10	1:2.5	Yes	Not required	Fluorimetric	Q 10 min	Yes
Plus anaerobic/F	25	10	1:2.5					BACTEC resin
ESP (Extra Sensing Power)—(Difco Laboratories)							
80A aerobic	80	10	1:8	Yes	Not Required	Pressure	Q 12 min—aer	Currently under FDA approval
80N anaerobic	80	10	1:8				Q 24 min—anaer	
EZ 40A aerobic	40	5	1:8	Yes	Not Required	Pressure	Q 12 min—aer	Currently under FDA approval
EZ 40N anaerobic	40	5	1:8				Q 24 min—anaer	
Vital 200, 300, 400 (BioMeriux)							
Aerobic	40	10	1:4	Yes	Not Required	Fluorescent	Q 15 nin	
Anaerobic	40	10	1:4	Yes	Not Required	Fluorescent	Q 15 min	
MicroScan (Microscan)							
Aerobic	60	10	1:6	Yes	Not Required	Fluorescent	Q 10 min	
Anaerobic	60	10	1:6	Yes	Not Required	Fluorescent	Q 10 min	

Table 2
Microbiology of Infective Endocarditis

Gram-positive cocci	Gram-negative bacilli
Viridans streptococci (α- and β-hemolytic)	*Campylobacter fetus*
S. mitis (S. mitior)	*Enterobacter* spp
S. mitis	*Escherichia coli*
S. sanguis	*Klebsiella* spp
S. angiosus	*Legionella micdadei*
S. mutans	*Legionella pneumophila*
S. salivarius	*Rahnella aquatilis*
S. bovis	*Pasteurella dagmatis*
S. pneumoniae	*Pasteurella gallinarum*
Beta-hemolytic streptococci	*Pasteurella multocida*
S. pyogenes (group A)	*Pasteurella ureae*
S. agalactiae (group B)	*Proteus* spp
S. equisimilis (group C)	*Pseudomonas aeruginosa*
S. angionosus (group F)	*Pseudomonas cepacia*
S. canis (group G)	*Salmonella* spp
Enterococci	*Serratia* spp
E. faecalis (group D)	*Yersinia enterocolitica*
E. faecium (group D)	Gram-negative coccobacilli
E. durans	HACEK microorganisms
E. solitarius	*Haemophilus influenzae*
E. avium (non-group D)	*H. parainfluenzae*
Other gram-positive cocci	*H. aphrophilus*
Abiotrophia defectiva (Streptococcus defectivus)	*H. paraphrophilus*
Abiotrophia adiacens (Streptococcus adjacens)	*Actinobacillus actinomycetemcomitans*
Abiotrophia elegans sp. no.	*Cardiobacterium hominis*
Aerococcus urinae	*Eikenella corrodens*
Gemella haemolysans	*Kingella denitrificans*
Gemella morbillorum	*Kingella kingae*
Lactococcus	Other gram negative coccobacilli
Pediococcus	*Acinetobacter* calcoaceticus
Staphylococci and related species	*Bordetella bronchiseptica*
S. aureus	*Bartonella*
S. epidermidis	*Brucella*
S. lugdunensis	Anaerobic Bacteria
Stomatococcus mucilaginous	*Anaerobiospirillum succiniproducents*
Micrococcus agilis	*Bacteroides fragilis*
Gram negative cocci	*Bacteroides oralis*
Neisseria gonorrhoeae	*Clostridium bifermentans*
N. meningitidis	*Clostridium innocuum*
N. subflava	*Clostridium perfringens*
Branhamella catarrhalis	*Fusobacterium necrophorum*
Gram-positive bacilli	*Lactobacillus*
	Peptococcus

(continued)

Table 2 *(continued)*

Gram-positive cocci	Gram-negative bacilli
Actinomyces pyogenes	Prevotella bivia
Arcanobacterium haemolyticum	Proprionibacterium acnes
Bacillus cereus	Proprionibacterium granulosum
Bacillus subtilis	Veillonella dispar
Corynebacterium and diphtheroids	Filamentous bacteria (gram +
C. diphtheriae	intracellular)
C. xerosis	Actinomyces israelii
C. pseudodiphtheriticum	Mycobacterium tuberculosis
C. jeikeium	M. chelonnei
CDC group GI (LD3), G2 (LD2), 11	M. fortuitum
Listeria monocytogenes	Nocardia asteroides
Oerskovia turbata	Intracellular Parasites
Rothia dentocariosa	Coxiella burnetii
	Chlamydia psittaci
	Chlamydia trachomatis

Table 3
Fungal Organisms Recovered in Infective Endocarditis

Frequently Identified Fungal Organisms	Incidence[49]
Candida spp	
Candida albicans	32%
Candida stellatoidea	
Candida parapsilosis	
Candida guillermondii	23%
Candida krusei	
Candida tropicalis	
Aspergillus spp	27%
Curvularia genuculata	
Hormondendrum dermatitidis	10%
Mucoracae	
Torulopsis glabrata	

Others (8%)

Acremonium (Cephalosporium)	Histoplasma capsulatum
Arnium leporiunum	Lecycthophora spp
Blastomyces dermatitidis	Paecilomyces spp
Blastoschizomyces capitatus	Penicillum spp
Chrysosporium spp	Phycomyces
Coccidiodes immitis	Rhodotorula
Coprinius spp	Saccharomyces cerevisiae
Crytococcus neoformans	Scedosporium spp
Fusarium spp	Trichosporon beigelli
Hansenula anomalia	Wangiella dermatitidis

Table 4

Organisms Recovered by Blood Culture in Cases of Definite Infective Endocarditis, 10-year Retrospective Review, Providence St. Vincent Medical Center, Portland, Oregon.[31]

Organism	Incidence
Streptococcus spp	58.7%
Staphylococcus aureus	21.4
No growth	9.3
Staphylococcus epidermidis	5.0
Actinobacillus	1.4
Actinomyces viscosus	0.7
Cardibacterium	0.7
Haemophilus parainfluenzae	0.7
Klebsiella pneumoniae	0.7
Lactobacillus casei	0.7
Propionibacterium	0.7

from indwelling intravascular devices.[28,33] The blood collection site (peripheral venous, vascular line, etc.) may be useful data in separating true positive culture results from false positive culture results.

Skin Antisepsis

Appropriate skin antisepsis cannot be overemphasized. Blood culture contamination occurs most frequently at the blood draw site. Bates reported that a single false positive blood culture resulted in over $4,000 in additional charges and lengthened hospital stay.[26] Skin antisepsis is the most important step in ensuring a low false positive blood culture rate.[23,26,33,34]

Tincture of iodine (2% iodine with 2.4% sodium iodide diluted in ethanol) is widely regarded as the gold standard for skin antisepsis.[34] The 2 misconceptions that have decreased tincture of iodine use are that iodine burns will occur and that hypersensitivity to the tincture is common. In truth, iodine burns are an unfortunate effect of the 7% tincture (though not of the 2% tincture) and hypersensitivity to iodine is rare.[34] Currently, skin antisepsis is widely performed by use of 70% isopropyl alcohol followed by an iodophore. Although iodophores such as povidine-iodine are excellent broad-spectrum antiseptics, they require 1.5 to 2 minutes of contact time for maximal antiseptic effect,[23] a requirement that may be ignored by the person drawing the blood for culture. Povidine-iodine has also been reportedly contaminated with *Pseudomonas cepacia* resulting in pseudobacteremia.[7]

Timing, Number of Culture Sets, Inoculation Volume, Length of Incubation and Media Selection

Some experimental evidence suggests that bacteremia precedes a febrile spike. In contrast to other types of bacteremia, the bacteremia of untreated infective endocarditis is continuous.[32] As such, timing blood culture with febrile episodes has no utility.

Various recommendations have been made regarding the number of blood culture sets to obtain. With the improved detection offered by continuous monitoring blood culture systems, the number of recommended cultures to evaluate bacteremia in general has been reduced to 2 within a 24-hour period.[23] The recommendation of 3 sets of blood cultures within a 24-hour time period continues to apply in cases of suspected endocarditis.[16,23,30,33,35] In consideration of Bayes' theorem, Aronson demonstrates concisely that with a high pre-test probability of 80% in patients with suspected endocarditis, slightly over one third of patients will have negative blood cultures if only 3 culture sets are drawn in the blood culture series. In light of this finding, he recommends 4 or even 5 blood cultures for completeness.[21]

The blood volume cultured is the single most important variable.[23,33] The quantity of inocula is partially determined by the blood culture system that is used and the blood volume accepted by the particular media bottle (Table 1). The microorganism concentration ranges from 1–100 colony forming unit/mL during endovascular related bacteremia in adults.[28,32] A direct relationship exists between blood volume and blood culture diagnostic yield. When larger volumes of blood are cultured, more bacteremias and fungemias are detected. Numerically, for each additional milliliter of blood cultured, a 3% increase in yield can be achieved.[10,28,33] This extrapolates to a 15% to 30% increase in bacterial detection with a 10mL increase in blood volume. Many of the current blood culture data are based on a minimum of a 10mL inoculant. Clinical practice may be guided by defining a blood culture "set" to be a minimum of 10mL blood inoculated into aerobic media. In the event that the standard blood cultures allow only a 5mL inoculant, it may be necessary to order additional aerobic culture bottles to define the "set." For adults, collection of 20 mL to 30 mL of blood per culture is optimal with division of the inoculant into aerobic, anaerobic and possibly fungal media.[10]

Microorganism concentration during bacteremia in infants and children exceeds that seen in adults.[36,37] Smaller blood volumes can be cultured from pediatric patients without compromising the blood culture yield, but the use of pediatric blood culture bottles is imperative. Inoculation of the smaller pediatric blood volume into adult blood culture bottles will result in a reduced blood-to-broth ratio that is outside the manufactur-

Table 5
Recommended Inocula Volume for Pediatric Blood Cultures[36,37]

Age	Inocula Volume
Neonatal	1–2 mL
Infants—1 month to 2 years	2–3 mL
Older children	3–5 mL
Adolescents	10–20 mL

er's recommendations and reduces diagnostic yield. Additionally, the growth of some organisms implicated in pediatric endocarditis that are not frequently recovered in adult endocarditis is inhibited by certain anticoagulants (e.g. sodium polyanetholsulfonate) in the standard blood culture media bottle. Guidelines for the blood volume to collect from neonatal and pediatric patients are compiled in Table 5.[36,37]

The length of culture incubation is dependent on the practice parameters within each microbiology laboratory. Longer incubation periods may result in recovery of additional microorganisms; however, pathogen recovery decreases over time with a greater proportion of contaminant organisms recovered late in the incubation period.[23,29,38] Generally, blood cultures are incubated for 5 to 7 days. A 5-day incubation period is sufficient with most automated systems.[23,28,29] Limiting incubation and testing to 5 days will recover most pathogens and will eliminate the recovery of many contaminating microorganisms.[29,33] It has been widely held that longer incubation periods may be warranted in patients with suspected endocarditis. Nevertheless, many of the implicated microorganisms (including the HACEK group) are usually recovered within the first 5 to 7 days.[29,33] Exceptions include blood cultures drawn following exposure to antimicrobials. In this case, it may be necessary to incubate for a longer time period and to perform blind or terminal subcultures on the blood culture broth.[23] Recent modifications in blood culture media may provide other options in this commonly encountered circumstance and are discussed below. Less commonly, a clinical suspicion of *Brucella, Legionella, Mycobacterium* and filamentous fungi warrants extended incubation, up to 4 to 6 weeks. Communication with the microbiology laboratory is necessary if the clinical scenario warrants an extended incubation or additional subcultures.

Empirical antibiotic therapy in patients who present with fever or vague symptoms suggesting a possible infectious etiology is widespread. Empirical antibiotic therapy prior to obtaining blood cultures may prolong detection of clinically significant microorganisms or result in a false negative blood culture. Resin-containing media (BACTEC resin media,

Becton Dickinson Diagnostic Instrument Systems, Spark, MD), blood pretreatment with a resin-based antimicrobial device (not widely used; Becton Dickinson Microbiology Systems, Cockeysville, MD), lysis centrifugation to separate microorganisms from serum (Isolator, Wampole Laboratories, Cranbury, NJ) and BacT/Alert FAN media (Organon Teknika, Durham, NC) can overcome the effects of serum antibiotics.[23,29,33,39,40,41] While FAN media was originally postulated to exert its enhanced recovery effect by reducing or inactivating antimicrobial substances in the culture bottle, it has since been observed that the improved detection may be due to absorption of toxic metabolites and serum inhibitors as well as a richer broth to support growth.[40]

BacT/Alert FAN and BACTEC resin media both show an increase in recovery of all microorganisms (particularly *S. aureus*), but no difference in the speed of detection between the 2 media when used in continuous monitoring blood culture systems. [20,23,41,42] The enhanced recovery was most apparent when patients were receiving antibiotics at the time of blood culture.[40] In addition, the BacT/Alert FAN system supports growth of fungal organisms without requiring separate fungal medium formulations that do not support bacterial growth.[40] A universal medium such as this one obviates the need for inoculum division. Detracting from the obvious advantages of these newer media, contaminant recovery rates are higher when compared to standard blood culture bottles.[23,39,40–42] Gram's stain interpretation was difficult with the original FAN formulation due to charcoal particle presence in the broth. This has been remedied in the newer formulations. Another limiting feature is cost. Enhanced media bottles cost 3 to 4 times as much as the standard counterparts.[33] Arguments in favor of using the enhanced media include routine antibiotic use in this patient group, improved *S. aureus* isolation and enhanced recovery of fastidious organisms.

Aerobic and anaerobic blood culture bottles form one blood culture set according to the guidelines of the College of American Pathologists. Despite this recommendation, routine anaerobic cultures for septicemia evaluations remain controversial.[23,43] Interestingly, the proportion of bacteremias due to obligate anaerobes has decreased substantially over time, and large studies document that anaerobic organisms are rarely the cause of endocarditis.[23,28,30] Sample division into separate culture bottles decreases the ability to recover the responsible pathogen. Weinstein and others recommend that anaerobic culture be used selectively for patients who are at high risk for anaerobic bacteremia.[40] For example, a female patient with a known bicuspid aortic valve who has undergone hysterectomy and subsequently becomes febrile would justify anaerobic blood cultures. In all other cases, the full inoculant should be used for aerobic and/or fungal media.

More rapid detection of pathogenic microorganisms in clinical specimens may result in earlier initiation of appropriate antimicrobial therapy and improved patient outcome.[22] To that end, continuous monitoring blood culture systems have been developed that assess blood culture growth every 10 to 24 minutes. The 3 continuous monitoring blood culture systems currently available in the United States are the BACTEC 9000 series, the Difco ESP, and the BacT/Alert system (Table 1). Comparative studies published to date have demonstrated that all 3 continuous monitoring blood culture systems detect growth sooner than earlier generation BACTEC instruments and manual systems.[28] The newer systems also include features that improve the overall diagnostic yield of the blood culture: sample agitation, compatibility with the newer media formulations and blood culture media bottles which accept a larger volume of blood.

Once a blood culture bottle is identified as positive, microorganism identification is pursued. A direct Gram's stain examination of the blood-broth mixture is the initial and possibly the most useful rapid test for blood cultures. Rapid or conventional methods for species identification are then performed on blood culture isolates. Frequently, this involves subculturing the blood culture onto solid media. Automated microbial identification systems can identify microorganisms from overnight subcultures within 8 to 13 hours while conventional methods may require 24 to 49 hours.[8,22] Some biochemical tests have been adapted for testing blood culture isolates directly from blood- broth mixtures allowing a presumptive identification within 2 to 4 hours.[8] This methodology has not yet supplanted either conventional or rapid routine methods. (Although molecular methods have been developed, they have not been approved for use on blood culture specimens and are unlikely to be available for organism identification in the near future.) The combination of continuous monitoring blood culture systems with rapid bacterial identification methods clearly decreases the time required to identify blood culture isolates. Despite this, further evaluation is necessary to document any positive effects on clinical outcome.

Although more rapid microorganism identification should result in earlier initiation of appropriate antimicrobial therapy and improved patient outcome, this translation is clinician-dependent.[22] In a recent study, Matsen documented that 72 hours following placement of antimicrobial susceptibility reports into the patient's chart nearly half of physicians were unaware of the results.[44] Furthermore, physicians who were oblivious to the results were also more likely to use inappropriate therapy based on antimicrobial susceptibility patterns.[44] In contrast, Chorny observed that rapid identification methods and timely antimicrobial susceptibility test results are more likely to result in initiation or alterations of antimicrobial therapy.[22] In addition, therapeutic changes are significantly more likely to be considered when direct test results are available.[22] Additional studies are needed to document the therapeutic benefit of rapid microbial identification systems.

A positive blood culture result raises 2 questions for interpretation: Is this a true positive culture? Does the positive culture represent infective endocarditis? No single clinical or microbiological criterion can differentiate true positive cultures from contaminants.[45] Microbiological parameters useful in interpreting the blood culture results include the recovered microorganism identity, subsequent positive blood cultures, the total number of positive blood cultures in the series and the presence of the same microorganism as that found in the blood cultured from another normally sterile site.[28,30] Clinically, known risk factors for bacteremia, such as the presence of prosthetic material, elevated inflammatory indices and a scenario consistent with sepsis will influence the interpretation of blood culture results.[45]

Microorganisms can be categorized according to their likelihood of representing a true infection (Table 6). Certain microorganisms almost always represent a true infection, while the diphtheroids and coagulase-negative staphylococci represent interpretive challenges. Contaminant blood cultures represent up to half of all positive blood cultures.[21,40,45] Generally, contaminants are present in a single bottle of the culture set

---

Table 6
Guidelines for Blood Culture Interpretation Based on Culture Results[21,23,26,45]

Microorganisms representing true infection
(>90% of isolates)

Staphylococcus aureus
Eschericia coli
Enterobacteriaceae
Pseudomonas aeruginosa
Streptococcus pneumoniae
Candida albicans

Microorganisms rarely representing true infection
(<5% of isolates)

Bacillus spp
Proprionibacterium acnes

Microorganisms with problematic interpretation
(5–15% represent true infection)

Corynebacterium spp and other diphtheroids
Coagulase-negative staphylococci

and are detected late in incubation.[21,40] Polymicrobial bacteremia is unusual, so multiple organisms isolated from one culture suggest contamination. To complicate matters, many microorganisms implicated in endocarditis are also the same commensal skin microbes that are frequently considered contaminants. Diphtheroids and coagulase- negative staphylococci culture isolates represent true infection in only 6% to 15% of cultures.[21,26,45] These "contaminants" represent true infection more frequently in the patient population with prosthetic valves and immune compromise.

A useful interpretive concept is the percentage of positive culture sets. If most cultures in a series are positive, there is a high probability that the organism is clinically relevant, as contaminants are rarely isolated in subsequent cultures.[38,45] Although the likelihood of a false positive culture increases with the number of cultures in a series, correct interpretation improves because individual blood culture results are reviewed within the context of the series and not independently.[21,40,45] Avoid assumptions when considering contaminant microorganism isolates which may be causative agents in endocarditis. Some investigators have assumed that all single bottles positive for coagulase-negative staphylococci are contaminants. [21,22,26,45] Peacock argues data suggesting that although a single positive bottle is unlikely to represent true infection, this is not invariably the case.[45] If clinical suspicion of endocarditis persists and only one blood culture bottle is positive, consider pre-culture antibiotic use or decreased inoculum size as possible explanations for the negative cultures.

Culture-Negative Endocarditis

Blood cultures are negative in 5% to 15% of patients with endocarditis.[11,15,30,46–49] Previous antimicrobial therapy is the most frequently associated factor. Some significant pathogens that are known to cause endocarditis require growth conditions that will not be met with standard blood culture systems (Table 7). The available epidemiological information, culture requirements, tissue examination, serological and molecular methods for these organisms are discussed separately below. Useful serological methods are summarized in Table 8.

Bartonella

Bartonella is a slow-growing gram-negative bacterium implicated in cat scratch disease, bacillary angiomatosis and other diseases. In a series of 22 cases, *Bartonella* endocarditis occurred in patients with pre-existing

Table 7
"Culture-Negative" Endocarditis Microorganisms Likely To Require
Specialized Recovery Culture Techniques[11,15,30,35,46,48,49]

Bacteria	Filamentous bacteria (Gram-positive intracellular parasites)
Bartonella spp	Actinomyces israelii
Brucella spp	Mycobacterium tuberculosis
Campylobacter fetus	Mycobacterium chelonnei
Corynebacterium spp	Mycobacterium fortuitum
Coxiella burnetti	Nocardia asteroides
HACEK group	**Non-bacterial organisms**
Legionella spp	Chlamydia spp
Listeria monocytogenes	Mycoplasma spp
Neisseria spp	**Fungi**
Nutritionally variant streptococci	Aspergillus spp
Anaerobic bacteria	Candida spp
Anaerobiospirillum succiniproducens	Curvularia genuculata
Peptococcus spp	Torulopsis glabrata
Veillonella dispar	
Fusobacterium necrophorum	

valvular disease or valve surgery (17 of 22), homeless patients (8 of 22), alcoholic patients (10 of 22) and cat fanciers (3 of 22).[50] Three species are associated with endocarditis: *B. henselae, B. quintana* and *B. elizabethae*. Body louse is the vector, correlating to the higher case numbers seen in homeless populations of the inner city.[7,11]

Cultures for *Bartonella* species may be performed on blood or valvular tissue.[7,8,10,11] *Bartonella* is difficult to grow by routine blood culture techniques, requiring a minimum incubation period of 4 to 8 weeks. Growth is sufficiently slow that the thresholds for detection in continuous monitoring blood culture systems will rarely be reached. Blind subculturing to fresh chocolate agar or sheep blood agar and incubation under increased CO_2 and humidity is often necessary. Acridine orange staining of blood culture media at time of subculture may provide another means of detecting organisms. Other methods have been reported to improve the yield and to shorten recovery time. These include adding endothelial cells to the culture media and cell line culture using the human endothelial ECV 304 cell line.[11,50] When available, the lysis centrifugation blood culture method can be used with the sediment plated directly onto chocolate agar and incubated under increased CO_2 and humidity.[7,50,51]

Light and electron microscopic evaluation is recommended for valvular tissue. Routine hematoxylin and eosin stains will show features of subacute endocarditis, but are unlikely to reveal *Bartonella* organisms. The

Table 8
Serologic Methods Useful in Establishing a Diagnosis in Cases of Culture-Negative Endocarditis

Organism	Technique	Interpretation and notes
Bartonella spp	Enzyme Immunoassay (EIA)	↑ 1:64 to 1:100—infection ↑ 1:1600 suggestive of endocarditis ↑ Cross reactivity with Chlamydia antibody assays
Brucella spp	Standard tube agglutination (STA)	↑ >1:160—infection ↑ ≥1:620—suggestive of endocarditis ↑ Titers remain ↑ up to 1 year post infection ↑ Cross reactivity to Yersinia, Francisella, and Vibrio
	STA with 2-mercaptoethanol (2-ME)	↑ IgG determination only ↑ 1:160—ongoing infection
	Enzyme immunoassay (EIA)	↑ IgA, IgG and IgM determinations ↑ See reference intervals provided by reference laboratory
	Microimmunofluorescence (MIF)	↑ IgA, IgG and IgM determinations ↑ See reference intervals provided by reference laboratory
Campylobacter fetus	Complement fixation antibody titers	↑ Limited utility—see reference intervals
Chlamydia spp	Microimmunofluorescence	↑ Titers correlating to endocarditis not reported ↑ Titers correlating to endocarditis not reported ↑ Cross reactivity seen with Bartonella spp

Organism	Test		Notes
Coxiella burnetii	Complement fixation antibody titers	↑	IgA, IgG antibody titers more useful for chronic infection
Legionella pneumophila	Microimmunofluorescence (MIF)	↑	Phase I antigen 1:200—chronic infection
		↑	Phase I antigen IgA = 320 - chronic infection
	Direct Fluorescent Antigen (DFA)	↑	Method available for urine and sputum—applicability to valve specimens is theoretical
	Indirect Fluorescent Antibody	↑	IgG and IgM titer determination available
		↑	1:512 diagnostic of Legionella infection
		↑	No defined titer diagnostic of endocarditis
Listeria monocytogenes	Complement fixation antibody titers	↑	No defined titer diagnostic of endocarditis
Mycoplasma pneumoniae	Complement fixation antibody titers	↑	1:8—evolving or resolving infection
		↑	1:32 or ≥4-fold increase over 2–3 weeks—evolving infection
		↑	≥1:64—recent infection
		↑	serial detections warranted
Neisseria gonorrheae	Complement fixation antibody titers	↑	No reference interval for endocarditis
	Enzyme immunoassay (EIA)	↑	Antigen detection currently available for genital swabs. Swab of excised valves have no standardized reference interval
Nocardia spp	Enzyme immunoassay (EIA)	↑	IgG antibody detection
		↑	No defined titer diagnostic of endocarditis

pleomorphic rods may be highlighted with Warthin-Starry stain. Electron microscopy of *B. quintana* demonstrates both intracellular and extracellular bacteria grouped in small clusters surrounded by a thin vacuolar membrane.[50,51]

A serological test using a microimmunofluorescence antibody has been reported. Titers of 1:64 to 1:100 by this method indicate *Bartonella* infection while a titer of 1:1600 or more had a positive predictive value of 0.884 for cases of *Bartonella* endocarditis.[50] Enzyme immunoassay on serum specimens is more widely available through reference laboratories. The diagnostic titers are dependent upon the methodology. Communication with the reference laboratory to determine the most appropriate specimen for analysis is recommended. Frozen, refrigerated and room temperature sera have been used for both IgG and IgM determinations. Diagnostic serologies are often requested as groups (i.e., as a battery) to evaluate a difficult case. Patients with *Bartonella* endocarditis may produce antibodies that react with *Chlamydia pneumoniae*, *C. psittaci* and *C. trachomatis*. The clinical history and *Bartonella* titers are helpful when chlamydial endocarditis is suspected. Although *Bartonella* titers are often useful, not all cases of endocarditis detected by culture, molecular methods or electron microscopy showed elevation of *Bartonella* titers.[51] Serological tests should not be relied upon exclusively to provide a diagnosis but have been suggested to be considered "minor" clinical criteria when using the Duke classification.[53,54] Molecular methods including DNA amplification of the 16S ribosomal RNA (rRNA) or the citrate synthase gene, have been developed. [11,35,50,52,53] Amplification can be performed on whole blood or valvular tissue (fresh frozen or paraffin-embedded).[50] A qualitative result is reported. Availability is limited to specialized reference laboratories.

Brucella

Brucellosis is a zoonotic disease associated with endocarditis in less than 2% of cases. Endocarditis, however, is the main cause of mortality in patients with brucellosis.[53] *Brucella* are slow-growing, gram-negative coccobacilli with *B. melitensis* and *B. abortus* most commonly associated with endocarditis. Residence in or travel to the Middle East or Mediterranean countries, with or without ingestion of unpasteurized milk products, may raise clinical suspicion for this entity.

Traditionally, culture for *Brucella* has been with biphasic media (Castaneda bottles). Over the last decade, technological improvements have increased the yield by automated blood culture to 70% to 90% in patients with known brucellosis.[11,51] Despite slow growth, newer blood culture methods and enriched media often allow recovery in 5 to 7 days. In some cases, or with prior antibiotic use, several weeks of incubation may be needed to detect growth. The growth rate may be insufficient to meet the threshold requirements in automated systems. Therefore, blind and/or terminal subcultures are frequently necessary. Improved recovery is seen with the lysis centrifugation method, followed by growth on *Brucella* media.[11,51] Tissue culture of excised valves can be particularly useful. Cultures of vegetations commonly yield *Brucella* despite antimicrobial therapy administered for up to 6 weeks.[53]

Patients with *Brucella* endocarditis develop an antibody response against the outer membrane lipopolysaccharide (O-specific fraction). The most commonly applied serological method is the standard tube agglutination test (STA). An elevated agglutinating *Brucella* antibody titer (usually >1:160) is indicative of *Brucella* infection, and a markedly elevated titer (1:620) indicates *Brucella* endocarditis. The STA is both sensitive and specific. Serological cross-reactions between *Brucella*, *Yersinia*, *Francisella* and *Vibrio* occur but rarely cause diagnostic confusion. Titers may remain elevated up to a year after the acute infection. IgM separation from IgG antibodies is achieved with addition of 2-mercaptoethanol to the STA test, allowing quantification of IgG antibodies. Ongoing infection is suggested by a titer of 1:160 in 2-mercaptoethanol treated samples.[53] Enzyme immunoassay and radioimmunoassays for IgA, IgG and IgM antibodies are available through reference laboratories. Despite the known antibody persistence, some authors recommend regular serological analysis to monitor therapeutic response.[11]

Ribosomal RNA sequence amplification with polymerase chain reaction performed on valvular tissue has been used to document *Brucella* infection but is currently limited to research facilities.[53]

Campylobacter

Campylobacter are curved, microaerophilic motile rods. Of the 3 groups of *Campylobacter*, *C. fetus* is associated with endocarditis. *Campylobacter* can be isolated from blood by a variety of blood culture systems, but most systems require blind subcultures to increase yield and decrease the time required for microbial growth detection. Subcultures are in a microaerophilic environment.

C. fetus complement fixation antibody determination is available through reference laboratories, although no reports correlating titers to occurrence of endocarditis were found in the literature.

Chlamydia

Three species of *Chlamydia* can cause endocarditis: *C. psittaci*, *C. trachomatis* and *C. pneumoniae*. *C. psittaci* accounts for most of these rare cases. Endocarditis may present in an acute, subacute or chronic manner with universal aortic valve involvement in reported cases. *Chlamydia* are obligate intracellular parasites and are not culturable with routine methods. Shell vial inoculation with valvular tissue followed by specific fluorescent monoclonal antibody testing documents infection. Significant infection risk to laboratory personnel limits use of this method.[53,55]

Microimmunofluorescent methods are available for determination of IgA, IgG, IgM and total antibodies for *C. pneumoniae*, *C. psittaci* and *C. trachomatis*. Absolute titers have not been defined as indicative of endocarditis. Complement fixing antibodies over 1:32 have been reported in isolated cases of *Chlamydia* endocarditis. Antibodies to *Bartonella* may cross-react, therefore, concomitant evaluation for *Bartonella* may be warranted. Direct fluorescent antibody technique, a technique standardized for genitourinary specimens, may be attempted on smears from valvular tissue. Sensitivity and specificity of this method have not been determined.

Polymerase and ligase chain reaction methods have been developed for *C. trachomatis*. Qualitative polymerase chain reaction techniques amplifying *C. pneumoniae* DNA are available through reference laboratories for use on sputum, bronchial lavage, cerebrospinal fluid or tissue (fresh frozen and paraffin-embedded).

Corynebacterium

Corynebacterium are generally regarded as culture contaminants but are proven pathogens in immunocompromised patients, intravenous drug users and patients with cardiac valve prostheses. *Corynebacteria* are implicated in both early and late prosthetic valve endocarditis and infrequently cause native valve endocarditis.[7,11] Time of incubation is the single most important factor in improving recovery. *Corynebacterium*, recovered in multiple blood cultures, indicates infection rather than contamination and warrants lengthening the incubation period of subsequent cultures.

Coxiella

Coxiella burnetii causes the worldwide zoonosis Q fever. Chronic infection results in endocarditis in roughly 11% of patients.[11,53] It occurs worldwide, but the highest prevalence is within the United Kingdom, France and Spain. Cases in the United States are rare. Transmission is possible via inhalation, ingestion, transfusion and transplacental transfer.

C. burnetii is an obligate intracellular parasite and, as such, cannot be cultured by routine methods. Conventional shell vial assays have been reported to propagate the organism but pose significant risk of infection to laboratory personnel and, for this reason, cannot be recommended.[20,56] Culture of valvular material is not recommended for the same reasons. Diagnosis is dependent upon serological tests in combination with tissue examination.

Light and electron microscopy are recommended for native valvular tissue or encrustations and vegetations from prosthetic material. Histological examination shows features of acute and subacute disease within the valve. *Coxiella* microorganisms can be demonstrated with Giemsa and Gimenez stains.[7,57,58] Immunohistological techniques have also been reported but are not widely available.[19,20,57,58] Characteristic electron microscopic findings include identification of 2 morphologic cell types, a small round cell variant and a larger rod-shaped variant, the combination of which may yield a conclusive diagnosis.[52,58]

Complement fixation and indirect microimmunofluorescence serological assays provide the cornerstone for *C. burnetii* diagnosis. Antigenic variation occurs with the phase of the disease. Phase I antibodies present in high titer during chronic disease and phase II antibodies are elevated during both acute and chronic disease.[54,59,60] Complement fixing antibodies to *Coxiella* phase I antigen of greater than 1 : 200 are indicative of chronic *Coxiella* infection.[11,54] By microimmunofluorescence, an IgA titer of 320 or higher against phase I antigen is indicative of chronic infection.[8,11] IgA and IgG antibody determinations are more reliable than IgM antibodies for documenting chronic infections.[54,59] Peacock suggests that the presence of a high phase I specific IgA antibody titer with microimmunofluorescence is diagnostic for endocarditis and differentiates between endocarditis and other forms of chronic Q fever.[59] In geographic areas where this infection is prevalent, high anti-phase I serological titers may be considered a major clinical criterion in the Duke classification system.[54]

Recently, polymerase chain reaction was used to amplify a DNA segment of the superoxide dismutase gene unique to *C. burnetii* from valve tissue.[11,61,62] This methodology may become available to reference laboratories.

HACEK Organisms

HACEK organisms (see Table 2) are fastidious gram-negative bacteria responsible for approximately 3% of endocarditis cases.[11] *Hemophilus* species account for half of these cases.[47,63]

Culture of HACEK microorganisms is often approached with trepidation. These slow-growing organisms require factors V and X (not present in standard media) and are best cultivated in 5% to 10% CO_2. Prospective data regarding the optimal media for recovering these bacteria, the duration of incubation, the optimal number of subcultures, and the use of specialized media are lacking. Conservative processing with lengthy incubation (7 to 14 days), blind subcultures at 2 and 7 days and terminal subcultures at the conclusion of incubation are recommended.[33,51] Subcultures must include a chocolate agar plate incubated aerobically with 5% to 10% CO_2. Following isolation, definitive speciation is often difficult due to metabolic or biochemical variability. Rapid commercial kits are available but may not identify all species.[63] HACEK organisms may be identified to the species level and sometimes strain by analysis of certain specific rRNA genes.[63] Currently, this method remains experimental.

Legionella

Legionella pneumophila is generally associated with community acquired pneumonia. However, rare cases of prosthetic valve endocarditis have been reported. The low case numbers prevent extrapolation of serological and molecular methods ordinarily used in the setting of pneumonia to endocarditis cases.

A variety of blood culture methods can isolate *L. pneumophila* but optimal recovery requires blind subcultures to 3 media that improve recovery: nonselective buffered charcoal yeast extract (BCYE) agar, semiselective *Legionella* medium (BCYE with additional antibiotics) and 5% sheep blood agar. Growth may be inadequate in automated blood culture systems to reach preset thresholds; consequently, blind subculture is required. Blood culture sensitivity is 50% to 80% with 100% specificity when the above subculture media are used.[11] Valvular tissue cultures should be directly plated to these 3 media as well.

Direct fluorescent antigen detection for sputum smears and enzyme immunoassay for urine specimens have been well studied.[7,8,64] Both may be used for valve material smears or culture. Antibody detection in the serum is limited by the lengthy time to seroconversion. An indirect fluorescent antibody titer of 1:512 is diagnostic of *Legionella* infection, with separate IgG and IgM determinations available. Serotyping is also available in the event nosocomial acquisition is suspected.

The DNA detector method for *Legionella* species is available through reference laboratories with standardization of the technique performed on sputum.[65] Other specimens, including valve tissue, may be acceptable for evaluation.

Listeria

Listeria monocytogenes has been implicated in fewer than 51 cases of endocarditis worldwide.[11] Blood culture recovery is improved with early and terminal blind subcultures to sheep blood agar.[7,8,51] Complement fixation tests for *Listeria* antibodies can be performed on serum samples.[64] There is no defined titer diagnostic of endocarditis.

Mycobacteria

Rare, but fulminant, cases of *Mycobacteria chelonei*, *M. fortuitum* and *M. avium* complex endocarditis have been reported. Blood cultures for *Mycobacteria* require specialized broth media and an extended incubation time. The BACTEC radiometric system with 13A media has excellent sensitivity. Cultures should be maintained for a minimum of 4 to 8 weeks. Periodic subculturing or tissue culture to Löwenstein Jensen agar may enhance recovery. The MB/Bact (Organon Teknika, Durham, NC), ESP (Accumed International, Chicago, IL) and BACTEC 9000 with Myco/F Lytic Medium (Becton Dickinson, Franklin Lakes, NJ) continuous monitoring systems are currently under investigation.[8,33] Qualitative DNA polymerase chain reaction is available through reference laboratories.[65]

Mycoplasma

Mycoplasma pneumoniae, an organism commonly implicated in atypical pneumonia, rarely causes endocarditis.[11] Diagnosis relies on the combination of tissue culture and serum antibodies. Conventional blood culture systems do not support *Mycoplasma* growth.[7,8] Enriched peptone basal agar with yeast extract and serum should be used for tissue culture.[7,8,51] Serological methods are supportive but cannot provide definitive diagnosis independently. Antibody levels to *M. pneumoniae* persist only a few weeks or months following infection. Lower titers (1:8 to 1:32) may provide evidence of evolving or resolving infection.[11] A fourfold or greater increase in complement fixation titer over a 2 to 3 week period implicates *M. pneumoniae* and single high titers (1:64 or greater) are suggestive of recent infection. Titer interpretation is guided by the results of several determinations. Qualitative DNA polymerase chain reaction assays (standardized on sputum specimens) are available through reference laboratories; application to valve material may be limited.

Neisseria

Neisseria endocarditis is a clinically aggressive infection. Once common in the pre-antimicrobial era, *Neisseria* endocarditis is now rare. Endocarditis occurs as a catastrophic complication in 1% to 2% of cases of disseminated gonococcal infection.[11,66] *N. gonorrhoeae* culture from blood is inhibited by a common anticoagulant, sodium polyanetholesulfonate (SPS), present in most blood culture bottles. The inhibitory effect of SPS may be reduced by adding 1.2% sterile gelatin to the media, although this may decrease the recovery of other pathogens.[7,8] Alternately, the lysis centrifugation method is effective for recovering *N. gonorrhoeae* from blood. Antimicrobial sensitivity testing is essential as antibiotic resistance is common. Enzyme immunoassay detection of *N. gonorrhoeae* antigens is currently available for use with genital swabs. Antibodies are detected by complement fixation of serum samples. Clinical experience with molecular techniques is limited with blood cultures. Ligase chain reaction is presently used with urine, cervical and urethral swabs. The method does not precisely translate to blood. The molecular techniques available are limited *to N. gonorrhoeae* and would not be sensitive or specific to other species of *Neisseria* that may be implicated in endocarditis.

Nocardia

The aerobic actinomycete *Nocardia* is an infrequent cause of endocarditis. *Nocardia* species characteristically cause suppurative infections of the lungs and central nervous system in patients with immune dysfunction. *Nocardia* most often involves prosthetic valves. Definitive diagnosis requires blood or tissue culture and so cannot be made presumptively based on serological status. Blood cultures are frequently negative. Recovery is enhanced by blind subcultures to blood agar, Sabouraud dextrose agar or BCYE agar.[7,8,11,51] Adequate growth on these solid media requires a prolonged incubation period of at least 72 hours. *Nocardia* IgG antibodies can be detected in serum by enzyme immunoassay. No reference interval or interpretive standardization for endocarditis is available.

Nutritionally Variant Streptococci (*Abiotrophia* spp)

The nutritionally variant streptococci (*S. adjacens, S. defectivus*) are commensal organisms of the upper respiratory tract, recently reclassified as *Abiotrophia adiacens* and *A. defectiva* based on 16S rRNA gene polymerase chain reaction and restriction fragment length polymorphism analysis.[67,68] A third species in this newly classified genus (*A. elegans* sp nov) has been implicated in culture-negative endocarditis.[69] Distinct from the viridans streptococci by restriction fragment length polymorphism patterns and pyridoxal requirements, they account for 10% of cases classified as viridans endocarditis.[11,70] While it is able to grow in most blood culture media, cultivation during routine subculture upon solid media poses significant difficulty. Wilson suggests that this detection of gram-positive cocci in blood culture with failure to grow on routine subculture should alert the laboratory to the possibility of nutritionally variant streptococci (*Abiotrophia* spp).[27] Agar media supplemented with 0.001% pyridoxal, brucella agar with sheep blood, or a standard blood agar supplemented with a staphylococcal streak will provide sufficient pyridoxal for growth.[11,27,70]

Fungal Organisms

The incidence of fungemia and fungal endocarditis is increasing.[11,13,15,16,47,49,71] Clinical suspicion should be raised and fungal cultures obtained in patients with prosthetic devices, indwelling catheters, those receiving hemodialysis or hyperalimentation. Intravenous drug users and immune compromised patients are also at significant risk.

A variety of fungal organisms may cause endocarditis (Table 3) with *Candida* sp and *Aspergillus* sp accounting for nearly 75% of cases.[13,16,49] Fungi are present in blood in much lower numbers than bacteria, making fungemia detection inherently difficult. The paucity of circulating organisms is particularly apparent when a yeast phase of the organism does not exist.[11] Consequently, fungi other than *Candida* rarely grow in conventional blood culture systems.[11,49] *Candida* sp endocarditis will yield positive blood cultures in 83% to 95% of cases.[11,49] The Isolator Lysis-centrifugation system (Wampole Laboratories, Cranbury, NJ) continues to be recommended for improved fungi recovery, especially filamentous fungi.[10,11,16,49] Instrumented blood culture systems with newer media formulations (BACTEC aerobic resin and BacT/Alert aerobic FAN medium) and high blood volume (HBV)cultures (BACTEC) perform well for the isolation of fungi other than *Cryptococcus*.[11,49]

Fungal endocarditis is frequently complicated by emboli. Culture of embolic sites is an essential supplementary means of recovering pathogenic fungi. *Aspergillus* endocarditis can frequently be documented by culture of skin emboli while blood cultures often remain negative.[49] All skin, vitreal, oropharyngeal and lung lesions should be carefully cultured.[49] Tissue not used for culture should be submitted for histological examination. Fungal organisms are not easily seen on routine hematoxylin and eosin stains. Fungal stains (Periodic Acid–Schiff [PAS] and Grocott's/Gomori Methamine Silver [GMS]) should be performed on all tissue blocks. These stains are quite sensitive and may allow for genus identification based upon differential histological features. Several commercial immunologic methods have been developed to detect fungal antigens and antibodies. Evaluation of these methods has failed to show any clinical usefulness in endocarditis.[11,49]

Molecular methods for fungal identification are limited to rRNA and DNA probes that will identify pure cultures submitted on an agar slant. Probes are available through reference laboratories for *Blastomyces dermatitidis*, *Coccidiodes immitis* and *Histoplasma capsulatum*.

Antimicrobial Susceptibility Testing

Empirical antibiotic therapy is instituted or adjusted based on the initial Gram's stain result from positive blood culture bottles. The final decision regarding the selection of antibiotics depends on the in vitro microorganism susceptibility.[13,15,30,46] Routine antibiotic susceptibility tests indicate minimum inhibitory concentrations (MIC) but provide no information on bactericidal activity. [35] Bactericidal therapy is necessary for effective treatment of endocarditis as demonstrated by experimental models and supported by clinical experience.[30,46,47,72,73] Bactericidal antibiotic concentrations that inhibit microorganism growth may lack bactericidal effect and fail to sterilize the vegetation.[72,73,74,75] Thus, susceptibility tests limited to MIC may not be sufficient to guide endocarditis therapy.[74] Bactericidal activity testing in endocarditis has been recommended, and the National Committee for Clinical Laboratory Standards has recently issued guidelines for standardization of bactericidal testing.[15,37,74,76,77] Nonetheless, quantitative correlation of in vitro test results to experimental models and clinical outcome remains difficult even when highly standardized, reproducible tests are used.[76,77]

Tests used to determine bactericidal activity are the minimum bactericidal concentration (MBC), serum bactericidal test (SBT) and time-kill curves (Table 9). Several physiologic and pharmacodynamic factors specific to endocarditis can influence antibiotic effectiveness including bacterial quantity within the vegetations, metabolic state, residence within endothelial cells, exopolysaccharide secretion and the antibiotic diffusion characteristics within the vegetation.[18,72,74] For many antibiotics, kill rate is proportional to growth rate. [11,75] Microorganisms on the vegetation surface are likely to be in the logarithmic growth phase while those deep within the vegetation will subsist in a stationary growth phase. Bactericidal testing is performed on subcultures during the logarithmic growth phase.[7,75,76] MBC, SBT and time-kill curves may reflect the antibiotic effect on actively reproducing microorganisms on the valve surface but not on the stationary-phase microorganisms deep within the vegetation or within endothelial cells.[18] Bactericidal assays also assume a uniform antibiotic concentration within the valve and vegetation following administration. In an elegant study using 14C-labeled antibiotics, Carbon et al showed 3

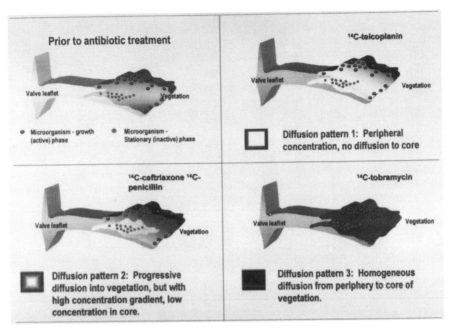

Figure 14. Diffusion characteristics of selected antimicrobial agents into vegetations. Adapted from text by Carbon, et al.[72,73]

distinct diffusion patterns into infected vegetations (Figure 14), therefore homogeneous diffusion of all antibiotics cannot be assumed.[72,73] Exopolysaccharide secretion may also impair antibiotic diffusion and is frequently encountered with *Staphylococcus aureus* and *Pseudomonas* species. Finally, microbial phenotypic variance in antibiotic tolerance is an additional factor that cannot be accounted for with in vitro testing.

Serum inhibitory and bactericidal titers have been well studied but fail to provide sufficient evidence for correlation to clinical outcome even when standardized methodologies are used.[35,76,77] While bacteriological cure can be predicted by the serum bactericidal test, bacteriological failure and clinical outcome cannot.[76,77] Although the in vitro evaluation of the bactericidal testing is attractive conceptually and appears to be necessary clinically, the results must be interpreted with caution.

Ancillary Laboratory Tests

Many laboratory indices may be abnormal in patients with endocarditis and therefore substantiate a clinical suspicion for the diagnosis.

Table 9
Antimicrobial Susceptibility Testing Terminology[7,74,76]

Inhibitory Tests	Definition	Clinical Utility
Minimum Inhibitory Concentration (MIC)	The lowest concentration of an antimicrobial agent that inhibits growth, as determined visually after a standard incubation period (usually 18 to 24 hours)	• Most commonly employed methodology for susceptibility testing • Disk and broth methods used • Does not provide information on bactericidal effect
Serum Inhibitory Titer (Schlichter Test)	The highest dilution of a serum sample taken from a patient receiving antimicrobial therapy that inhibits visible growth after incubation (usually 18 to 24 hours)	• Indirect quantification of serum antibiotic levels • Requires use of log phase subculture • Contact clinical microbiology laboratory

Bactericidal Tests	Definition	Clinical Utility
Minimum Bactericidal Concentration (MBC)	The lowest concentration of an antibacterial agent that causes at least a 3 $\log_{10}$ reduction in the number of surviving cells after a standard incubation period (usually 18 to 24 hours)	• Microdilution technique recommended • Some automated systems available • Requires use of log-phase subculture • Contact clinical microbiology laboratory

Serum Bactericidal Titer (SBT)	The highest dilution of a serum sample taken from a patient receiving antimicrobial therapy that causes at least a 3 $\log_{10}$ reduction in the number of surviving cells after incubation (usually 18 to 24 hours)	• Until recently, poorly standardized • Clinical utility uncertain • Requires use of log-phase subculture • Requires serum at peak and trough intervals • Contact clinical microbiology laboratory
Killing Curve (Time-Kill Study)	A single antibiotic concentration (usually near the mean achievable level in blood) is studied for its effect on the killing rate on a log phase subculture. Subcultures to antibiotic-free agar are performed at specific intervals during a 24-hour incubation.	• Labor intensive • Permits graphical extrapolation of the bactericidal rate • Serum effects not studied with this method • Contact clinical microbiology laboratory
Checkerboard (Synergy) Test	Combinations of two antimicrobial agents studied. Doubling dilutions of each agent are prepared with one increasing along the vertical axis and the other along the horizontal axis (12 by 12 configuration). The appearance of bacteriostatic or bactericidal activity is typically determined for each tube in the set with the result indicating the optimal concentrations of each drug in combination for inhibitory and bactericidal effects.	• Labor intensive • Serum effects not studied • Clinical utility in complicated patients who are not good candidates for surgical therapy • Contact clinical microbiology laboratory

Hematologic Indices

The complete blood count may be normal; however, the white blood cell count is generally increased in acute endocarditis with an increase in segmented neutrophils.[15,16,35] Decreased or normal white cell counts are more likely present in subacute endocarditis, the immune compromised hosts and the elderly.[15,35] Normocytic, normochromic anemia is found in 70% to 90%, with or without concomitant iron indices suggesting anemia of chronic disease.[15,16,35] Platelet abnormalities with reactive thrombocythemia or thrombocytopenia related to disseminated intravascular coagulation are seen less frequently.[30]

Indices of Hemolysis

Immune-mediated and mechanical hemolysis may contribute significantly to anemia and lead to positive direct and indirect antihuman globulin tests (DAT, Coomb's). Hemolysis usually improves with effective endocarditis treatment. Urine hemosiderin may give a relative indication of the degree of hemolysis.[35] Serum haptoglobin levels increase with the acute phase response, thus normal serum haptoglobin levels do not rule out significant hemolysis.[78]

Coagulation Indices

Prothrombin and partial thromboplastin times are useful screening tests but may not accurately reflect the complex abnormalities associated with endovascular infections. The risk of disseminated intravascular coagulation (DIC) with endocarditis is significant and may precede endocarditis or develop as sequelae of the infectious process.[30] Fibrinogen levels may be increased, normal or decreased. Fibrinogen levels increase with the acute phase response (Figure 15) and with chronic compensated DIC. With uncompensated DIC, fibrinogen levels decrease. Fibrin split products or D-dimer, will be elevated in both compensated and uncompensated DIC.

Erythrocyte Sedimentation Rate

Erythrocyte sedimentation rate (ESR) is reportedly elevated in 67% to 100% of endocarditis cases.[15,16,35,79] Recent studies have shown a substantial proportion of endocarditis with an ESR within the normal limits.[79,80] Although no statistical correlation with the duration of the disease could be made, a tendency for the ESR to be lower in more aggressive cases

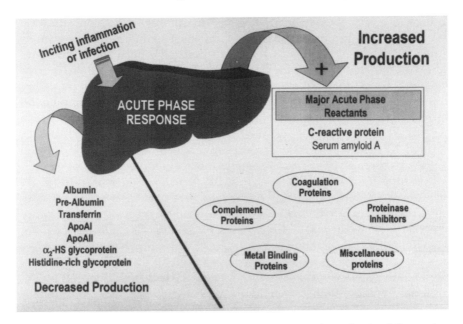

Figure 15. The acute phase response results in increased synthesis of C-reactive protein, a clinically useful marker of the inflammatory process.

was evident.[79,80] Patients with congestive heart failure, renal failure and DIC may not show an increase in the ESR.[78] Although ESR value declines with effective therapy, the rate of decline is sufficiently slow to preclude its use as a therapeutic monitoring tool.[16,35,79,80] Further, ESR values do not differentiate between uneventful and complicated cases of endocarditis, particularly those managed surgically.[79,80,81]

C-reactive Protein

C-reactive protein (CRP) is a pentraxin protein which functions as a major acute phase reactant. CRP is an opsonin for bacteria, parasites and immune complexes.[78,82] CRP can activate complement and bind to chromatin, histones and small nuclear ribonucleoprotein particles.[78,82] Standardized serum immunochemical assay methods are rapid and widely available.[80,83] Under normal conditions, CRP is present only in trace amounts.[78,82,84] Within individuals, CRP levels are tightly regulated with minimal variability when studied over a 6-month period.[84] During the acute phase response, acute phase reactant biosynthesis is increased while synthesis of other plasma proteins decreases (Figure 15).[78,82] The plasma concentrations of individual acute phase reactants are variable with most induced slightly above normal levels.[78] In contrast, CRP concentration may increase up to a thousand times in response to inflammation or infection.[78,82,84] The magnitude of the CRP response has been shown to correlate with the severity of tissue damage.[83] The half-life of CRP is approximately 8 to 12 hours; therefore, when the inflammatory or infectious stimulus is removed, CRP levels quickly decline.[78,79,82] The marked response and short half-life make CRP an attractive clinical marker. A rise in serum CRP is nonspecific and is not diagnostic of infection or endocarditis. Serum CRP levels support the diagnosis of endocarditis, give an indication of the infection severity and are invaluable in therapeutic monitoring.

In long-term prospective studies, CRP levels are increased in nearly all cases of endocarditis.[79,80,83] Generally, a serum CRP level above 10 mg/L is considered to be indicative of a clinically significant inflammatory process.[78,80,84] In strictly defined cases of endocarditis, serum levels of 90–110 mg/L at presentation are reported.[79,80] In contrast to ESR, increases in CRP occur early in the disease process with an elevated CRP level at presentation in 96% of patients.[79,80,83] The CRP level is influenced by the bacterial etiology, with higher levels reported for *Staphylococcus aureus* endocarditis.[79,80] In one study, the initial CRP levels in culture-negative and prosthetic valve endocarditis were reportedly less than those with native valve endocarditis (56 mg/L versus 94 mg/L respectively).[79] In a subsequent study, no difference in CRP levels was appreciated between native and prosthetic valve endocarditis both at presentation and during treatment.[80] Neonates and the elderly both show significant increases in CRP with endocarditis.[79,80,85] The reference range for normal in neonates is below 1 mg/dL with increases to 1.5 mg/dL to 27 mg/dL reported.[85] Cirrhotic patients may not respond with a rise of CRP.[80]

Immunologic Assays

Bacteremia stimulates humoral and cellular immune responses, resulting in circulating immune complex formation. Immune complexes, precipitating the systemic immune mediated processes historically associated with endocarditis, are often detectable with subacute endocarditis.[15,35] The circulating immune complex titer falls with effective antibiotic therapy and rises or reappears with therapeutic failure.[16,35] McCartney et al compared circulating immune complexes to serum CRP in patients with streptococcal endocarditis and found that circulating immune complex determination was more time-consuming and a less sensitive indicator of treatment response.[86] Elevated rheumatoid factor levels may be present in up to 51% of patients with subacute endocarditis.[15,35] Comparable to other inflammatory indices, rheumatoid factor levels will decrease with effective therapy.[15,35] Serological markers for systemic diseases may be drawn in the course of the diagnostic work-up. Antineutrophil cytoplasmic antibodies with a perinuclear pattern (p-ANCA) can be seen in isolated cases of endocarditis without systemic vasculitis. The perinuclear pattern corresponds to several antigens, with myeloperoxidase specificity favoring vasculitis. Determination of proteinase-3 and myeloperoxidase titers will clarify the results of the p-ANCA serology. Antiphospholipid antibodies will be present in up to one third of patients with endocarditis.[14]

Urinalysis

Urinalysis may detect proteinuria and microscopic hematuria, reflecting immunologic renal injury.[15,16,35]

Monitoring Therapy

A recent study of endocarditis within our institution showed a recurrence rate of approximately 1 in 7 cases (23 of 140 patients), with a corresponding mortality of 22% with recurrences.[31] These figures highlight the importance of monitoring therapy. The most critical component of monitoring the adequacy of antimicrobial therapy is careful and frequent clinical assessment. While periodic blood cultures to ensure blood sterility have been recommended,[16,35] serial measurements of CRP provide more clinically useful information.[79,80,83] Serum antibiotic levels and bactericidal testing are discussed above.

Bacteremia due to endovascular infection is characteristically continuous in the untreated state. Prior to antimicrobial therapy, microorganisms on the vegetation surface are shed into the circulation (Figure 16). Bactericidal antibiotics eradicate surface microorganisms rapidly and blood cultures become negative. Sterilization of the vegetation surface does not guarantee complete eradication of the infection. Latent microorganisms within the vegetation and endothelial cells may persist and are a potential source for recurrence. Treatment with bacteriostatic antibiotics, or bacteriostatic doses of bactericidal antibiotics, arrests growth and replication. Circulating and tissue inflammatory cells then eliminate the non-replicating microorganisms. Early in the course of therapy, surface microorganisms may persist and result in positive blood cultures. Despite an initial positive blood culture, however, therapy may over time be effective in eradicating the organisms. Discontinuation of therapy based upon initial surface sterilization by bactericidal agents will inevitably lead to recurrence. Alteration of therapy based upon an early positive culture under

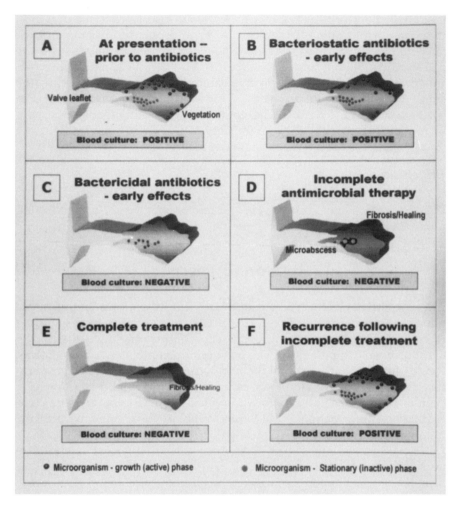

Figure 16. Potential responses to antimicrobial therapy in valvular endocarditis and the corresponding blood culture findings based on therapeutic response and stage of treatment. Therapeutic monitoring with blood cultures does not provide clinically relevant information.

bacteriostatic conditions may not be warranted either. Thus, repeat blood cultures early in the course of therapy provide little useful information.

Blood cultures do not differentiate between complete and incomplete courses of antimicrobial therapy for several weeks following therapy cessation. With incomplete treatment, vegetations may be smaller but still contain deeply seated viable bacteria. Despite residual endocarditis, blood cultures taken immediately after the cessation of therapy will be negative.

Recurrence becomes evident once the vegetation reaches a critical size and surface microorganisms are again shed. Symptoms suggestive of recurrence should guide the use of repeat blood cultures.

Repeated blood cultures are clearly warranted for evaluation of early prosthetic valve endocarditis. Residual endocarditis can be differentiated from nosocomial endocarditis if the repeated blood culture recovers a different organism than that implicated in the initial endocarditis.

Serial CRP determinations are valuable in monitoring antimicrobial therapy effectiveness. CRP levels will be elevated in 96% of endocarditis patients prior to therapy, and should decrease within 24 hours after effective therapy is begun.[79,80] In endocarditis patients studied by McCartney et al, the mean time to CRP normalization was 13 days (range 6 to 30 days).[83] Persistently elevated CRP concentrations corresponded to treatment failure.[80] Transient increases in CRP during in the course of medical therapy denote allergic drug reactions and/or complicating infections.[80,83]

Postoperative CRP measurements are also valuable. Cardiac surgery itself results in a characteristic CRP rise on the second and third postoperative days.[81,86–91] A persistently elevated CRP is more sensitive for detecting postoperative infectious complications than fever and increased white blood cell counts.[80,83,87,89] Patients undergoing valve replacement surgery for endocarditis showed the characteristic CRP rise which normalized by 17 days (range 8 to 24 days) postoperatively when no infectious complications developed.[80,83] Complications, including early prosthetic valve endocarditis, other infections and death, were accompanied by persistently elevated CRP levels.[80,83]

In summary, persistently elevated CRP levels indicate an ongoing inflammatory process and provide more clinically useful information than bactericidal assays and repeated blood cultures. While persistently increased CRP levels are not specific for persistent or recurrent endocarditis, they warrant further evaluation, a change in antimicrobial management and surgical consultation.[83]

References

1. Lukes AS, Bright DK, Durack DT. Diagnosis of infective endocarditis. *Infect Dis Clin North Am* 1993;7:1–8.
2. Durack DT, Lukes AS, Bright DK, et al. New criteria for diagnosis of infective endocarditis: Utilization of specific echocardiographic findings. *Am J Med* 1994;96:200–209.
3. VonReyn CF, Levy BS, Arbeit RD, et al. Infective endocarditis: An analysis based on strict case definitions. *Ann Intern Med* 1981;94:505–518.
4. Bayer AS. Revised diagnostic criteria for infective endocarditis. *Cardiol Clin* 1996;14:345–350.

5. Bayer AS, Ward JI, Ginzton LE, et al. Evaluation of new clinical criteria for the diagnosis of infective endocarditis. Am J Med 1994;96:211–219.
6. Hoen B, Selton-Suty C, Danchin N, et al. Evaluation of the Duke criteria versus the Beth Israel criteria for the diagnosis of infective endocarditis. Clin Infect Dis 1995;21: 905–909.
7. Koneman EW, Allen SD, Janda WM, et al (eds.) Color Atlas and Textbook of Diagnostic Microbiology, 4th ed. Philadelphia, PA, JB Lippincott Co., 1992.
8. Forbes BA, Sahm DF, Weissfeld AS (eds.) Diagnostic Microbiology, 10th ed. St. Louis, MO, Mosby-Yearbook, Inc., 1998.
9. Miller JM, Harvey TH. Specimen collection, transport and storage. In Murray PR, Baron EJ, Pfaller MA, et al (eds.) Manual of Clinical Microbiology, Washington, DC, American Society for Microbiology Press; 1995. pp 19–32.
10. Forbes BA, Granato PA. Processing specimens for bacteria. In Murray PR, Baron EJ, Pfaller MA, et al. (eds.) Manual of Clinical Microbiology, Washington DC, American Society for Microbiology Press, 1995. pp 265–281.
11. Berbari EF, Cockerill FR III, Steckelberg JM. Infective endocarditis due to unusual or fastidious microorganisms. Mayo Clin Proc 1997;72:532–542.
12. Giladi M, Szold O, Elami A, et al. Microbiological cultures of heart valves and valve tags are not valuable for patients without infective endocarditis who are undergoing valve replacement. Clin Infect Dis 1997;24:884–888.
13. Weinstein J, Brusch JL. Infective Endocarditis. New York, NY, Oxford University Press, 1996. pp 123–164.
14. Silver MD. Infective endocarditis. In Silver MD (ed.) Cardiovascular Pathology. New York, NY, Churchill Livingstone, 1991. pp 895–931.
15. Bansal RC. Infective endocarditis. Med Clin North Am 1995;79:1205–1239.
16. Karchmer A. Infective endocarditis. In Braunwald E (ed.) Heart Disease: A Textbook of Cardiovascular Medicine, 5th ed. Philadelphia PA, WB Saunders, 1997. pp 1077–1099.
17. Billingham ME. Normal heart. In Sternberg S (ed.) Histology for Pathologists. New York, NY, Raven Press, 1992. pp 215–231.
18. Dariouche RO, Hamill RJ. Antibiotic penetration of and bactericidal activity within endothelial cells. Antimicrob Agents Chemother 1994;38:1059–1064.
19. Brouqui P, Dumler JS, Raoult D. Immunohistologic demonstration of Coxiella burnetii in the valves of patients with Q fever endocarditis. Am J Med 1994; 97:451–458.
20. Muhlemann K, Matter L, Meyer B, et al. Isolation of Coxiella burnetii from heart valves of patients treated for Q fever endocarditis. J Clin Microbiol 1995; 33:428–431.
21. Aronson MD, Bor DH. Blood cultures. Ann Intern Med 1987;106:246–253.
22. Chorny JA, Wilson ML. Rapid detection and identification of microorganisms from blood cultures. Clin Lab Med 1994;14:181–195.
23. Weinstein MP. Current blood culture methods and systems: Clinical concepts, technology and interpretation of results. Clin Infect Dis 1996;23:40–46.
24. Burnie JP, Clark I. Immunoblotting in the diagnosis of culture-negative endocarditis caused by streptococci. J Clin Pathol 1995;48:1130–1136.
25. Kjerulf A, Tvede M, Hoiby N, et al. Crossed immunoelectrophoresis used for bacteriological diagnosis in patients with endocarditis. APMIS 1993;101: 746–752.
26. Bates DW, Boldman L, Lee TH. Contaminant blood cultures and resource

utilization: The true consequences of false-positive results. *JAMA*, 1991;265: 365–369.

27. Wilson M. Blood cultures: Introduction. *Clin Lab Med* 1994;14:1–7.

28. Weinstein MP, Mirrett S, Wilson ML, et al. Controlled evaluation of 5 versus 10 milliliters of blood cultured in aerobic BacT/Alert blood culture bottles. *J Clin Microbiol* 1994;32:2103–2106.

29. Wilson ML, Weinstein MP, Reller LB. Automated blood culture systems. *Clin Lab Med* 1994;1:149–169.

30. Saccente M, Cobbs CG. Clinical approach to infective endocarditis. *Cardiol Clin* 1996;14:351–362.

31. Vlessis AA, Hovaguimian H, Jaggers J, et al. Infective endocarditis: Ten-year review of medical and surgical therapy. *Ann Thorac Surg* 1996;61:1217–1222.

32. Werner AS, Cobbs CG, Kaye D, et al. Studies on the bacteremia of bacterial endocarditis. *JAMA* 1967;202:127–131.

33. Wilson ML, Weinstein MP. General principles in the laboratory detection of bacteremia and fungemia. *Clin Lab Med* 1994;14:69–82.

34. Washington JA. Collection, transport and processing of blood cultures. *Clin Lab Med* 1994;14:59–68.

35. James P. Laboratory aspects of infective endocarditis. *Br J Biomed Sc* 1993;50: 249–257.

36. Daher AH, Berkowitz FE. Infective endocarditis in neonates. *Clin Pediatr* 1995; 2:198–206.

37. Paisley JW, Lauer BA. Pediatric blood cultures. *Clin Lab Med* 1994;14:17–30.

38. Weinstein MP, Reller LB, Murphy JR, et al. The clinical significance of positive blood cultures: A comprehensive analysis of 500 episodes of bacteremia and fungemia in adults. I. Laboratory and epidemiologic observations. *Rev Infect Dis* 1983;5:35–53.

39. McDonald LC, Fune J, Gaido LB, et al. Clinical importance of increased sensitivity of BacT/Alert FAN aerobic and anaerobic blood culture bottles. *J Clin Microbiol* 1996;34:2180–2184.

40. Weinstein MP, Mirrett S, Wilson ML, et al. Controlled evaluation of BacT/Alert standard aerobic and FAN aerobic blood culture bottles for detection of bacteremia and fungemia. *J Clin Microbiol* 1995;33:978–981.

41. Jorgensen JH, Mirrett S, McDonald LC, et al. Controlled clinical laboratory comparison of BACTEC Plus Aerobic/F Resin medium with BacT/Alert FAN medium for detection of bacteremia and fungemia. *J Clin Microbiol* 1997;35: 53–58.

42. Levin PD, Yinnon AM, Hersch M, et al. Impact of the resin blood culture medium in the treatment of critically ill patients. *Crit Care Med* 1996;24:5: 797–801.

43. Goldstein EJC. Anaerobic bacteremia. *Clin Infect Dis* 1996;23 (Suppl 1):97–101.

44. Matsen JM. Rapid reporting of results: Impact on patients, physician and laboratory. In Tilton, RC (ed.) *Rapid Methods and Automation in Microbiology.* Washington, DC, American Society for Microbiology Press, 1984. pp 98–102.

45. Peacock SJ, Bowler CJW, Crook DWM. Positive predictive value of blood cultures growing coagulase-negative staphylococci. *Lancet* 1995;346:191–192.

46. Bayer AS. Infective endocarditis: State of the art. *Clin Infect Dis* 1993:313–322.

47. Oakley CM. The medical treatment of culture-negative infective endocarditis. *Eur Heart J* 1995;16 (Suppl B): 90–93.

48. Stratton CW. The role of the microbiology laboratory in the treatment of infective endocarditis. *J Antimicrob Chemother* 1987;20 (Suppl A):41–49.
49. Rubenstein E, Lang R. Fungal endocarditis. *Eur Heart J* 1995;16 (Suppl B): 84–89.
50. Raoult D, Fournier PE, Drancourt M, et al. Diagnosis of 22 new cases of Bartonella endocarditis. *Ann Intern Med* 1996;125:646–652.
51. Wilson ML, Mirrett S. Recovery of select rare and fastidious microorganisms from blood cultures. *Clin Lab Med* 1994;14:119–131.
52. Jalava J, Kotilainen P, Nikkari S, et al. Use of the polymerase chain reaction and DNA sequencing for detection of Bartonella quintana in the aortic valve of a patient with culture-negative infective endocarditis. *Clin Infect Dis* 1995; 21:891–896.
53. Fernandez-Guerrero ML. Zoonotic endocarditis. *Infect Dis Clin North Am* 1993; 7:135–152.
54. Fournier PE, Casalta JP, Habib G, et al. Modification of the diagnostic criteria proposed by the Duke endocarditis service to permit improved diagnosis of Q fever endocarditis. *Am J Med* 1996;100:629–633.
55. Shapiro DS, Kenney SC, Johnson M, et al. *Chlamydia psittaci* diagnosed by blood culture. *N Engl J Med* 1992;326:1192.
56. Gil-Grande R, Aguado JM, Pastor C, et al. Conventional viral cultures and shell vial assay for diagnosis of apparently culture-negative *Coxiella burnetii* endocarditis. *Eur J Clin Microbiol Infect Dis* 1995;14:64–67.
57. Raoult D, Laurent JC, Mutillod M: Monoclonal antibodies to *Coxiella burnetii* for antigenic detection in cell cultures and in paraffin-embedded tissues. *Am J Clin Pathol* 1994;101:318–320.
58. Stein A, Raoult D. Q fever endocarditis. *Eur Heart J* 1995;16 (Suppl B):19–23.
59. Peacock MG, Philip RN, Williams JC, et al. Serological evaluation of Q fever in humans: Enhanced phase I titers of immunoglobulins G and A are diagnostic for Q fever endocarditis. *Infect Immun* 1983;41:1089–1098.
60. Williams JC, Johnston MR, Peacock MG, et al. Monoclonal antibodies distinguish phase variants of *Coxiella burnetii*. *Infect Immun* 1984;43:421–428.
61. Frazier ME, Mallaria LP, Samuel JE, et al. DNA probes for the identification of *Coxiella burnetii* strains. *Ann NY Acad Sci* 1990;590:445–448.
62. Stein A, Raoult D. Detection of *Coxiella burnetii* by DNA amplification using polymerase chain reaction. *J Clin Microbiol* 1992;30:2462–2464.
63. Hamed KA. Haemophilus parainfluenzae endocarditis: Application of a molecular approach for identification of pathogenic bacterial species. *Clin Infect Dis* 1994;19:677–683.
64. Hermann JE. Immunoassays for the diagnosis of infectious diseases. In Murray PR, Baron EJ, Pfaller MA, et al (eds.) *Manual of Clinical Microbiology*, Washington DC, American Society for Microbiology Press; 1995. pp 19–32.
65. Podzorski RP, Persing DH. Molecular detection and identification of microorganisms. In Murray PR, Baron EJ, Pfaller MA, et al (eds.) *Manual of Clinical Microbiology*, Washington DC, American Society for Microbiology Press; 1995. pp 130–154.
66. Kubak BM, Nimmagadda AP, Holt CD. Advances in medical and antibiotic management of infective endocarditis. *Cardiol Clin* 1996;14:405–436.
67. Kawamura Y, Hou XG, Sultana F, et al. Transfer of *Streptococcus adjacens* and *Streptococcus defectivus* to *Abiotrophia* gen nov as *Abiotrophia adjacens* comb nov

and *Abiotrophia defectiva* comb nov, respectively. *Int J Syst Bacteriol* 1995;45: 798–803.

68. Ohara-Nemoto Y, Tajika S, Sasaki M. Identification of *Abiotrophia adjacens* and *Abiotrophia defectiva* by 16S rRNA gene PCR and restriction fragment length polymorphism analysis. *J Clin Microbiol* 1997;35:2458–2463.

69. Roggenkamp A, Abele-Horn M, Trebesius KH, et al. *Abiotrophia elegans* sp nov, a possible pathogen in patients with culture-negative endocarditis. *J Clin Micro* 1998;36: 100–104.

70. Bouvet A. Human endocarditis due to nutritionally variant streptococci: *Streptococcus adjacens* and *Streptococcus defectivus*. *Eur Heart J* 1995;16 (Suppl B): 24–27.

71. Stratton CW. Blood cultures and immunocompromised patients. *Clin Lab Med* 1994;14:31–49.

72. Carbon C. Experimental endocarditis: A review of its relevance to human endocarditis. *J Antimicrob Chemother* 1993;31 (Suppl D):71–85.

73. Carbon C, Cremieux AC, Fantin B. Pharmacokinetic and pharmacodynamic aspects of therapy of experimental endocarditis. *Infect Dis Clin North Am* 1993; 7:37–51.

74. Stratton CW. Serum bactericidal test. *Clin Microbiol Rev* 1988;1:19–26.

75. Mulligan MJ, Cobbs CG. Bacteriostasis versus bactericidal activity. *Infect Dis Clin North Am* 1989;3:389–398.

76. Peterson LR, Shanholtzer CJ. Tests for bactericidal effects of antimicrobial agents: Technical performance and relevance. *Clin Microbiol Rev* 1992;5: 420–432.

77. Weinstein MP, Stratton CW, Ackley A, et al. Multicenter collaborative evaluation of a standardized serum bactericidal test as a prognostic indicator in infective endocarditis. *Am J Med* 1985;78:262–271.

78. Steel DM, Whitehead AS. The major acute phase reactants: C-reactive protein, serum amyploid P component and serum amyloid A protein. *Immunol Today* 1994;15:81–89.

79. Hogevik H, Olaison R, Andersson R, et al. C-reactive protein is more sensitive than erythrocyte sedimentation rate for diagnosis of infective endocarditis. *Infection* 1997;25:82–85.

80. Olaison L, Hogevik H, Alestig K. Fever, C-reactive protein and other acute-phase reactants during treatment of infective endocarditis. *Arch Intern Med* 1997;157:885–892.

81. Berger D, Bolke E, Huegel H, et al. New aspects concerning the regulation of the post- operative acute phase reaction during cardiac surgery. *Clin Chim Acta* 1995;239:121–130.

82. Szalai AJ, Agrawal A, Greenhough TJ, et al. C-reactive protein: Structural biology, gene expression and host defense function. *Immunologic Res* 1997;16: 127–136.

83. McCartney AC, Orange GV, Pringle SD, et al. Serum C-reactive protein in infective endocarditis. *J Clin Pathol* 1988;41:44–48.

84. Macy EM, Hayes TE, Tracy RP. Variability in the measurement of C-reactive protein in healthy subjects: Implications for reference intervals and epidemiological applications. *Clin Chem* 1997;43:52–58.

85. Daher AH, Berkowitz FE. Infective endocarditis in neonates. *Clin Pediatr* 1995; 2: 198–206.

86. McCartney AC, McGovern T, Cobb S, et al. The measurement of C-reactive

protein and immune complexes in endocarditis caused by coagulase-negative staphylococci. *J Infect* 1987;15:213–219.

87. Ghoneim ATM, McGoldrick J, Ionescu MI. Serial C-reactive protein measurements in infective complications following cardiac operation: Evaluation and use in monitoring response to therapy. *Ann Thorac Surg* 1982;34:166–175.

88. Milholic J, Hudec M, Muller MM, et al. Early prediction of deep sternal wound infection after heart operations by alpha-1 acid glycoprotein and C-reactive protein measurements. *Ann Thorac Surg* 1986;42:429–433.

89. Verkkala K, Valtonen V, Javinen A, et al. Fever, leucocytosis and C-reactive protein after open heart surgery and their value in the diagnosis of postoperative infections. *Thorac Cardiovasc Surg* 1987;35:78–82.

90. Aronen M. Value of C-reactive protein in detecting complications after closed-heart surgery in children. *Scand J Thor Cardiovasc Surg* 1990;24:147–151.

91. Boralessa H, DeBeer FC, Manchie A, et al. C-reactive protein in patients undergoing cardiac surgery. *Anaesthesia* 1986;41:11–15.

Chapter 3
Epidemiology of Native Valve Endocarditis

David C. Stuesse, M.D.
Angelo A. Vlessis, M.D., Ph.D.

Epidemiology of infective endocarditis has been the subject of numerous publications since 1909.[1] The estimated incidence and mortality rates in these studies, based primarily on retrospective reviews of medical records, have varied widely. Interestingly, the epidemiological data on endocarditis have evolved in the last 25 years as health care and disease patterns have changed. Although infective endocarditis is not contagious, epidemiological information is useful for determining populations at risk and for quantifying the threat of the disease to a population. To report the most contemporary epidemiological data on infective endocarditis, large series published within the last 15 years are reviewed in this chapter.

Obtaining accurate demographic data on infective endocarditis is difficult for several reasons. Foremost, endocarditis is difficult to diagnose definitively. In patients treated medically, the diagnosis of endocarditis is not always completely objective. Unequivocal diagnoses are made only histopathologically, at the time of surgery or at autopsy. Thus, a number of cases will go undiscovered while the disease may be incorrectly diagnosed in others. In addition, most epidemiological studies are based on retrospective reviews. As such, these studies are susceptible to selection and observer bias.[2] Several recent epidemiological studies have been performed prospectively to obtain more accurate information.[3–7] Most of these prospective studies rely on information reported by other physicians. In one unique study, however, inter-observer bias was eliminated

From: Vlessis AA, Bolling S (eds): *Endocarditis: A Multidisciplinary Approach to Modern Treatment.* © Futura Publishing Co., Armonk, NY, 1999.

by having one physician personally visit all patients identified as having endocarditis.[3] Undoubtedly, geographic variation in the incidence of infective endocarditis exists as well. Factors such as access to dental and medical care as well as the prevalence of intravenous drug use and immune compromise affect the incidence of native valve endocarditis from one population to the next. These elements contribute to the variation in data among the different studies listed below and should be kept in mind when interpreting the conclusions drawn from individual studies.

Many modern studies of endocarditis use the diagnostic criteria published by von Reyn in 1981.[8] Von Reyn and his colleagues separated endocarditis cases into definite, probable or possible categories. Cases defined as *definite* are based on histological confirmation. Cases defined as *probable* or *possible* are based on blood culture results, plus the presence of fever, regurgitant heart murmurs, predisposing heart disease, vascular emboli and the lack of evidence for extracardial sources of bacteremia (See Chapter 5, Table 1). These categories have standardized the diagnosis of endocarditis and provided uniformity to the reports published since 1981. Others have modified von Reyn's criteria to include evidence of valvular vegetations on echocardiography.[4,7,9–11] Most studies reviewed here use a derivative of these criteria for diagnosis.

Basic epidemiological information on infective endocarditis is reported in Table 1. The reported crude incidence of native valve endocarditis ranges from 12 to over 80 cases per million person-years.[3–7,11,12] Most studies report incidences between 12–24 cases per million person-years.[3–5,11,12] These figures generally include patients in the definite, probable and possible endocarditis groups combined. Mean age for diagnosis of endocarditis ranges from 48 to 64 years. Women with the disease tend to be older than their male counterparts, 70 years versus 59 respectively.[11] The male sex predominates on the order of 1.2:1 to 2.0:1.[3,4,10–14] Infective endocarditis in children is extremely rare, with reported incidences of 3.0 to 3.9 cases per million child-years.[3,15]

Table 1
Incidence and Mortality of Endocarditis

Reference	3	4	5	6	7	10	11	12	13	14	Weighted Average
Cases per 1,000,000 person-years	12	14	21	>80 45***	53		14	24			34
Mean age	47*	48*			62*		64		51*	57*	53
Male: female	1.6:1	1.3:1			1:1.3	1.4:1	1.2:1	1.4:1	2:1	1.9:1*	1.5:1
Mortality, %	20	12*	18		23*	27	33 18**	35*	45*	37*	24

* Combined native and prosthetic valve; ** Treated group only; *** Excluding intravenous drug use cases.

The reported mortality rate of native valve endocarditis varies. In series that report mortality rates for native valve infections separately from prosthetic valve infections (Table 2), mortality ranges from 18% to 33%.[3,5,10] When untreated cases identified at autopsy are excluded, the reported mortality rate is 18% to 27%.[3,5,10] Mortality rates as high as 45% have been reported from combined native and prosthetic valve infections.[13] It is unclear, however, whether the mortality rate for native valve infection is truly lower than that for prosthetic valve infection. Watanakunakorn and Burkert[10] report a lower mortality rate for prosthetic valve endocarditis compared to native valve disease while Van der Meer et al[3] describe similar rates. Despite these epidemiological reports, most clinical case studies clearly show a higher mortality with prosthetic valve endocarditis as compared to the native valve counterpart.[5,13,14] Other factors that correlate positively with increased mortality are older patient age,[10] *Staphylococcus aureus* infection,[10-12,14] the presence of embolic phenomena,[4,12] and the degree of heart failure at the time of presentation.[14] Treatment with combined medical and surgical therapy may lead to lower mortality than cases treated with medical therapy alone.[5,11,14] Valve replacement is performed in approximately 13% to 41% of patients with endocarditis.[4,5,7,11-14] Additional factors contributing to death in patients with endocarditis are heart failure, peripheral emboli, and uncontrolled infection.[13,14]

The most common presenting symptoms for endocarditis are fever, fatigue, malaise and dyspnea (Table 2). Pyrexia, heart murmur and microscopic hematuria are the most common clinical signs. Evidence of central nervous system embolization is found in 10% to 26% of patients with

Table 2
Presenting Signs and Symptoms of Endocarditis*

Reference	4	5	7	10	11	12	13	14	Weighted Average
Fever		79		66	85		63	76	74
Malaise Fatigue		79	50	40			71	49	56
Dyspnea		42	49			43	44	16	37
Arthralgia/Myalgia			37		16		15	20	21
Pyrexia	97	84	89	77		93	82		85
Murmur	57			81			83		76
CNS (stroke)	13			26	11	27	10		19
Splinter hemorrhage		26			17	8			20
Embolic, generalized	35			45		35			41
Micro. hematuria		28		60		70	27	13	39

* Values in the table represent percentages of the patients studied.

Table 3
Valvular Involvement in Endocarditis*

Reference	7	10	11	12	13	14	Weighted Average
Aortic	44	22	58	43	44	31	38
Mitral	29	29	32	42	35	42	34
Aortic and Mitral	15	7	5	11	15	4	8
Tricuspid	7	5	2	3	0	5	4

* Values in the table represent percentages of the patients studied.

endocarditis.[4,10–13] Splinter hemorrhages were commonly reported in several studies[5,11] but Osler's nodes and Janeway's lesions are infrequently discovered. There are few specific symptoms and signs of endocarditis. As a result, premortem diagnosis usually hinges on a constellation of clinical signs, symptoms and laboratory studies.

The affected valve in infective endocarditis can be elucidated by physical exam, echocardiography and by direct visualization at surgery or autopsy. Mitral and aortic valves are affected with nearly the same frequency (Table 3). Simultaneous involvement of both the mitral and aortic valves occurs in 5% to 15% of cases.[7,10–14] It is reasonable to assume that the incidence of tricuspid valve infection is related to the prevalence of intravenous drug use in the population studied. Mortality rates and the incidence of embolic phenomena are similar in patients with mitral versus aortic valve involvement.[3,11–13] Due to associated heart failure, cases of native aortic valve endocarditis are treated with surgery more often than mitral valve endocarditis.[11,13,14]

Gram-positive bacteria predominate in infective endocarditis (Table 4). Unfortunately, because many of the studies combine native and pros-

Table 4
Commonly Reported Microorganisms*

Reference	4	7	10	11	12	13	14	Weighted Average
Staphylococcus aureus	35	31	48	28	21	13	21	31
Alpha-hemolytic Streptococcus	25	28	11	22	16	42	59**	28
Enterococcus	9	6	5	8	17	9		8
Gram negative bacilli	3	9	3	2		1		4
Fungi	3	1	1					1

* Values in the table represent percentages of the patients studied; ** Includes all *Streptococcus* spp.

thetic valve infections, the spectrum of bacteria reported may not accurately reflect native valve cases alone. *Staphylococcus aureus* and alpha-hemolytic streptococcus are by far the most frequently cultured organisms in this disease.[4,7,10-14] Of the alpha-hemolytic streptococci, *S. viridans* is the most common isolate. Enterococcus has been reported in 5% to 17% of cases.[4,7,10-13] Gram-negative rods are relatively rare, comprising 1% to 9% of cases.[4,7,10,11,13] Fungal endocarditis is also rare, comprising 3% to 5% of endocarditis.[4,7,10] Infection with *S. aureus* has been associated with a shorter interval from onset of symptoms to diagnosis[8,10,16] and with a higher morbidity,[8,14,15,17] implicating a more virulent course with the organism.

Pre-existing heart disease was discovered in 42% to 98% of patients in the reviewed studies (Table 5). Congenital heart disease was identified in 4% to 13% of patients with endocarditis.[3,11-14] A history of rheumatic heart disease was present in 1.5% to 44% of endocarditis patients in the publications reviewed.[5,7,11-14] A history of previous endocarditis was identified as a significant risk factor in 3 studies; 11% to 15% of patients with endocarditis had a prior history of the same illness.[3,4,7] In the study by Van der Meer and colleagues,[3] each patient was personally reviewed by the authors and 98% of patients were identified as having pre- existing heart disease. One could, of course, argue that the prevalence of heart disease in Van der Meer's study was overreported because of bias in this direction. However, the severity of heart disease is not given and may not have been noted in the other studies unless it was moderate to severe. Regardless, it is likely that Van der Meer's study more accurately represents the relationship between pre-existing heart problems and endocarditis than the retrospective studies. According to Van der Meer and his colleagues, 32% of patients had underlying aortic valve disease, while 36% had underlying mitral valve disease. Valvular regurgitation was the most common abnormality found. In the same study, the prevalence of mitral valve prolapse in patients with endocarditis was 8%. The preva-

Table 5
Predisposing Cardiac Abnormalities*

Reference	3	5	7	11	12	13	14
Mitral valve prolapse	8	19	18	0	2		16
Congenital heart disease	10			4.5	13	4	3.5
Rheumatic disease		18	18	1.5	11	44	16
All cardiac lesions	98	71**		42	66		

* Values in the table represent percentages of the patients studied; ** Includes prosthetic valves.

lence of mitral valve prolapse in the other endocarditis studies ranges from 2% to 19%. Interestingly, several studies have found the prevalence of mitral valve prolapse in the general population to be 4% to 8%.[16–19] Therefore, although mitral valve prolapse has been previously identified as a significant risk factor for endocarditis,[20,21] based on the above data, the incidence of coexisting mitral valve prolapse and endocarditis appears similar to the incidence of mitral valve prolapse in the general population.

The pathogen's portal of entry in endocarditis is often difficult to ascertain. Any condition leading to bacteremia can cause endocarditis. Commonly reported portals of entry include dental infection and procedures, surgery, endoscopy, intravenous catheters, intravenous drug abuse, and infection of the skin, lungs, bowel, and urinary tract. In 3 epidemiological reports on endocarditis, the percentage of patients who had undergone a dental procedure within 3 months of the known onset of the disease was 13%, 14%, and 21% respectively.[5,13,11] The overall percentage of control patients who had undergone a dental procedure within 3 months was not reported; however, in 57% to 66% of these patients, organisms consistent with a dental source were cultured.[11,13] Alpha-hemolytic streptococcus is the organism most commonly associated with bacteremia from dental infections or procedures. Of patients with native valve endocarditis, known valvular heart disease, natural dentition, and a dental procedure within 180 days of onset, a relative risk of 4.9 for identifying alpha-hemolytic streptococcus as the etiologic organism as compared to patients without these 3 risk factors has been found.[22] *Staphylococcus aureus* is the most common pathogen found in patients with endocarditis and skin lesions[7] while *Streptococcus fecalis* is commonly associated with a urinary tract source.[5,7] The actual portal of entry is difficult to elucidate since there is a variable incubation period between the bacteremic episode and the onset of symptoms.[22] In all reports reviewed herein, the majority of endocarditis cases had no known entry portal.

Intravenous drug use is a known risk factor for developing infective endocarditis. In the studies reviewed, the percent of cases thought to be caused by intravenous drug use ranges from 7% to 44%. The tricuspid valve is the most commonly affected valve in these cases with tricuspid valve involvement identified in 46% to 92% of endocarditis in intravenous drug users.[3–5,10] In one study of 12 patients with endocarditis secondary to intravenous drug use, *Staphylococcus aureus* was the most commonly isolated organism (69%).[5] In another study of 32 patients with a history of narcotic abuse, *S. aureus* was implicated in 92% of right side heart endocarditis and 29% of left heart endocarditis.[3] The median age for patients with drug abuse-induced endocarditis is much lower than the mean age of patients with community acquired endocarditis, 31 years versus 64 years respectively.[10] The mortality rate for intravenous drug use-induced endocarditis in a series of 21 patients was 9% versus 21% in patients with no history of intravenous drug use.[10] The lower observed mortality likely reflects the younger mean age of the population using intravenous drugs and their resilience to the effects of acute valvular insufficiency.

Native valve endocarditis still causes significant morbidity and mortality worldwide. The mortality rate of infectious endocarditis remains high despite modern treatments and medical advances. However, since endocarditis is a treatable disease, physicians must be cognizant of the signs and symptoms of the disease in order to diagnose and treat the disease in earlier stages. Based on the studies reviewed, mitral valve prolapse is not a significant risk factor for developing endocarditis; however, congenital and acquired valvular heart disease should be considered risk factors. It is notable that mitral and aortic valve endocarditis occur at nearly the same frequency and are associated with similar mortality rates. The presence of congestive heart failure, increased patient age, the presence of embolic phenomena, and infection with *S. aureus* are indicators of a poor prognosis. Timely surgical intervention decreases the mortality of the disease, especially in aortic endocarditis. Patients with a history of intravenous drug use are especially susceptible to endocarditis. In most patients, the source of the pathogen cannot be ascertained. However, dental disease is probably one of the leading portals of entry for pathogens in endocarditis.

References

1. Horder T. Infective endocarditis with an analysis of 150 cases with special reference to the chronic form of the disease. *QJM* 1909;2:289–324.

2. Lilienfeld AM. *Foundations of Epidemiology*. New York, NY. Oxford University Press, 1976. pp 164–187.

3. Van der Meer JTM, Thompson J, Valkenburg HA, et al. Epidemiology of bacterial endocarditis in the Netherlands. I. Patient characteristics. *Arch Intern Med* 1992;152:1863–1868.

4. King JW, Nguyen VQ, Conrad SA. Results of a prospective statewide reporting system for infective endocarditis. *Am J Med Sci* 1988;295(6):517–527.

5. Skehan JD, Murray M, Mills PG. Infective endocarditis: Incidence and mortality in the northeast Thames region. *Br Heart J* 1988;59:62–68.

6. Berlin JA, Abrutyn E, Strom BL, et al. Incidence of infective endocarditis in the Delaware Valley, 1988–1990. *Am J Cardiol* 1995;76:933–936.

7. Hogevik H, Olaison L, Andersson R, et al. Epidemiologic aspects of infective endocarditis in an urban population: A 5-year prospective study. *Medicine* 1995;74(6):324–339.

8. Von Reyn CF, Levy BS, Arbeit RD, et al. Infective endocarditis: An analysis based on strict case definitions. *Ann Intern Med* 1991;94(1):505–518.

9. Durack DT, Lukes AS, Bright DK. New criteria for diagnosis of infective endo-

carditis: Utilization of specific echocardiographic findings. Duke Endocarditis Service [see comments]. *Am J Med* 1994;96:200–209.

10. Watanakunakorn C, Burkert T. Infective endocarditis at a large community teaching hospital, 1980–1990: A review of 210 episodes. *Medicine* 1993;72(2): 90–102.

11. Nissen H, Nielsen PF, Frederiksen M, et al. Native valve endocarditis in the general population: A 10-year survey of the clinical picture during the 1980s. *Eur Heart J* 1992;13:872–877.

12. Benn M, Hagelskjaer LH, Tvede M: Infective endocarditis, 1984 through 1993: A clinical and microbiological survey. *J Intern Med* 1997;242:15–22.

13. Whitby M, Fenech A. Infective endocarditis in adults in Glasgow, 1976–81. *Int J Cardiol* 1985;7:391–403.

14. Vlessis AA, Hovaguimian H, Jaggers J, et al. Infective endocarditis: Ten-year review of medical and surgical therapy. *Ann Thorac Surg* 1996;61:1217–1222.

15. Schollin J, Bjarke B, Wesstrom G. Infective endocarditis in Swedish children. I. Incidence, etiology, underlying factors and port of entry of infection: *Acta Paediatr Scand* 1986;75:993–998.

16. Bairate I, Briancon S, Danchin N, et al. Screening for a frequent cardiac disorder: Mitral valve prolapse. *Can J Public Health* 1991;82(6):425–428.

17. Zuppiroli A, Favilli S, Risoli A, et al. Mitral valve prolapse: A prevalence study using bidimensional echocardiography in a young population. *G Ital Cardiol* 1990;20(6):161–166.

18. Bryhn M, Persson S. The prevalence of mitral valve prolapse in healthy men and women in Sweden: An echocardiographic study. *Acta Med Scand* 1984; 215(2):157–160.

19. Hickey AJ, Wolfers J, Wilcken DE. Mitral valve prolapse: Prevalence in an Australian population. *Med J Aust* 1981;1(1):31–33.

20. Baddour LM, Bisno AL. Infective endocarditis complicating mitral valve prolapse. *Rev Infect Dis* 1986;8:117–137.

21. McKinsey DS, Ratts TE, Bisno AL. Underlying cardiac lesions in adults with infective endocarditis. *Am J Med* 1987;82:681–688.

22. Van der Meer JTM, Thompson J, Valkenburg HA, et al. Epidemiology of bacterial endocarditis in the Netherlands. II. Antecedent procedures and use of prophylaxis. *Arch Intern Med* 1992;152:1869–1873.

Chapter 4

Epidemiology and Risk Factors for Prosthetic Valve Endocarditis

Gary L. Grunkemeier, Ph.D.
Hui-Hua Li, M.D.

Introduction

Prosthetic valve endocarditis (PVE) is arguably the most dreaded complication of artificial heart valves. The complications affecting heart valves have been specified in the reporting guidelines produced by an ad hoc committee of the Society of Thoracic Surgeons and the American Association for Thoracic Surgery. These were first published in 1988[1-3] and have been recently updated and endorsed by 4 cardiac surgery journals.[4-7] The guidelines include 6 major categories of complications: structural valvular deterioration, nonstructural dysfunction, thrombosis, thromboembolism, bleeding and endocarditis. Importantly, the authors note that all of the other complications may occur secondary to endocarditis. Endocarditis is fatal in 25–60% of cases, depending on factors such as timing (early or late), infecting organism and mode of treatment. It can be cured medically with aggressive antibiotic treatment, but often requires valve replacement, and in some patients 2 or more sequential "re-replacements" have been required. It has been proposed[8] that the term "replacement device endocarditis" should be used instead of PVE since all replacement devices are not prostheses; however, we will use the term PVE to include all replacement devices (including homografts), as is commonly done.

From: Vlessis AA, Bolling S (eds): *Endocarditis: A Multidisciplinary Approach to Modern Treatment.* © Futura Publishing Co., Armonk, NY, 1999.

PVE is a neo-disease, one that by definition appeared only when heart valve replacement became a clinical reality. Our candidate for the first reported case of PVE occurred in Starr's classic paper on the first successful series of mitral valve replacements.[9] The seventh patient in that series, reported as "under treatment" in 1961, eventually died from PVE, along with 2 of the other 16 patients in that series, within 60 days of valve replacement.[10] Early descriptions of this new complication were given by cardiologists and their surgical colleagues.[11,12]

This chapter describes the results of a current (1998) literature review of the risk of PVE. Some parts of this review were reported in a recent article that dealt with several other aspects of PVE, including pathophysiology, etiology, diagnosis, treatment and prophylaxis.[13] Here, we will briefly review the methods used to gather the data and generate the statistics, and then present the results.

Methods

Selection of Valve Series

Published articles, primarily those abstracted on MedLine, the World Wide Web database (available at: www.nlm.nih.gov/databases/medline.html) were reviewed. To be used, reports had to meet certain selection criteria. The total patient-years of follow-up, or information from which this could be calculated, must be present. Data must be given separately by position and by valve model. Articles reporting particular subsets of patients, such as those of a certain age range, valve size or indication for surgery, were usually excluded. Only the most recent report of a given series from a given institution was included.

Information on PVE was abstracted from the qualifying reports and entered into a database written in Microsoft Access (Microsoft Corp., Redmond, WA). From this database, information was extracted on series published within the last 10 years (since 1987) that had a minimum follow-up of 300 patient-years by position (aortic, mitral).

Statistical Methods

Linearized rates were calculated by dividing the number of PVE cases by the total follow-up years and multiplying by 100. This gives units of events per 100 patient-years, often abbreviated as percent per year. When possible, only late events were used to calculate the rates, with the total follow-up being reduced appropriately.[13]

Confidence intervals for these rates were computed using an approximation suggested by Cox,[14] which was recently recommended by a paper that compared the properties of several alternative methods.[15] Two-sided 90% confidence intervals were used so that the upper limits correspond to one-sided 95% upper limits, as required by the FDA guidance document for the clinical evaluation of new heart valves.[16,17] The FDA requirement is that this upper confidence limit falls below 2.4% per year: this represents 2 times the "objective performance criterion" of 1.2% per year, which is meant to represent the current average rate for all valves in both positions.

Cumulative hazard functions were used to examine the assumption of constant hazard, necessary to justify the use of linearized rates. These are rarely given directly, but can be easily computed as the negative logarithm of the actuarial or Kaplan-Meier event- free curve. If the cumulative hazard is a straight line (*linear* function of postoperative time), then its slope is equal to the (instantaneous) PVE hazard, which in this case is called the *linearized* rate.

To aid in interpretation of the relationship of scatterplots of PVE rates versus continuous variables such as age, we fit a line of central tendency using a scatterplot smoothing function called a local weighted regression smoother, or LOWESS.[18] All statistical calculations and graphics were performed using the S-PLUS statistical program (MathSoft, Seattle, WA).

Results

PVE Risk: The Case for Constancy

Early Versus Late Risk

The FDA heart valve guidance document states that "complications which occur in the early post-operative period must not be included in the calculation of linearized rates."[16] This is because the risk of complication is higher, and would not fit the assumption of approximately constant risk (early events are summarized using simple percentages). The "early" period for postoperative complications is traditionally the first 30 days after surgery. But for PVE, the period of early increased risk is considered to be within 60 days of implantation, and it has been found to extend to about 3 to 6 months[19–21] or even one year[22–26] by some investigators.

In some papers it is possible to exclude early events when they are given separately, but these are for events within 30 days only, and in most series even this is not possible. Thus, the late constant hazard is contaminated by early events with a higher risk. Nevertheless we feel that linearized rates provide a good first approximation, and are not too highly influenced by the early risk, especially in larger series where the overwhelming amount of follow-up is late, thus diluting the effect of the early, possibly higher, risk.

Cumulative Hazard for PVE

As evidence to support the use of linearized rates, we looked at the relatively few cumulative hazard curves for PVE. Some of these curves were derived from series other than those summarized by linearized rates in the risk factors section below. These are shown in Figures 1 and 2 for aortic and mitral series, respectively. The longest series (25 years) in each figure are from our own experience with mostly mechanical caged ball valves, and they are approximately linear. Information about the series plotted in Figures 1 and 2 is contained in Tables 1 and 2, respectively.

The solid line "N" in Figure 1 is from a detailed study of PVE which featured software specifically designed to model the shape of the hazard

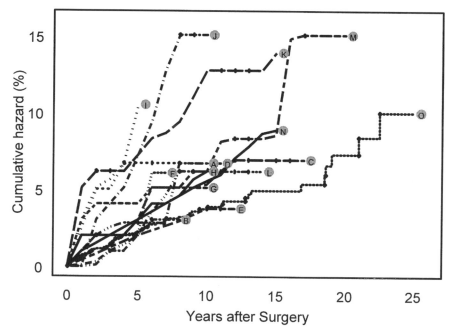

Figure 1. Cumulative hazard curves for PVE from 15 aortic valve series. The 9 shortest are from recent publications and the longest (to 25 years) is from our series. The relative linearity of these curves implies that the risk is relatively constant and can therefore be summarized by a single number, the "constant hazard" which is called the "linearized rate" in the cardiac surgical literature.

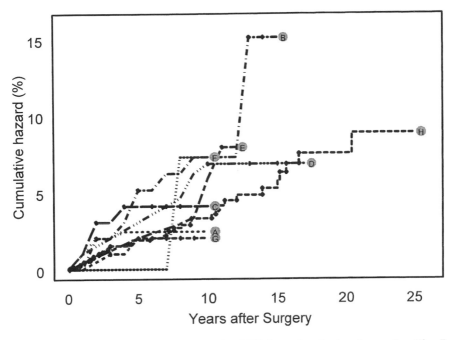

Figure 2. Cumulative hazard curves for PVE from 8 mitral valve series. The 5 shortest are from recent publications and the longest (to 25 years) is from our series. The relative linearity of these curves implies that the risk is relatively constant and can therefore be summarized by a single number, the "constant hazard" which is called the "linearized rate" in the cardiac surgical literature.

function.[21] This software detects 3 potential components of risk: early, intermediate steady state, and late.[27] This study found an early risk that peaked between 2 and 3 months, at a momentary maximum of about 3.2% per year, but disappeared after about 6 months. The late component was missing entirely, so that the rate was constant after the early risk period, at about 0.5% per year. In spite of the high but relatively brief spike, the actuarial event-free curve, or its cumulative hazard counterpart (Figure 1), did not deviate noticeably from a straight line.

The other cumulative hazard functions in Figures 1 and 2 do not deviate in a consistent way from linearity. In Figure 1, the few curves that rise steeply and do not conform to the pattern of the others include an early ("I") and a discontinued ("J") model of pericardial valves, and a discontinued treatment method of homograft valves ("K"). These valves were associated with earlier than average structural valve deterioration, suggesting a possible link between tissue valve failure and endocarditis. The steep jumps in some of the curves in Figures 1 and 2 display the

Table 1
References for Aortic Valve Cumulative Hazard Functions

Code	Ref	Model	Valves	Valve-years
A	35	Bileaflet	254	1111
B	67	Porcine	376	1474
C	68	Porcine	578	5187
D	69	Porcine	395	1264
E	70	Porcine	1335	6809
F	71	Pericardial	482	835
G	72	Pericardial	416	1872
H	73	Pericardial	310	2290
I	74	Pericardial	194	471
J	75	*Pericardial	476	2189
K	76	*Homograft	210	2520
L	77	Homograft	410	1054
M	77	Homograft	124	890
N	29	Mixed	2443	16,857
O	PDX	Mixed	2983	18,482

* = Discontinued models or preservation methods; PDX = Combined series from authors' institution. See Figure 1 for further information.

disproportionate effect of late events occurring when relatively few patients are still at risk.

This examination of the appropriateness of the constant hazard assumption for PVE includes only the first occurrence of PVE for each valve, which is all that is considered by event-free analyses and cumulative hazard functions (Figures 1 and 2). Yet the linearized rates include subsequent events for each valve, which are known to occur with a risk greater than

Table 2
References for Mitral Valve Cumulative Hazard Functions

Code	Ref	Model	Valves	Valve-years
A	35	Bileaflet	202	962
B	78	Porcine	121	1010
C	67	Porcine	195	747
D	68	Porcine	512	3877
E	70	Porcine	938	4784
F	72	Pericardial	115	518
G	75	*Pericardial	234	1076
H	PDX	mixed	1524	10,524

* = discontinued models; PDX = Combined series from authors' institution. See Figure 2 for further information.

that of an initial event. This effect, then, also violates the assumption of linearized rates; however, it is small, involving only a percentage of a percentage of patients. Thus, linearized rates may still be used as an acceptable first approximation to PVE risk.

Risk Factors for PVE

If the (late) PVE risk is assumed constant, we can summarize the risk for a given series by the linearized rate. We have done this for 115 series selected from the literature as described above. We are interested in assessing the relationships between PVE and certain factors related to the valve models and the series (Figures 3–11). These figures represent qualitative comparisons of many series, which differ with respect to important risk factors. Thus we do not attempt to draw statistical conclusions regarding similarities or differences; nevertheless, viewing the totality of information from these sources does lead to some clinical impressions and conclusions. We also examine the effect of previous endocarditis on the risk of subsequent PVE.

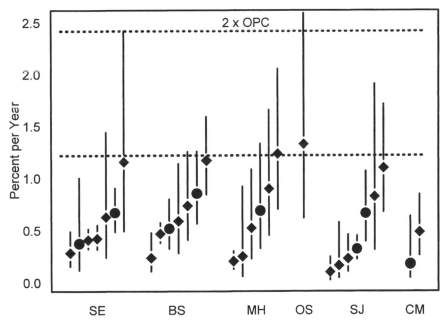

Figure 3. PVE rates for mechanical aortic valves, with 90% confidence intervals. Circles indicate that late PVE events only were used; diamonds indicate that all events were used because early and late events were not given separately. Modified with permission from *Journal of Heart Valve Disease.*[13]

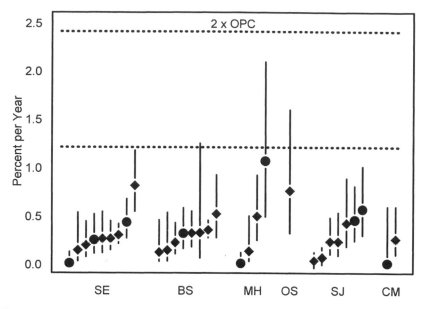

Figure 4. PVE rates for mechanical mitral valves, with 90% confidence intervals. Symbols, source: see legend to Figure 3.

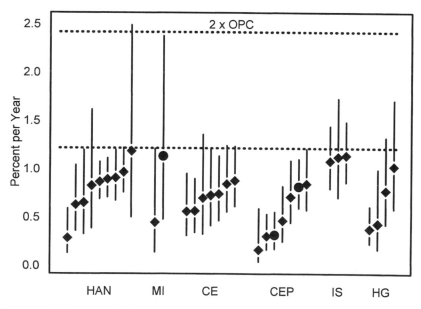

Figure 5. PVE rates for biological aortic valves, with 90% confidence intervals. Symbols, source: see legend to Figure 3.

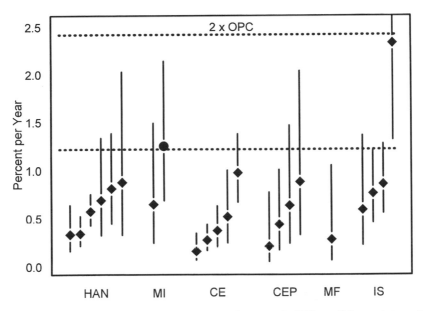

Figure 6. PVE rates for biological mitral valves, with 90% confidence intervals. Symbols, source: see legend to Figure 3.

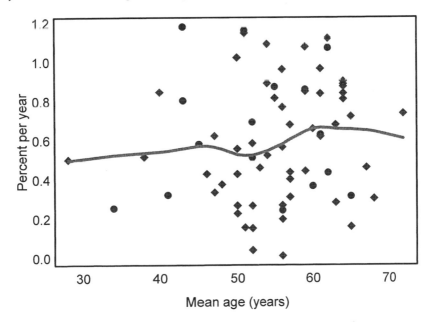

Figure 7. PVE rates according to mean age at implant. The line represents a LOWESS fit (see methods section of text). There does not seem to be a relationship with mean age. Symbols, source: see legend to Figure 3.

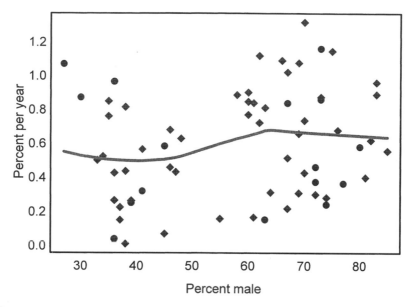

Figure 8. PVE rates according to patient sex (percent male). The line represents a LOWESS fit (see methods section of text). The series to the right of 50% are aortic, to the left are mitral. Thus the slight relationship with percent male is due to position. Symbols, source: see legend to Figure 3.

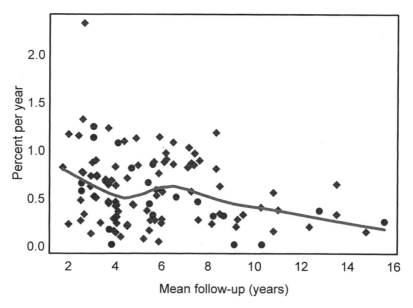

Figure 9. PVE rates according to mean follow-up time. The line represents a LOWESS fit (see methods section of text). There seems to be a trend toward decreased rates with very long mean follow-up times (beyond 8 years). Symbols, source: see legend to Figure 3.

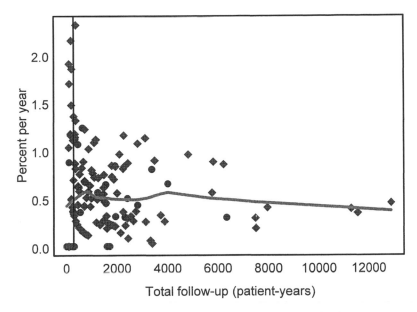

Figure 10. PVE rates according to total follow-up time. The line represents a LOWESS fit (see methods section of text). This figure includes series with less than 300 patient-years of follow-up, to show the instability of the estimates in the smaller series (to the left of the vertical line). Symbols, source: see legend to Figure 3.

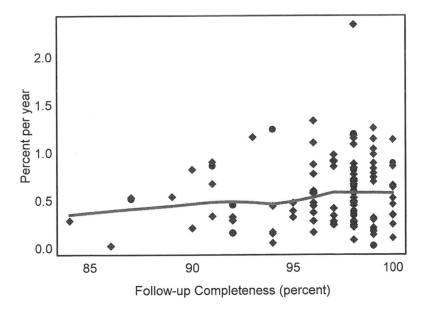

Figure 11. PVE rates according to completeness of follow-up. The line represents a LOWESS fit (see methods section of text). There appears to be a slight average increase in PVE rate with higher follow-up completeness. Symbols, source: see legend to Figure 3.

Valve Factors

The valve-related factors associated with a series are: type of valve (mechanical, biological), position (aortic or mitral) and model. Comparative linearized rates are plotted by valve model for mechanical aortic (Figure 3), mechanical mitral (Figure 4), biological aortic (Figure 5) and biological mitral (Figure 6) valves. These figures are adapted from Vlessis et al,[13] where the individual references for each series are given. For each valve model in each position these rates vary widely; thus these rates must depend on factors other than the valve model itself. The range of values for different models are surprisingly similar, and mostly range from very small up to the OPC value of 1.2% per year, shown by a dashed horizontal line in each figure. Mechanical valves in the mitral position (Figure 4) seem to have a somewhat lower range of values than for the other 3 combinations of position and valve type.

Previously, PVE risk has been found to be higher in the aortic than the mitral position[28] and higher for porcine than for mechanical valves.[28,29] This is consistent with our finding of no overall difference in the aortic position (Figures 3 and 5), but some difference in favor of mechanical valves in the mitral position (Figures 4 versus 6). However, other authors found no difference in the risk of PVE by model, position or type of valve (mechanical versus bioprosthesis).[20,30,31]

The homograft series in the aortic position exhibit PVE rates similar to other biological and mechanical aortic valves. Thus, although the homograft enjoys a lower risk of early PVE[29] it may be comparable to other valves with regard to late PVE. The discontinued Ionescu-Shiley pericardial valve has somewhat higher average PVE rates than other bioprostheses (Figures 5 and 6), and it was discontinued because of unsatisfactory durability. This could be evidence of a relationship between PVE and tissue valve deterioration. It could be that tissue deterioration is a risk for PVE, or that PVE, even after being cured, hastens tissue deterioration.[32]

Series Factors

There are several factors other than valve model and position which differ among these series, and which could potentially influence the risk of PVE. Patient age and gender are patient-related but are only available in aggregate as mean values for a series. Other factors that are available pertain to follow-up. We examined the PVE rates for all models and positions as a function of mean patient age (Figure 7), percent male (Figure 8), mean follow-up time (Figure 9), total patient-years of follow-up (Figure 10) and percent completeness of follow-up (Figure 11). Not all of these figures have the same number of symbols, because not all of these variables were available for every series.

There appears to be no relationship with mean age (Figure 7), although one study found an increased risk with young age.[21] The slight increase in risk apparent with percentage of male patients (Figure 8) reflects the fact that percentages above 50% are aortic series, with slightly higher rates, for tissue valves at least, and below 50% are mitral series. The slight fall-off in rates with reduced follow-up completeness (Figure 11) could be expected. Plotting PVE rates versus mean follow-up (Figure 9) is another way of assessing the constancy of risk over time, since if the rate went down over time, series with longer mean follow-up would in general have lower rates. It appears that to a mean follow-up of about 8 years the rates are similar, with a possible reduction thereafter.

Comparing rates over total patient-years of follow-up (Figure 10) reveals an interesting point. The estimates tend to cluster more along the average as the series gets larger, as expected, since the standard error is inversely proportional to the square root of the total follow-up years. Figure 10 alone includes series with less than 300 patient-years of follow-up, to show the instability of the estimates in the smaller series. The vertical line represents the cutoff (300 patient-years) used for series in Figures 3–10. The rates to the left of that line vary greatly, and many have a rate of 0. Of the series with >300 patient-years, the one with the highest PVE rate has just slightly more than 300 patient-years.

Previous Endocarditis

Patient factors that have been associated with PVE risk are renal dysfunction, young age and previous endocarditis,[29] and perioperative factors such as wound infections.[21,30] The most significant predictor of PVE is previous endocarditis, carrying a relative risk found to be sevenfold (p = 0.0001)[28] and eightfold (p = 0.001).[30] We therefore review some of the results with this special subset of high-risk patients, those with an indication of previous endocarditis.

As a measure of the relative size of this risk group, we extracted the percentages of valve replacement patients with endocarditis as the indication for surgery from several valve series, including some other than those summarized by linearized rates above. The percentage of endocarditis in the aortic series ranged from 2% to 13%, with a weighted mean of 6.3%.[33–38] Percentages in the mitral series ranged from 1% to 9%, with a weighted mean of 4%.[33–36,39,39A]

In studies of subseries of patients with endocarditis as the indication for surgery, several factors have been found to affect the outcome.[40] Combinations of risk factors have been used to create subgroups of endocarditis patients with survival ranging from 0% at 30 days to 100% at 5 years.[41] There is not a consensus on the exact set of risk factors, but they include the following variables.

- Valve position. Both aortic[42] and mitral[43] valve positions have been found to have a higher risk.
- PVE versus native valve endocarditis (NVE). PVE is considered more difficult to control than NVE, but one study claims that, because of the superior diagnostic capability of transesophageal (versus transthoracic) echocardiography, late PVE now has no worse prognosis than NVE.[44]
- Early versus late PVE. Early PVE has worse outcomes than late PVE,[42-45] related to the fact that staphylococcus organisms are more virulent than streptococci.[29]
- Active versus remote endocarditis. Active endocarditis (AE) has a worse prognosis than remote (RE) or healed endocarditis as an indication for surgery,[29,45] at least initially. A recent study that examined the hazard functions in great detail[21] showed that indications of both AE and RE had a higher risk of recurrent PVE than did other indications. But until about 10 years postoperation AE did worse than RE, and, in fact, until about 3 years after operation, RE had the same result as for other indications.
- Surgical versus medical treatment. Several papers have shown that for PVE surgical or combined medical/surgical therapy provides better outcomes than medical therapy alone,[42,46-49] especially for *S. aureus* infections or complicated PVE.[42,50] The comparison between medical and surgical therapy is a bit unfair, however, since the patient groups are largely selected based on the outcome of medical therapy: medical successes are not operated on, while medical failures are. One paper suggests that "evaluation in controlled clinical trials is appropriate."[48] However, it is difficult to consider these comparable therapies appropriate for randomized evaluation, since they should not be regarded as competing but rather collaborating, in fact sequential, therapies. Thus, a proposal like that of Dr. Alsip and colleagues for a "point system. . .to assist in decision- making concerning surgery in patients with active infective endocarditis"[51] may be a better course.
- Replacement device. Many physicians prefer to use homograft valves to replace infected prostheses[52-56] especially for severe cases involving annular abscess.[54,57-62] However, some prefer mechanical valves,[28,63,64] and still others prefer bioprostheses.[40,43,65] The Ross procedure has also been advocated.[66]

Conclusions

The risk of PVE appears to be approximately constant, permitting a "linearized rate" to adequately summarize the rate for a given series. Linearized PVE rates for each valve model exhibit a wide range, from around 0 to the 1.2% per year that the FDA document proposes as a performance standard. The range of rates for all models, types and positions varies little, except for the mechanical mitral valves, which have somewhat lower rates on average. These facts imply that the risk of PVE is mostly related to factors other than the valve model itself. Among tissue valves, PVE rates are somewhat higher for discontinued or other tissue valves which had higher than average structural deterioration, suggesting a relationship between PVE and tissue valve degeneration. The subset of heart valve patients who have endocarditis as the indication for surgery have a relatively high risk of subsequent PVE. There are factors within this subset of patients, related to their previous endocarditis and subsequent therapy, which further increase their risk.

Acknowledgements: We are indebted to Mr. John B. Thiel for programming the literature extraction database, to Ms. Cindy L. Fessler for reviewing the manuscript, and to Ms. Juanita Solis for helping in maintaining the database.

References

1. Clark RE, Edmunds LH Jr, Cohn LH, et al. Guidelines for reporting morbidity and mortality after cardiac valvular operations. *Eur J Thorac Surg* 1988;2(5): 293–295.
2. Edmunds LH Jr, Clark RE, Cohn LH, et al. Guidelines for reporting morbidity and mortality after cardiac valvular operations. *J Thorac Cardiovasc Surg* 1988; 96(3):351–353.
3. Edmunds LH Jr, Clark RE, Cohn LH, et al. Guidelines for reporting morbidity and mortality after cardiac valvular operations. *Ann Thorac Surg* 1988;46: 257–259.
4. Edmunds LH Jr, Clark RE, Cohn LH, et al. Guidelines for reporting morbidity and mortality after cardiac valvular operations. *Eur J Thorac Surg* 1996;10: 812–816.
5. Edmunds LH Jr, Clark RE, Cohn LH, et al. Guidelines for reporting morbidity and mortality after cardiac valvular operations. *J Thorac Cardiovasc Surg* 1996; 112(3):708–711.
6. Edmunds LH Jr, Clark RE, Cohn LH, et al. Guidelines for reporting morbidity and mortality after cardiac valvular operations. *Ann Thorac Surg* 1996;62(3): 932–935.
7. Edmunds LH Jr, Clark RE, Cohn LH, et al. Guidelines for reporting morbidity and mortality after cardiac valvular operations. *Asian Cardiovascular Thoracic Annual* 1996;4:126–129.

8. Kirklin JW, Barrett-Boyes BG. Replacement device endocarditis. In Kirklin JW, Barratt-Boyes BG (eds.) *Cardiac Surgery.* New York, NY, Churchill Livingstone, Inc., 1993. pp 545–547.

9. Starr A, Edwards M. Mitral replacement: Clinical experience with a ball valve prosthesis. *Ann Surg* 1961;154:726–740.

10. Starr A, Edwards ML, Griswold H. Mitral replacement: Late results with a ball valve prosthesis. *Prog Cardiovasc Dis* 1962;5(3):298–312.

11. Stein PD, Harken DE, Dexter L. The nature and prevention of prosthetic valve endocarditis. *Am Heart J* 1966;71(3):393–407.

12. Block PC, DeSanctis RW, Weinberg AN, Austen WG. Prosthetic valve endocarditis. *J Thorac Cardiovasc Surg* 1970;60(4):540–548.

13. Vlessis AA, Khaki A, Grunkemeier GL, et al. Risk, diagnosis and management of prosthetic valve endocarditis: A review. *J Heart Valve Dis* 1997;6(5):443–465.

14. Cox DR. Some simple approximate tests for poisson variates. *Biometrika* 1953; 40:354–360.

15. Grunkemeier GL, Anderson WN Jr. Clinical evaluation and analysis of heart valve substitutes. *J Heart Valve Dis* 1998;7(2):163–169.

16. Draft Replacement Heart Valve Guidance, Food and Drug Administration, Division of Cardiovascular, Respiratory, and Neurological Devices, Center for Devices and Radiological Health, October 14, 1994,Version 4.1.

17. Grunkemeier GL, Johnson DM, Naftel DC. Sample size requirements for evaluating heart valves with constant risk events. *J Heart Valve Dis* 1994;3(1):53–58.

18. Cleveland WS. LOWESS: A program for smoothing scatterplots by robust locally weighted regression. *Am Statistician* 1981;35:54.

19. Ivert TS, Dismukes WE, Cobbs CG, et al. Prosthetic valve endocarditis. *Circulation* 1984;69(2):223–232.

20. Rutledge R, Kim BJ, Applebaum RE. Actuarial analysis of the risk of prosthetic valve endocarditis in 1598 patients with mechanical and bioprosthetic valves. *Arch Surg* 1985;120(4):469–72.

21. Agnihotri AK, McGiffin DC, Galbraith AJ, et al. The prevalence of infective endocarditis after aortic valve replacement. *J Thorac Cardiovasc Surg* 1995; 110(6):1708–20; discussion 1720–4.

22. Calderwood SB, Swinski LA, Waternaux CM, et al. Risk factors for the development of prosthetic valve endocarditis. *Circulation* 1985;72(1):31–37.

23. Chastre J, Trouillet JL. Early infective endocarditis on prosthetic valves. *Eur Heart J* 1995;16(Suppl B):32–8.

24. Freeman R. Prevention of prosthetic valve endocarditis. *Journal of Hospital Infection* 1995;30(Suppl):44–53.

25. Lytle BW, Priest BP, Taylor PC, et al. Surgical treatment of prosthetic valve endocarditis. *J Thorac Cardiovasc Surg* 1996;111(1):198–207; discussion 207–210.

26. Dossche KM, Defauw JJ, Ernst SM, et al. Allograft aortic root replacement in prosthetic aortic valve endocarditis: A review of 32 patients. *Ann Thorac Surg* 1997;63:1644–1649.

27. Blackstone EH, Naftel DC, Turner ME Jr. The decomposition of time-varying hazard into phases, each incorporating a separate stream of concomitant information. *J Amer Stat Assoc* 1986;81:615–624.

28. Arvay A, Lengyel M. Incidence and risk factors of prosthetic valve endocarditis. Eur J Cardiothorac Surg 1988;2(5):340–346.

29. Agnihotri AK, McGiffin DC, Galbraith AJ, et al. The prevalence of infective endocarditis after aortic valve replacement. *J Thorac Cardiovasc Surg* 1995; 110(6):1708–20; discussion 1720–4.

30. Grover FL, Cohen DJ, Oprian C, et al. Determinants of the occurrence of and survival from prosthetic valve endocarditis: Experience of the Veterans Affairs Cooperative Study on valvular heart disease. *J Thorac Cardiovasc Surg* 1994; 108(2):207–214.

31. Cortina JM, Martinell J, Artiz V, et al. Surgical treatment of active prosthetic valve endocarditis: Results in 66 patients. *Thorac Cardiovasc Surg* 1987;35(4): 209–214.

32. Tornos P, Sanz E, Permanyer-Miralda G, et al. Late prosthetic valve endocarditis. Immediate and long-term prognosis. *Chest* 1992;101(1):37–41.

33. Akins CW. Long-term results with the Medtronic-Hall valvular prosthesis. *Ann Thorac Surg* 1996;61(3):806–813.

34. Louagie Y, Noirhomme P, Aranguis E, et al. Use of the Carpentier-Edwards porcine bioprosthesis: Assessment of a patient selection policy. *J Thorac Cardiovasc Surg* 1992;104(4):1013–1024.

35. Kratz JM, Crawford FA, Jr., Sade RM, et al. St. Jude prosthesis for aortic and mitral valve replacement: A ten-year experience. *Ann Thorac Surg* 1993;56(3): 462–8.

36. Aupart MR, El Hammami S, Diemont F, et al. The Carbomedics prosthetic heart valve: Four year follow-up in 100 patients. *J Cardiovasc Surg (Torino)* 1996;37(6):597–601.

37. Aupart MR, Sirinelli AL, Diemont FF, et al. The last generation of pericardial valves in the aortic position: ten-year follow-up in 589 patients. *Ann Thorac Surg* 1996;61(2):615–20.

38. Pellerin M, Mihaileanu S, Couetil JP, et al. Carpentier-Edwards pericardial bioprosthesis in aortic position: long-term follow-up 1980 to 1994. *Ann Thorac Surg* 1995;60(2 Suppl):S292–5; discussion S295–6.

39. Isomura T, Hisatomi K, Hirano A, et al. The St. Jude medical prosthesis in the mitral position. *Eur J Cardiothorac Surg* 1994;8(1):11–4.

39A. Aupart MR, Neville PH, Hammami S, et al. Carpentier-Edwards pericardial valves in the mitral position: Ten-year follow-up. *J Thorac Cardiovasc Surg* 1997; 113(3):492–498.

40. Pansini S, di Summa M, Patane F, et al. Risk of recurrence after reoperation for prosthetic valve endocarditis. *J Heart Valve Dis* 1997;6(1):84–87.

41. Kimose HH, Lund O, Kromann-Hansen O. Risk factors for early and late outcome after surgical treatment of native infective endocarditis. *Scand J Thorac Cardiovasc Surg* 1990;24(2):111–120.

42. Calderwood SB, Swinski LA, Karchmer AW, et al. Prosthetic valve endocarditis: Analysis of factors affecting outcome of therapy. *J Thorac Cardiovasc Surg* 1986;92(4):776–783.

43. Farina G, Vitale N, Piazza L, et al. Long-term results of surgery for prosthetic valve endocarditis. *J Heart Valve Dis* 1994;3(2):165–171.

44. Schulz R, Werner GS, Fuchs JB, et al. Clinical outcome and echocardiographic findings of native and prosthetic valve endocarditis in the 1990's. *Eur Heart J* 1996;17(2):281–288.

45. Gagliardi C, Di Tommaso L, Mastroroberto P, et al. Bioprosthetic valve endocarditis: Factors affecting bad outcome. *J Cardiovasc Surg (Torino)* 1991;32(6): 800–806.

46. Vlessis AA, Hovaguimian H, Jaggers J, et al. Infective endocarditis: Ten-year review of medical and surgical therapy. *Ann Thorac Surg* 1996;61(4):1217–1222.
47. Olaison L, Hogevik H, Myken P, et al. Early surgery in infective endocarditis. *QJM* 1996;89(4):267–278.
48. Yu VL, Fang GD, Keys TF, et al. Prosthetic valve endocarditis: superiority of surgical valve replacement versus medical therapy only. *Ann Thorac Surg* 1994; 58(4):1073–1077.
49. Nihoyannopoulos P, Oakley CM, Exadactylos N, et al. Duration of symptoms and the effects of a more aggressive surgical policy: Two factors affecting prognosis of infective endocarditis. *Eur Heart J* 1985;6(5):380–390.
50. Wolff M, Witchitz S, Chastang C, et al. Prosthetic valve endocarditis in the ICU: Prognostic factors of overall survival in a series of 122 cases and consequences for treatment decision. *Chest* 1995;108(3):688–694.
51. Alsip SG, Blackstone EH, Kirklin JW, et al. Indications for cardiac surgery in patients with active infective endocarditis. *Am J Med* 1985;78(6B):138–148.
52. Kirklin JK, Pacifico AD, Kirklin JW. Surgical treatment of prosthetic valve endocarditis with homograft aortic valve replacement. *J Card Surg* 1989;4(4): 340–347.
53. McGiffin DC, Galbraith AJ, McLachlan GJ, et al. Aortic valve infection: Risk factors for death and recurrent endocarditis after aortic valve replacement. *J Thorac Cardiovasc Surg* 1992;104(2):511–520.
54. McGiffin DC, Kirklin JK. The impact of aortic valve homografts on the treatment of aortic prosthetic valve endocarditis. *Semin Thorac Cardiovasc Surg* 1995; 7(1):25–31.
55. Petrou M, Wong K, Albertucci M, et al. Evaluation of unstented aortic homografts for the treatment of prosthetic aortic valve endocarditis. *Circulation* 1994; 90(5 Pt 2):II198–204.
56. Haydock D, Barratt-Boyes B, Macedo T, et al. Aortic valve replacement for active infectious endocarditis in 108 patients: A comparison of freehand allograft valves with mechanical prostheses and bioprostheses. *J Thorac Cardiovasc Surg* 1992;103(1):130–139.
57. Camacho MT, Cosgrove DM III. Homografts in the treatment of prosthetic valve endocarditis. *Semin Thorac Cardiovasc Surg* 1995;7(1):32–37.
58. Pagano D, Allen SM, Bonser RS. Homograft aortic valve and root replacement for severe destructive native or prosthetic endocarditis. *Eur J Cardiothorac Surg* 1994;8(4):173–176.
59. Miller DC. Predictors of outcome in patients with prosthetic valve endocarditis (PVE) and potential advantages of homograft aortic root replacement for prosthetic ascending aortic valve-graft infections. *J Card Surg* 1990;5(1):53–62.
60. Glazier JJ, Verwilghen J, Donaldson RM, et al. Treatment of complicated prosthetic aortic valve endocarditis with annular abscess formation by homograft aortic root replacement. *J Am Coll Cardiol* 1991;17(5):1177–1182.
61. Donaldson RM, Ross DM. Homograft aortic root replacement for complicated prosthetic valve endocarditis. *Circulation* 1984;70(3 Pt 2):1178–1181.
62. Bedi HS, Farnsworth AE. Homograft aortic root replacement for destructive prosthetic endocarditis. *Ann Thorac Surg* 1993;55(2):386–388.
63. Reul GJ, Sweeney MS. Bioprosthetic versus mechanical valve replacement in patients with infective endocarditis. *J Card Surg* 1989;4(4):348–351.
64. Gaudino M, De Filippo C, Pennestri F, et al. The use of mechanical prostheses in native aortic valve endocarditis. *J Heart Valve Dis* 1997;6(1):79–83.

65. Magilligan DJ Jr. Bioprosthetic valve replacement of aortic valve endocarditis: Detroit experience. *J Card Surg* 1990;5(1):73–75.
66. Joyce F, Tingleff J, Pettersson G. The Ross operation in the treatment of prosthetic aortic valve endocarditis. *Semin Thorac Cardiovasc Surg* 1995;7(1):38–46.
67. David TE, Armstrong S, Sun Z. Clinical and hemodynamic assessment of the Hancock II bioprosthesis. *Ann Thorac Surg* 1992;54(4):661–667; discussion 667–668.
68. Jamieson WR, Munro AI, Miyagishima RT, et al. Carpentier-Edwards standard porcine bioprosthesis: Clinical performance to seventeen years. *Ann Thorac Surg* 1995;60(4):999–1006.
69. Wilson ES, Jamieson MP. Carpentier-Edwards supra-annular bioprosthesis in the aortic position. Has altered design affected performance? *J Heart Valve Dis* 1996;5(1):40–44.
70. Jamieson WR, Burr LH, Tyers GF, et al. Carpentier-Edwards supraannular porcine bioprosthesis: Clinical performance to twelve years. *Ann Thorac Surg* 1995;60(2 Suppl):S235–40.
71. Torka MC, Salefsky BE, Hacker RW. Intermediate clinical results after aortic valve replacement with the Carpentier-Edwards pericardial bioprosthesis. *Ann Thorac Surg* 1995;60(2 Suppl):S311–5.
72. Pelletier LC, Carrier M, Leclerc Y, et al. The Carpentier-Edwards pericardial bioprosthesis: Clinical experience with 600 patients. *Ann Thorac Surg* 1995; 60(2 Suppl):S297–302.
73. Cosgrove DM, Lytle BW, Taylor PC, et al. The Carpentier-Edwards pericardial aortic valve: Ten-year results. *J Thorac Cardiovasc Surg* 1995;110(3):651–662.
74. Jamieson WR, Pelletier LC, Gerein AN, et al. The Mitroflow pericardial bioprosthesis: Comparison of early clinical performance in aortic and mitral positions. *Can J Surg* 1992;35(2):159–164.
75. Masters RG, Pipe AL, Bedard JP, et al. Long-term clinical results with the Ionescu Shiley pericardial xenograft. *J Thorac Cardiovasc Surg* 1991;101(1): 81–89.
76. Khaghani A, Dhalla N, Penta A. Patient status 10 years or more after aortic valve replacement using antibiotic sterilized homografts. In Bodnar EM (ed.) *Biologic and Bioprosthetic Valves.* New York, NY. Yorke Medical Books, 1986. pp 38–46.
77. O'Brien MF, McGiffin DC, Stafford EG, et al. Allograft aortic valve replacement: Long-term comparative clinical analysis of the viable cryopreserved and antibiotic 4 degrees C stored valves. *J Card Surg* 1991;6(suppl4):534–543.
78. Kawachi Y, Tanaka J, Tominaga R, et al. More than ten years' follow-up of the Hancock porcine bioprosthesis in Japan. *J Thorac Cardiovasc Surg* 1992; 104(1):5–13.

II

Diagnosis

Chapter 5
Clinical Diagnosis of Infective Endocarditis

Wendy S. Armstrong, M.D.
Michael Shea, M.D.

Introduction

The clinical diagnosis of infective endocarditis (IE) is often difficult. IE has a wide variety of clinical manifestations caused by 4 distinct processes: valvular pathology with local infection, embolic events, persistent bacteremia and features related to the immune response.[1] When manifestations of each of these processes are present, the diagnosis is clear. In most patients, however, fewer manifestations are seen, each with many potential etiologies. Since its initial description, the presentation of IE has changed substantially. Many of the classic manifestations of IE described by Osler are now rarely present, because prolonged untreated disease has largely been eliminated by antibiotic therapy. Furthermore, the character of the disease is changing with the addition of new risk factors that cause new patterns of disease. For example, intravenous drug use (IVDU) often results in right-sided endocarditis, which was infrequent in the past. While the decline in classic signs of IE has made diagnosis by physical examination alone more difficult, diagnosis has been aided by technology. Echocardiography, particularly transesophageal echocardiography, is now firmly established as an important diagnostic procedure for IE. The role of other technologies such as radionuclide imaging studies, computerized tomography and magnetic resonance imaging has yet to be determined.

From: Vlessis AA, Bolling S (eds): *Endocarditis: A Multidisciplinary Approach to Modern Treatment.* © Futura Publishing Co., Armonk, NY, 1999.

In the following 2 chapters, we will attempt to outline a systematic approach to the diagnosis of IE in the modern era.

In the past, endocarditis has been divided into 2 types, acute and subacute. These classifications described different patterns of disease seen with more or less virulent organisms, and were carefully tied to the identity of the causative organism. This classification system has become less useful with the recognition of new etiologic agents and with reports of fulminant disease caused by organisms previously thought to cause only subacute disease and vice versa. Presently of historical interest, these terms also describe patterns of disease that may have relevance to the urgency of therapy and the risk of complications. They do not identify the causative organism or dictate specific therapy.

Clinical Features

General Symptoms

Although some patients with IE present with fulminant symptoms, most describe nonspecific protean symptoms, often present for weeks prior to diagnosis. These symptoms include fever, chills, sweats, malaise, anorexia and weight loss. Fever is the most ubiquitous symptom of endocarditis and was seen in a large percentage of cases (between 64% and 93%) of native valve endocarditis in 6 large series.[2–7] Fever is also common in early prosthetic valve endocarditis, appearing in approximately 85% of cases.[4,5] In late prosthetic valve endocarditis, fever is noted in 58% to 79% of patients, and in endocarditis in the setting of IVDU, fever is seen in 75% to 88%. The degree of temperature elevation is variable. Fever over 102°F is seen in more than one third of patients with native valve endocarditis, with a trend toward higher fevers in patients with early prosthetic valve endocarditis and with a history of IVDU. In one series, patients over 60 were noted to have lower average initial temperatures (101.4°F) than patients under 40 (102.3°F).[8] Patients over 60 were also less likely to report fever and chills. In addition, fever may be absent in elderly patients or those with congestive heart failure, renal failure, a terminal disease or previous antibiotic therapy.[1] Despite reporting fever less frequently, the elderly were more likely to complain of anorexia and weight loss than their younger counterparts.

The duration of symptoms prior to presentation is also variable. A recent series of 135 patients with IE found that the mean time to presentation after the onset of symptoms in patients with native valve endocarditis was 29 days.[5] Patients with early prosthetic valve endocarditis and patients with a history of IVDU presented earliest (mean of 13 days and

11 days respectively), a trend supported in other series.[4] Pelletier and Petersdorf[6] noted that patients with pneumococcal and staphylococcal endocarditis presented earlier than those with streptococcal, enterococcal, anaerobic and culture-negative endocarditis. The same series of 125 cases noted that the duration of illness prior to presentation in patients who died was twice as long (61 days) as in those who survived (32 days).

The duration of fever after the initiation of therapy for endocarditis may be an important prognostic sign. In one series of 123 patients, more than half were afebrile after 72 hours of antibiotic therapy, 72% had defervesced after one week of therapy and 84% were afebrile after 2 weeks of therapy. [9] In multivariate analysis, prolonged fever was associated with large vessel embolization and evidence of microvascular phenomena on admission. Mortality in patients with persistent fever after 1 week of therapy was significantly higher than in those who defervesced (18% versus 2%). Blumberg et al[10] evaluated 26 patients with fever of more than 2 weeks' duration. Of these patients, 27% had myocardial abscesses. Other patients in whom the etiology of fever was discovered had nosocomial infections, drug fever or persistent infection as demonstrated by positive blood cultures or defervesence after cardiac surgery.

Cardiac Manifestations

The cardiac manifestations of endocarditis are numerous and vary depending on the infected valve. The aortic and mitral valves are consistently the most frequently involved. In 3 large series published in the 1970s, the aortic valve was involved in 39% of patients, the mitral valve was involved in 29% to 35% and both in 13% to 18%. The frequency of tricuspid infection ranged from 1% to 11%. Earlier series consistently showed mitral valve involvement more often than aortic valve involvement.[2-6] Because the disease spectrum is changing due to factors such as the declining prevalence of rheumatic heart disease and increasing prevalence of IVDU, the relative involvement of the heart valves is likely to continue to change. Aortic valve endocarditis and multivalvular involvement are associated with a poorer prognosis. In one study, patients with multivalvular endocarditis and a new regurgitant murmur had a 97% mortality rate.[6]

The physical examination finding of a new or changing murmur is often thought to be common. In fact, a cardiac murmur is absent in as many as 15% of patients with endocarditis,[11] a new murmur is appreciated in only 3% to 5% of cases, and a changing murmur is present in only 5% to 10% of patients.[1] Murmurs are most likely to be absent in endocarditis caused by a virulent organism associated with an acute course and in right-sided endocarditis.[2,3,11] In fact, tricuspid murmurs are appreciated in only one third of cases in which this valve is involved.[12] Changing murmurs can be difficult to interpret, and may be attributed to fever and/or anemia, both of which are often present in endocarditis and can produce hemodynamic changes. For that reason, detection of a *new* murmur, particularly one of valvular insufficiency, is more specific for endocarditis, despite being an infrequent finding. Finally, endocarditis can result from infection of the mural endocardium without valvular involvement; thus, there is no detectable murmur.

The most common cardiac complication of infective endocarditis is congestive heart failure (CHF). Cardiac decompensation is seen in 15% to 65% of patients and, in the present antibiotic era, is the most frequent cause of death.[13] In one series the survival rate at 1 year was 4 times greater for patients with normal cardiac function as compared to those with abnormal function.[14] However, these studies have not been done in the modern era of treatment for heart failure. Aortic insufficiency is the most common cause of CHF, followed by myocarditis. At times, acute mitral insufficiency develops in patients with aortic insufficiency due to hemodynamic rather than infectious processes. The jet from the regurgitant aortic valve can cause erosion or perforation of the anterior leaflet of the mitral valve or can rupture the chordae tendineae. Patients with this complication are at higher risk of refractory cardiac failure. Valve leaflet destruction or perforation and rupture of the papillary muscles or chordae tendineae can also occur due to effects from the vegetation itself. Occasionally, valvular stenosis can be caused by obstruction due to a large vegetation, typically in the setting of fungal endocarditis. Myocarditis in the setting of endocarditis may have many possible etiologies including microabscesses, coronary vasculitis, immune complex deposition and injury from microbial toxin production.[15]

Another feared complication of IE is the development of a myocardial abscess. Typically seen in infective endocarditis caused by virulent organisms such as *Staphylococcus aureus*, myocardial abscesses are reported in approximately 20% of autopsies, and are multiple in 20% of fatal cases.[12,13] They can be isolated within the myocardium due to metastatic infection or can arise from direct extension of infection around the valve. Perivalvular abscesses are common in prosthetic valve endocarditis and are adjacent to the prosthesis. In native valve endocarditis, perivalvular or annular abscesses involve the aortic valve more frequently than the mitral valve or atrioventricular ring. Complications of myocardial abscesses include further valvular compromise, conduction defects, fistulae and pericarditis. The type of conduction defect can offer clues to the location of the abscess.[11] New bundle-branch block suggests extension of a perivalvular aortic abscess, while heart block suggests extension of mitral valve abscesses into the atrioventricular node. Premature ventricular contractions can be caused by ventricular myocardial abscesses. Rupture of an aortic root abscess into the right atrium will lead to a left to right shunt, as will rupture of a septal abscess. Suppurative pericarditis is a consequence of rupture of an aortic valvular abscess through the pericardial wedge located between the aortic and pulmonary artery roots or can be secondary to aortic root dissection due to a valvular abscess.

In addition to abscess rupture and dissection, rupture of a mycotic aneurysm at the sinus of Valsalva can lead to suppurative pericarditis. Further complications can include cardiac tamponade or pyohemopericardium. Nonsuppurative pericarditis is also noted in infective endocarditis and can have many etiologies. These include pericardial immune complex deposition, seen in 10% of cases, an acute rheumatic fever flare, uremia due to renal failure related to glomerulonephritis, and as a sequela of myocardial infarction.

Emboli to the coronary arteries can lead to a myocardial infarction (MI). In fact, endocarditis is the most common cause of embolic MI. Such infarcts are typically small, occasionally multiple and frequently silent. Autopsy series show an incidence of 40% to 60% in fatal cases.[12] Emboli are more likely to originate from the aortic valve than from the mitral valve. Myocardial infarction can also result from coronary thrombosis due to adjacent inflammation from a myocardial abscess or pericarditis, or it can be caused by a coronary artery mycotic aneurysm.

Cutaneous/Peripheral Vascular Manifestations

Several peripheral vascular phenomena and other cutaneous signs bear a well-known association with infective endocarditis. Splinter hemorrhages are recognized as red, black or brown linear lesions with the long axis parallel to the nailbed. They are nonblanching, but are at times associated with finger swelling and pain. The association of endocarditis with subungual splinter hemorrhages was first reported in 1920 by Horder. Since then, studies of the overall prevalence of splinter hemorrhages in hospitalized patients suggest that the lesions are common, occurring in approximately 19% of patients.[16] The specificity of splinter hemorrhages for endocarditis is low, with the lesion often seen in patients with mitral stenosis, trichinosis, renal failure on peritoneal dialysis or in those with a history of frequent trauma to the hands, e.g. carpenters or mechanics.[16,17]

Janeway's lesions are painless, erythematous or hemorrhagic macules classically seen on the palmar surfaces and soles of the feet but occasionally found on the fingertips as well. They frequently appear in crops. Biopsies of the lesions show microabscesses without endarteritis, and the microorganism has been cultured from the lesions. These characteristics suggest that Janeway's lesions are predominantly a result of septic emboli rather than an immunologic phenomenon.[18]

Osler's nodes are painful, erythematous nodules, 1.0 mm to 1.5 mm in diameter, located most commonly on the pads of the fingers or toes, the thenar and hypothenar eminences or the sides of the fingers. Pain or parasthesias often precede the development of a visible lesion. Although endocarditis is the most frequent clinical setting in which they are encountered, Osler's nodes have been described in patients with other diseases, for example bacteremia, septic endarteritis and systemic lupus erythematosis (SLE). Osler's nodes are uncommon in acute bacterial endocarditis, prosthetic valve endocarditis and endocarditis caused by gram-negative organisms. They are more common in patients with fungal endocarditis and subacute bacterial endocarditis (SBE), particularly when caused by alpha-hemolytic streptococcal species. Overall the incidence of Osler's nodes in endocarditis has declined in the antibiotic era from a prevalence of 40% to 90% to only 10% to 23%,[19] likely because of the changing microbiological spectrum and the institution of early and effective antimicrobial therapy. The etiology of Osler's nodes is strongly debated. Biopsy data have demonstrated microabscesses favoring a microembolic etiology as well as evidence of perivasculitis favoring an immunologic mechanism. Proponents of a microembolic etiology argue that biopsy material demonstrating vasculitis was obtained several days after the appearance of the lesions, which does not eliminate the possibility that the vasculitis is a secondary phenomenon. Indirect evidence favors a microembolic etiology including the appearance of lesions in crops, an association with macrovascular emboli, and the development of lesions after clearance of bacteremia when immunologic phenomena should be quiescent.[19] In addition, organisms have been cultured from biopsy material providing direct evidence of a septic embolic pathogenesis.[20] Although good evidence favors a role for microemboli, coincident immunologic mechanisms cannot be ruled out.

Petechiae, seen in as many as 85% of patients with endocarditis in the preantibiotic era, are now present in only 19% to 40% of cases, but remain one of the most common cutaneous manifestations.[12] They are most frequently seen on the extremities, oral mucosa, soft palate and conjunctivae. As with Osler's nodes and Janeway's lesions, they often appear in crops. The finding lacks specificity for endocarditis and can be seen in other conditions such as renal failure, thrombocytopenia and bacteremia, and may be a complication of cardiopulmonary bypass. In the latter case, they represent fat microembolism.[13] At least one case report has described leukocytoclastic vasculitis in a patient with endocarditis. [21]

Clubbing of the nails was once a frequent feature of SBE, occurring in 76% of cases in the preantibiotic era, but now is only seen in 12% to 52% of cases.[12,22] Once again, the most likely explanation for this reduction is early therapy of the disease, as a prolonged time course is necessary to produce clubbing.

Ophthalmologic Manifestations

The classic ophthalmologic manifestation of endocarditis is the Roth spot. In 1872, Moritz Roth described small white spots on the retina seen in patients with sepsis, which are now known to consist of cytoid bodies in the nerve fiber layer resulting from infarction. He also described separate areas of retinal hemorrhage. In 1878, Litten reported an association between white-centered retinal hemorrhages and endocarditis, and incorrectly called these lesions Roth spots. It is these latter lesions that are most commonly referred to as Roth spots today.[22] Pathological analysis of these lesions shows an accumulation of lymphocytes with surrounding hemorrhage in the nerve fiber layer most likely due to septic emboli. Neither Roth's original lesions nor Roth spots are common findings in endocarditis, occurring in less than 5% of cases.[12] Roth spots have also been described in many clinical settings, including in patients with connective tissue diseases like SLE, leukemia, multiple myeloma, anemia, diabetes and HIV disease.[23]

Retinal artery or branch artery occlusion due to acute embolism causing sudden blindness are known complications of endocarditis. Other ophthalmologic manifestations include conjunctival petechiae as noted in the preceding section, premacular hemorrhage,[24] anterior ischemic optic neuropathy due to posterior ciliary artery occlusion, acute endophthalmitis and bilateral macular hole formation.[25] Papilledema can be seen in conditons associated with elevated intracranial pressure such as intracranial hemorrhage after rupture of a mycotic aneurysm or from a brain abscess resulting from metastatic infection.

Musculoskeletal Manifestations

Musculoskeletal complaints are common in endocarditis. They tend to occur early, often preceding other manifestations by months leading to misdiagnosis.[26] Low back pain is a common presenting musculoskeletal symptom and is often the patient's chief complaint. Seen in up to 33% of cases,[5-7] the pain tends to be severe and may be associated with radicular findings. In the majority of cases, no evidence of disk space infection is present, and symptoms resolve with therapy. Features favoring an etiology different from muscle strain, degenerative joint disease or disc disease include no history of injury or previous back pain, and radiographs without evidence of degenerative arthritis.[26]

In a series of 192 patients with endocarditis, arthralgias were the most common complaint at some point during the illness, and were found in 17% of cases.[26] The shoulder joint was most frequently involved, followed by the knee and hip. Both monoarticular and polyarticular involvement was noted. Synovitis was noted in 14% of the additional cases, again in a monoarticular or asymmetric oligoarticular pattern.[26] Like arthralgias, involved joints tended to be proximal and in the lower extremities, but the most frequently involved joint was the ankle. Synovial fluid shows an inflammatory pattern and positive cultures are infrequent.[22] Nonetheless, acute septic arthritis has been documented, particularly in association with staphylococcal endocarditis.[27]

Diffuse myalgias or myalgias limited to the calves and thighs were seen in 14% of patients. Cases of osteomyelitis and paraspinal abscesses have also been reported.[27]

Renal Manifestations

Renal involvement in endocarditis is common. The presence of renal insufficiency denotes a poorer prognosis. In patients with *S. aureus* endocarditis, the mean blood urea nitrogen (BUN) in patients who died of the disease was significantly higher than in survivors (62 mg/dl versus. 31.2 mg/dl respectively).[6] One series from France demonstrated a 70% mortality rate in individuals with significant renal failure in comparison to 35% mortality in all patients.[28] Several patterns of renal involvement have been described, often with coincident lesions in any individual patient.

The most common lesion is renal infarction, seen in as many as two thirds of cases at autopsy, though few are clinically suspected.[14] Although large emboli to the renal arteries have been described, infarcts typically result from smaller emboli. Renal insufficiency is infrequent unless a significant percentage of the kidneys is compromised. Renal abscess formation from septic emboli can occur but is not common, and is typically associated with virulent organisms causing metastatic infection at other sites as well. Surprisingly, renal infarction is seen in 10% to 15% of cases of right-sided endocarditis.[28] The presumed source of emboli are thrombosed pulmonary vessels at sites of septic pulmonary emboli. On gross inspection, the kidneys are often characterized as having a "flea-bitten" appearance with subcapsular petechiae present in the area of infarct.

Both focal and diffuse glomerulonephritis are associated with infective endocarditis. Focal glomerulonephritis is more common, although the incidence has declined in the antibiotic era from approximately 50%

before antimicrobial therapy to 18% to 25% presently.[28] The pathogenesis of this lesion is not definitively understood. Microscopic analysis reveals areas of focal glomerulonephritis limited to the edges of renal infarcts, suggesting an embolic source. In other patients, focal glomerulonephritis has been described as occurring independently of regions of infarct. In these cases, immunofluorescent microscopy supports an immunologic mechanism of injury.

Diffuse glomerulonephritis is less common than focal glomerulonephritis, occurring in 30% to 60% of cases prior to the advent of antibiotic therapy and in less than 15% of treated cases.[28] The histopathology of this lesion mimics that of postinfectious glomerulonephritis and is believed to be immunologically mediated. This subset of patients is more likely to develop renal failure than those with focal glomerulonephritis or renal infarcts. Antibiotic therapy can lead to complete recovery of renal function. Membranoproliferative glomerulonephritis has been described in association with *S. epidermidis* endocarditis but is unusual.[29]

In addition to these renal lesions, other etiologies of renal failure commonly occur in the setting of endocarditis. Antibiotic therapy can cause interstitial nephritis or acute tubular necrosis in the setting of endocarditis. Prerenal azotemia can occur in the setting of decreased cardiac output related to sepsis or valvular or myocardial compromise. Thrombotic microangiopathy is a known complication of sepsis associated with disseminated intravascular coagulation.

Pulmonary Manifestations

Pulmonary manifestations of endocarditis, with the exception of pulmonary edema due to congestive heart failure, are the predominant symptoms in patients with right-sided endocarditis. Although this group is predominantly composed of intravenous drug users, immunosupressed hosts and even normal hosts can develop right-sided disease. In the majority of patients with tricuspid valve infection, pulmonary symptoms, typically pleuritic chest pain, cough and shortness of breath, are the presenting features. Hemoptysis is also a frequent complaint. The chest radiograph is abnormal in 75% to 85% of patients.[1] The most common manifestations are septic pulmonary emboli with infarcts occurring in at least 87% of patients during the course of right-sided endocarditis.[1] In these cases, the chest radiograph shows nodular infiltrates. Recurrent pulmonary emboli should raise the suspicion of endocarditis. Other manifestations include pneumonia with evidence of cavitation, lung abscess, empyema due to rupture of an abscess into the pleural space or due to hematologic seeding, pneumothorax or pleural effusions.[30] Rarely, mycotic aneurysms of the pulmonary artery may be present.[15]

Splenic Manifestations

Splenomegaly has been reported in 23% to 57% of patients with endocarditis.[14] The incidence of splenomegaly is greater in patients with disease of longer duration, but may be declining in the antibiotic era.[1] Though 40% to 60% of autopsies show evidence of splenic infarct secondary to emboli, the majority are clinically asymptomatic.[22] Symptomatic emboli may cause left upper quadrant abdominal pain, left-sided pleuritic chest pain or left-sided pleural effusions. Splenic infarcts may be single or multiple and are frequently the only manifestations of systemic embolization in a particular patient.[31] Splenic abscesses are rare, with an incidence of 10% in the preantibiotic era and few reported since the introduction of antibiotics. Abscess should be suspected in the individual with persistent fever despite appropriate antibiotic therapy or recurrence of fever after the discontinuation of therapy. Splenic rupture is a potentially fatal complication of infarct or abscess and can occur as a late complication.[32]

Neurological Manifestations

Infective endocarditis is associated with many different neurological complications including cerebral infarct, mycotic aneurysm, brain abscesses and meningitis. A full discussion of these manifestations can be found in Chapter 7.

Other Vascular Manifestations

Extracranial mycotic aneurysms and large artery emboli are seen in IE. Mycotic aneurysms of the abdominal aorta and celiac axis as well as the superior mesenteric artery have been described. Emboli to large arteries of the extremities, most commonly the radial, brachial, pedal and popliteal arteries, can cause limb ischemia. This complication is most commonly seen in fungal endocarditis in which vegetations tend to be larger and more friable than bacterial endocarditis.[14]

Laboratory Evaluation

The diagnosis of endocarditis is made on the basis of clinical features, imaging studies and culture data. Aside from results of microbiological testing, laboratory abnormalities are generally nonspecific but can lend support to clinical features to suggest a diagnosis of infective endocarditis. These abnormalities are generally hematologic and immunologic.

Hematologic Testing

Anemia is seen in 50% to 80% of patients with endocarditis[4,11] and is typically normochromic and normocytic. Iron studies are usually consistent with the anemia of chronic disease. Anemia is more often associated with the subacute pattern of endocarditis and tends to be more pronounced in patients with a prolonged duration of disease.[6] The presence and degree of anemia are not correlated with any particular etiologic organisms. Hemolytic anemia is uncommon but can result from abnormal valvular flow. In patients with IE, it is usually seen in individuals with prosthetic valve endocarditis.

Leukocytosis is frequently absent in patients with subacute disease, but typically present in those with an acute pattern of endocarditis. More than half of the 107 patients with native valve endocarditis in one series had white blood counts greater than 10,000[4] with more than 90% of patients demonstrating a left shift. In their series of 125 patients at the University of Washington Hospitals, Pelletier and Petersdorf reported that the mean white blood count was 12,700. Leukocytosis was most pronounced in patients with pneumococcal, S. aureus and gram-negative endocarditis.[6] Leukopenia is present in 5% to 15% of patients. Splenomegaly is usually present in this subgroup.

Thrombocytopenia has been described in 5% to 15% of patients with IE and may be caused by splenomegaly and/or disseminated intravascular coagulation (DIC) due to sepsis. In addition, this hematologic abnormality is more common in cases of neonatal endocarditis.

Large mononuclear cells, or histiocytes, are seen in 25% of peripheral blood samples obtained by ear lobe puncture in patients with IE. The cells contain vacuoles and intracellular debris but may also demonstrate phagocytosed organisms. They are seen in many infections such as malaria, typhus, tuberculosis and typhoid fever and are therefore nondiagnostic.[1]

More than 90% of individuals with endocarditis have an elevated erythrocyte sedimentation rate (ESR). Congestive heart failure, renal failure and DIC can lower or normalize the ESR. In the absence of these clinical factors, a normal ESR should bring the diagnosis of IE into question. In one series, the mean ESR in all patients with IE was 57 mm/hr. In this series, a low ESR in patients with S. aureus endocarditis was a significant adverse prognostic factor, with a mean ESR in fatal cases of 40.7 mm/hr as compared to a mean in survivors of 77.5 mm/hr.[6] This difference could not be solely explained by the relationship of a low ESR to CHF, also a known adverse prognostic factor. Another indicator of inflammation is elevated C-reactive protein. In one study, CRP was elevated in 96% of patients with a mean of 110 mg/L. This study suggested that CRP falls more rapidly with treatment than ESR. The authors proposed that CRP may be a more sensitive indicator to detect complications when followed to assess response to therapy.[33]

Immunologic Testing

Rheumatoid factor (RF) is elevated in as many as 50% of patients with IE and has been reported in very high titers.[22,34] Elevations are correlated with a duration of disease greater than 6 weeks. Only 6% of patients with disease for less than 6 weeks have a positive RF. The titer usually falls with therapy and patients may become seronegative after weeks to months.[14] RF (anti-IgG IgM antibody) may impair the immune response to bacterial infection by inhibiting opsonization, but this remains unproven.[15]

Also present in IE are increased levels of circulating immune complexes (ICs) seen in 63% to 97% of patients.[5,35] Elevated levels of ICs (greater than 12 μg/mL) are nonspecific and are seen in 32% of patients with sepsis, 40% of intravenous drug users and 10% of normal controls.[22] However, in one study 35% of patients with IE and no patients with other etiologies of disease had levels greater than 100 μg/mL. Higher levels of ICs were seen in patients with extravalvular manifestations of disease. Titers fall with therapy.

Mixed cryoglobulinemia has been reported in as many as 84% to 95% of cases of IE and hyperglobulinemia is seen in 20% to 30% of patients.[1] Occasionally a monoclonal pattern has been noted.[36] A positive antinuclear antibody is noted in 8% to 30% of cases and a false positive VDRL is unusual, reported in only 0.2% of patients in one series.[6]

Serum complement levels can be low in IE, as was seen in one series in 47% of patients. In the same series, 78% of patients with glomerulonephritis (as determined by biopsy or urinary sediment) or azotemia had depressed complement levels as compared to only 11% with positive results with no evidence of renal disease, although the number of patients in whom complement levels were determined was small. As with most other immunologic abnormalities, complement levels return to normal with antimicrobial therapy.[6]

Urinalysis

Most patients with IE will have an abnormal urinalysis. Proteinuria is common and is seen in 50% to 80% of cases.[28] Hematuria is present in 50% to 60% of patients and is most often microscopic.[28] Gross hematuria can be present. No definitive studies are available to determine if gross hematuria is indicative of renal infarct. Pyuria has been reported in 50% to 60% of patients as well with a positive urine culture in only 15% to 30%.[28] Red blood cell casts are present in 10% to 12%.[28] White blood cell casts can also be seen. In the antimicrobial era, azotemia is present in only 10% to 33% of patients.[28]

Blood Cultures

Determining the infecting organism in endocarditis is not only vital to choosing an appropriate antimicrobial regimen, but is also important (although not necessary) for the diagnosis. Blood cultures are therefore the most important laboratory test. One feature of IE is a continuous bacteremia due to the intravascular location of infection. The degree of bacteremia over time is variable; however, in more than 80% of cases, less than 100 colony forming units are present per milliliter of blood.[37] Most studies suggest that, in the absence of previous antimicrobial therapy, 1 of the first 2 blood cultures will be positive more than 90% of the time. The optimal number of blood culture sets is not known, but in one series the number of cultures required to yield positive results in 77 of 82 cases was 5.[14] Arterial blood has not been demonstrated to improve the yield of organisms in IE and, therefore, venous blood is the recommended source of blood cultures. Blood cultures should be obtained from different venipuncture sites to decrease the risk of contamination of multiple culture bottles thereby confusing the practitioner. Patients with an acute pattern of disease should have multiple sets of cultures drawn over a short period of time to limit delaying antimicrobial therapy. In stable patients, drawing cultures over a longer period of time may be beneficial, particularly in those with recent antimicrobial therapy likely to sterilize immediate cultures.

Prior antimicrobial therapy significantly limits the likelihood of positive cultures. In one study from New York Hospital-Cornell Medical Center, the incidence of positive blood cultures in patients with streptococcal endocarditis was decreased from 97% to 91%.[37] Another series showed that of 58 patients with endocarditis and negative blood cultures, 62% had received prior antibiotic therapy.[38] Finally, while 100% of cultures were positive in 15 patients with endocarditis who had not received prior antibiotic therapy, only 64% of cultures were positive in those with previous antibiotic therapy.[39]

Blood culture bottles with antibiotic binding resins may improve microbial yield but have disadvantages as well.[40] Fastidious organisms and organisms with specific nutritional requirements can be difficult to isolate and can lead to negative culture results in endocarditis patients with appropriately obtained cultures. The HACEK organisms (*Hemophilus parain-fluenzae, H. aphrophilus, Actinobacillus, Cardiobacterium, Eikenella* and *Kingella*) are slow growing and may require 3 to 4 weeks before growth can be detected. Nutritionally deficient streptococci require media supplemented with L-cysteine or pyridoxal hydrochloride for growth. Other organisms that have been known to cause IE and which require special conditions for growth include *Legionella* and *Brucella*. Negative cultures are seen in as many as 50% of cases of fungal endocarditis.[41] Although *Candida* species are easily isolated in conventional cultures, *Aspergillus* species are rarely isolated. The lysis-centrifugation culture system may improve the yield of some fungal pathogens but these species often must be diagnosed by other means. Because fungal vegetations are large and can cause embolism to large arteries in the extremities, embolectomy specimens should be stained and cultured for organisms.

Although culture-negative endocarditis has been reported in as many as 30% of cases, carefully handled cultures from patients not previously on antimicrobial therapy should be negative in less than 5% of cases.[42] In this setting, other possible etiologies include *Coxiella burnetii* and *Chlamydia* species. Although there is one reported case of *C. psittaci* endocarditis diagnosed by blood cultures,[43] in general, these agents do not grow in culture and the diagnosis must be pursued through serological testing.

As noted, serological studies can aid in the diagnosis of endocarditis in which infection with an organism that cannot be cultured is suspected. Other alternative approaches include culturing other material such as bone marrow, urine, skin lesions and embolectomy specimens. To aid in the diagnosis of *S. aureus* endocarditis, the use of antibodies to the teichoic acid component of the organism's cell wall has been investigated. Because of imperfect sensitivity of this test, it remains largely an investigational tool.[36] In patients with persistently negative cultures, the noninfectious causes of endocarditis should be entertained, including marantic or nonbacterial thrombotic endocarditis, endocarditis associated with SLE, atrial myxoma and acute rheumatic fever.

Imaging Studies

Chest Radiography

The chest radiograph can provide limited nonspecific information in the work-up of the patient with IE. Cardiomegaly may indicate cardiac failure or pericardial involvement. The presence of a mechanical prosthetic valve can be detected in the patient unable to provide the history of valve replacement. Evidence of pulmonary congestion consistent with CHF can be noted, as can nodular infiltrates consistent with septic emboli. Other less common findings include effusions, pneumothoraces and cavitary lesions.

Electrocardiography

Electrocardiography (ECG) also provides nonspecific information, but may aid in the identification of individuals with significant previously unsuspected cardiac complications. Conduction defects are seen in patients with myocardial abscesses and can signify extension from a perivalvular focus. For example, a prolonged PR interval, a new left bundle branch block and a new right bundle branch block with left anterior hemiblock are all suggestive of abscess extension from the aortic valve into the ventricular septum. Extension of a perivalvular mitral abscess often affects the atrioventricular node and proximal bundle of His and can be associated with nonparoxysmal junctional tachycardia, first or second degree heart block or, less commonly, third degree heart block with a narrow QRS complex.[11,44] Transient heart block (including bundle branch block and hemiblock) may reflect edema in the perivalvular conduction tissue. Fixed heart block, or heart block present for more than 3 to 5 days, is more concerning for perivalvular abscess. In one study, the finding of unstable conduction abnormalities had a sensitivity of 28% and specificity of 89% for paravalvular extension of infection.[44] Other ECG findings can be helpful in patients with IE. ST segment elevation may indicate infarct or pericarditis. Ventricular premature beats can be seen with a myocardial abscess or myocarditis. T wave inversions suggestive of CNS pathology may also be present.

Echocardiography

Transthoracic and transesophageal echocardiography has become a valuable tool in the diagnosis of endocarditis, as well as an aid to evaluate complications and progression of disease. Its use will be discussed at length in Chapter 6.

Radionuclide Imaging

Radionuclide imaging has not been well studied in the evaluation of endocarditis. One study of gallium-67 myocardial imaging reported that 7 of 11 patients with IE had positive scans at 72 hours. In these scans, accumulation of tracer was seen within the cardiac borders but identification of the involved valve could not be made.[45] Indium scans also lack sensitivity for the diagnosis of IE.[46] Scattered reports suggest that technetium scanning may aid in identification of embolic complications of IE with demonstration of renal, splenic and cerebral infarcts in selected patients,[47,48] and may aid in the diagnosis of perivalvular abscess.[44] Cardiac imaging with technetium-99m–labeled antigranulocyte antibodies in 33 patients with IE showed a sensitivity of 79% and showed a specificity of 82% in 39 patients without IE. Although the sensitivity compared favorably to transesophageal echocardiography (TEE) in this study, the sensitivity of TEE was unusually low, likely due to a high percentage of cases in the study population with prosthetic valve endocarditis. Technetium imaging could not identify the involved valve or provide additional functional information. Nonetheless, the authors argued that together TEE and technetium imaging had a sensitivity of 100% and that radionuclide imaging may have a role in the treatment of patients with equivocal echocardiographic findings.[46] Overall, the role of radionuclide imaging in endocarditis has not been fully defined, and awaits further studies for clarification.

Computerized Tomography

Similarly, the role of computerized tomography (CT) has not been well studied. Only one case of an aortic root abscess diagnosed by CT has been reported.[49] The use of CT in the identification of abdominal complications has been better established. Serial abdominal CT evaluation of patients with IE revealed an incidence of splenic infarcts or abscesses in 24%, of which two thirds were asymptomatic.[31] In another study, 38% of asymptomatic patients had splenic infarcts or abscesses.[32] In these cases, CT allowed evaluation of the size of the abnormality affecting the decision to perform splenectomy based on the risk of splenic rupture. CT demonstration of renal infarcts and a superior mesenteric artery mycotic aneurysm have been reported.[50,51] Of course, the role of CT in evaluating intracranial pathology due to complications of IE is well understood.

Magnetic Resonance Imaging

The evaluation of cardiac pathology by magnetic resonance imaging (MRI) has been studied more extensively. Caduff and colleagues[52] have reported the successful use of MRI in 2 patients to visualize aortic valve vegetations and have suggested that this procedure may have particular utility in pediatric patients too small for the TEE scope. Five cases of perivalvular pseudoaneurysm were detected in another series with cardiac MRI, as compared to 2 detected by transthoracic echocardiography.

TEE was not performed in this series, however.[53] Single reports of detection of an aortic root abscess with fistula formation to the right ventricular outflow tract, of an aneurysm of the mitral- aortic intervalvular fibrosa and of a ventricular septal defect with ECG-gated imaging to add information about the flow jet have been published as well.[54–56] Like CT, MRI is a well-established imaging modality in the evaluation of central nervous system complications.

Cardiac Catheterization and Cineangiography

The utility and safety of cardiac catheterization with cineangiography in patients with IE have been debated. Catheterization has been used to aid in the identification of the infected valve(s) in both left- and right-sided endocarditis. In these instances, quantitative blood cultures are obtained from various cardiac chambers, from the great vessels and from peripheral sites, including the hepatic artery in cases where abdominal abscess is under consideration. A consistent increase in the number of organisms in culture is sought. Although this procedure has been used successfully to determine the infected valve,[57,58] false localization of the involved valve has been reported,[59] most likely because of spontaneous bacterial showers during the procedure. Catheterization can also provide information about the severity of valvular dysfunction and about left ventricular function. At times, catheterization can identify an involved valve when the clinical examination is unclear or can demonstrate myocardial involvement or fistula formation.[58,60] Finally, in patients who require surgery, angiography can define the coronary anatomy and allow determination of the need for concomitant coronary artery bypass grafting.

Many studies reporting the value of the clinical exam and noninvasive testing were performed before the advent of routine echocardiography on all patients. One study by Hosenpud and Greenberg[58] evaluated catheterization versus noninvasive assessment of patients with IE. Transthoracic echocardiography was performed in 14 of 19 patients studied. They found an equivalent sensitivity and specificity between noninvasive assessment and angiography in determining the site of valvular infection. Sensitivity was again identical in identifying myocardial invasion, however catheterization had an improved specificity (92% versus 100%). Finally, the clinical evaluation of left heart failure showed a 90% sensitivity and specificity. They concluded that catheterization had the greatest clinical utility in patients whose valvular involvement was uncertain or in whom the noninvasive assessment was ambiguous, but catheterization was not an absolute preoperative requirement. Since then, the routine use of TEE has undoubtedly increased the ability of the clinician to evaluate valvular and left ventricular function noninvasively.

The safety of cardiac catheterization has also been debated. Welton et al[61] evaluated the safety of catheterization during IE in 35 patients. Atrial fibrillation developed in one patient and there were no major complications. Other authors have reported respiratory and cardiac arrests,[58,60] pulmonary edema and brachial artery thrombosis, but such complications are infrequent. In general, infected valves should not be crossed if at all possible. Supravalvular injections of the aortic valve can often provide adequate information about valvular function and left ventricular function when aortic insufficiency is present. Overall, few patients suffer complications in experienced hands, and the feared complication of systemic emboli is extremely rare at worst.

Cardiac catheterization is a low risk procedure which can provide useful information to the clinician. In surgical candidates with a significant risk of atherosclerotic disease, coronary angiography is necessary if simultaneous bypass grafting is considered. In other patients, echocardiography and the clinical examination may provide adequate information for proper patient management, but in cases of ambiguity, catheterization can be considered. Because the procedure does carry some risks, it should not be performed routinely.

Diagnostic Criteria

In 1981 a series of diagnostic criteria for IE were proposed by von Reyn and colleagues[62] in an effort to aid in diagnosis and to provide a uniform population in studies of IE. The criteria were based on the characteristic features of IE described by Osler including predisposing valvular disease, bacteremia, embolic phenomena and evidence of an active endocardial process. Cases were rated as *definite, probable, possible* or *rejected* regarding the likelihood of IE (Table 1). Classification as *definite* required direct evidence of IE based on histology or bacteriology of valvular vegetations or peripheral emboli. As a result, the *definite* classification could be applied primarily to those patients who underwent surgery or died from their disease. The *probable* classification was reserved for individuals with (1) persistently positive blood cultures and either a new regurgitant murmur or predisposing heart disease and vascular phenomena; or (2) negative or intermittently positive cultures with fever, a new regurgitant murmur and vascular phenomena. Persistently positive blood cultures were defined as those positive in more than 70% of cases when more than 4 cultures were drawn or 100% positive when 2 or 3 cultures were drawn. The conditions fulfilling the criteria of vascular phenomena are listed in Table 1. Cases rated as *possible* fulfilled some but not all the criteria listed above. An exception was made for those individuals with streptococcal infections

Table 1
The Von Reyn Criteria, 1981[62]

Definite
Direct evidence of infective endocarditis based on histology from surgery or autopsy, or on bacteriology (Gram stain or culture) of valvular vegetation or peripheral embolus.

Probable
A. Persistently positive blood cultures[1] plus one of the following:
   1. New regurgitant murmur, or
   2. Predisposing heart disease[2] and vascular phenomena[3]
B. Negative or intermittently positive blood cultures[4] plus all three of the following:
   1. Fever
   2. New regurgitant murmur, and
   3. Vascular phenomena

Possible
A. Persistently positive blood cultures plus one of the following:
   1. Predisposing heart disease, or
   2. Vascular phenomena
B. Negative or intermittently positive blood cultures with all three of the following:
   1. Fever
   2. Predisposing heart disease, and
   3. Vascular phenomena
C. For viridans streptococcal cases only: at least two positive blood cultures without an extra-cardiac source, and fever.

Rejected
A. Endocarditis unlikely, alternate diagnosis generally apparent
B. Endocarditis likely, empiric antibiotic therapy warranted
C. Culture negative endocarditis diagnosed clinically, but excluded by postmortem

---

[1] At least two blood cultures obtained, with two of two positive, three of three positive, or at least 70% of cultures positive if four or more cultures obtained.
[2] Definite valvular or congenital heart disease, or a cardiac prosthesis (excluding permanent pacemakers).
[3] Petechiae, splinter hemorrhages, conjunctival hemorrhages, Roth spots, Osler's nodes, Janeway lesions, aseptic meningitis, glomerulonephritis, and pulmonary, central nervous system, coronary or peripheral emboli.
[4] Any rate of blood culture positivity that does not meet the definition of persistently positive.

in the viridans group due to the frequent association of this species with IE. In these cases patients with fever and 2 positive blood cultures without an extracardiac source were identified as *possible* cases of IE. Finally, cases were described as *rejected* if they fulfilled none of the criteria above.

Since publication of these criteria, both the clinical setting of IE and the use of noninvasive diagnostic testing for IE have evolved. Therefore, a modification of the von Reyn criteria known as the Duke criteria[63] was proposed in 1994 (Table 2). These criteria recognize that IE is now seen in patients without cardiac pathology often in the setting of IVDU, and have added IVDU as a predisposing condition. In addition, the utility of

---

Table 2
The Duke Criteria, 1994[63]

Definite
  Pathological criteria
    Microorganism: demonstrated by culture or histology in a vegetation, *or* in a vegetation that has embolized, *or* in an intracardiac abscess, *or*
    Pathological lesions: vegetation or intracardiac abscess present, confirmed by histology showing active endocarditis
  Clinical criteria, using specific definitions as listed
    2 major criteria, *or*
    1 major and 3 minor criteria, *or*
    5 minor criteria
Possible
  Findings consistent with infective endocarditis that fall short of *definite* but not *rejected*
Rejected
  Firm alternate diagnosis for manifestations of endocarditis, *or*
  Resolution of manifestations of endocarditis, with antibiotic therapy for 4 days or less, *or*
  No pathologic evidence of infective endocarditis at surgery or autopsy, after antibiotic therapy for 4 days or less

Definitions used in the Duke criteria
Major Criteria
  • Positive blood cultures for infective endocarditis
    —Typical microorganisms for IE from two separate blood cultures
      Viridans streptococci†, *Streptococcus bovis,* HACEK group, *or*
      Community-acquired *Staphylococcus aureus* or enterococci, in the absence of a primary focus, *or*
    —Persistently positive blood culture, defined as recovery of microorganisms consistent with IE from:
      (i) Blood cultures drawn more than 12 hours apart, *or*
      (ii) All of three or a majority of four or more separate blood cultures, with first and last drawn at least 1 hour apart
  • Evidence of endocardial involvement
    —Positive echocardiogram for IE
      (i) Oscillating intracardiac mass, on valve or supporting structures, *or* in the path of regurgitant jets, *or* on implanted material, in the absence of an alternative anatomic explanation, *or*
      (ii) Abscess, *or*
      (iii) New partial dehiscence of a prosthetic valve, *or*
    —New valvular regurgitation (increase or change in pre-existing murmur not sufficient)

(continued)

Table 2 *(continued)*

Minor Criteria
- Predisposition: predisposing heart condition or intravenous drug use
- Fever: ≥ 38.0°C (100.4°F)
- Vascular phenomena: major arterial emboli, septic pulmonary infarcts, mycotic aneurysm, intracranial hemorrhage, conjunctival hemorrhages, Janeway's lesions
- Immunologic phenomena: glomerulonephritis, Osler's nodes, Roth spots, rheumatoid factor
- Microbiological evidence: Positive blood culture but not meeting major criterion as noted previously* or serological evidence of active infection with organism consistent with IE
- Echocardiogram: consistent with IE but not meeting major criterion as noted previously

† including nutritional variant strains; * excluding single positive cultures for coagulase-negative staphylococci and organisms that do not cause endocarditis.

echocardiography in the diagnosis of IE has been added to the criteria and the importance of isolating organisms typically implicated in IE has been expanded. In the Duke classification, cases can be designated as *definite* using both pathological and clinical criteria, replacing the *probable* category created by von Reyn. Clinical findings are weighted as "major" or "minor" analogous to the Jones criteria for the diagnosis of rheumatic fever. According to the Duke system, major clinical criteria include (1) persistently positive blood cultures or 2 cultures of a typical organism as defined in Table 2; or (2) evidence of endocardial involvement as defined by echocardiographic findings or a new regurgitant murmur. Minor criteria include fever, predisposition, vascular phenomena, immunologic phenomena, microbiological evidence and echocardiographic findings. The latter 2 criteria include those findings which do not meet the definition of a major criterion. Cases with 2 major criteria, 1 major and 3 minor criteria or 5 minor criteria are classified as clinically *definite*. Cases are rejected if a firm alternate diagnosis has been made, if the manifestations consistent with IE resolve after 4 days or less of antibiotic therapy or if no pathological evidence of IE is present in cases treated with antibiotics for 4 days or less. All other cases are classified as *possible*.

Ten studies (including the original cohort) have been published comparing the von Reyn and Duke criteria[5,63-71] and one study has compared the Duke criteria to the clinical opinion of a panel of infectious disease specialists.[72] These studies are limited by the lack of a large "gold standard" group with pathologically confirmed infective endocarditis. Despite this, the sensitivity of the Duke criteria has been consistently greater than that of the von Reyn criteria. For example, Heiro et al[67] evaluated

243 patients with a clinical course suspicious for IE. Of these, 64 had a pathologically proven diagnosis. Forty-six of these patients (72%) were classified as *definite* by the Duke criteria based on clinical features only. The remaining 18 patients (28%) were classified as *possible* and none were *rejected*. In contrast, only 33 (51%) were classified as *probable* by the von Reyn criteria and 26 (41%) were *rejected*. In this subset of patients with a pathologically confirmed diagnosis, the Duke criteria had a sensitivity of 72% versus 52% for the von Reyn criteria. Of these patients, 75% fulfilled major echocardiographic criteria in the Duke classification. Of the entire 243 patients (including those with and without a pathological diagnosis), 114 (47%) were classified as *definite* using the Duke criteria compared to only 64 (26%) of patients using the von Reyn criteria. Only 37 (15%) were *rejected* using the Duke system versus 115 (47%) using the von Reyn criteria. No patients in this population admitted to intravenous drug use, a setting in which the Duke criteria are expected to be more sensitive. Similar results have been seen in populations with rates of IVDU as high as 50%.[64] Overall, the sensitivity of the Duke criteria has ranged from 71% to 100% in various series.[63–71]

These series demonstrate that the Duke criteria classify more patients as *definite* or *possible* than the von Reyn criteria classify as *definite*, *probable* or *possible*. This led to concern that the specificity of the Duke criteria may be low with a trend toward overdiagnosis based on false positive echocardiography results. Subsequently, other studies have evaluated either the specificity[68,69,72,73] or the negative predictive value[74] of the Duke criteria. The results suggest that the specificity ranges from 77% to 99%, although the highest specificity was identified in a population with a very low prior probability of IE. When compared, these rates are not significantly lower than rates achieved with the von Reyn criteria. Finally, Dodds et al[74] followed the initial cohort tested by Durack et al[63] and found the Duke criteria to have a negative predictive value of 92% to 98%.

The ability of these criteria to successfully identify patients with prosthetic valve endocarditis has been questioned. Two recent small studies have attempted to address this issue. Lamas et al[69] evaluated 118 patients with pathologically proven IE. Eighteen of these patients had prosthetic valve endocarditis. Of these, 50% were classified as *probable* using the von Reyn criteria and an identical number were classified as *definite* using the Duke criteria. They proposed modifying the Duke criteria to increase the sensitivity for prosthetic valve endocarditis by adding the following clinical and laboratory features to the list of minor criteria: newly diagnosed clubbing, splenomegaly, splinter hemorrhages, petechiae, an elevated ESR, an elevated C-reactive protein, microscopic hematuria, central non-feeding venous lines and peripheral venous lines. Using these criteria, 89% of patients with proven prosthetic valve endocarditis were classified as *definite* by the Duke criteria based on clinical features alone. In contrast, Nettles et al[70] evaluated 25 cases of pathologically confirmed prosthetic valve endocarditis. In this series, 19 (76%) were classified as *definite* using the Duke criteria as compared to 6 (24%) classified as *probable* in the von Reyn scheme when clinical parameters alone were considered. These results suggest that the Duke criteria are more sensitive than the von Reyn criteria in cases of prosthetic valve endocarditis. Clearly, larger series of patients with prosthetic valve endocarditis are required to adequately assess the Duke criteria in this setting as well as the proposed modifications.

In summary, the Duke criteria are more sensitive and appear to have equivalent specificity to the von Reyn criteria. The Duke criteria are especially useful in patients with culture-negative and right-sided endocarditis as well as endocarditis due to *S. aureus*.[75] These series have demonstrated that the advantage of the Duke criteria is closely related to the addition of echocardiographic criteria. One persistent criticism of the Duke criteria is related to the *possible* classification.[66,75] Patients classified as possible have insufficient objective data to be classified as having *definite* endocarditis but an alternate diagnosis has not been established. Therefore this classification group does not represent a group with a clear intermediate likelihood of having endocarditis, which leaves the implications for treatment confusing. Although these 2 classification schemes may aid in diagnosis, they were developed to create consistent populations for clinical studies. Overall, the Duke criteria represent a step forward in the classification of cases of suspected endocarditis and are certainly more relevant to current practice.

Summary

The clinical diagnosis of IE requires a multifaceted approach. Physical examination findings, microbiological results, laboratory testing and invasive and noninvasive imaging procedures all combine to aid in the diagnosis of IE. Technological advances are likely to add to these options in the future. The development of clinical criteria is important both clinically and for research purposes but requires periodic reassessment.

References

1. Scheld WM, Sande MA. Endocarditis and intravascular infections. In Mandell GL, Bennett JE, Dolin R (eds.) *Principles and Practice of Infectious Diseases.* New York, NY, Churchill Livingstone, 1995. pp 740–752.

2. Pankey GA. Subacute bacterial endocarditis at the University of Minnesota Hospital, 1939 through 1959. *Ann Intern Med* 1961;55:550–561.

3. Pankey GA. Acute bacterial endocarditis at the University of Minnesota Hospitals, 1939–1959. *Am Heart J* 1962;64:583–591.

4. Garvey GJ, Neu HC. Infective endocarditis–an evolving disease: A review of endocarditis at the Columbia-Presbyterian Medical Center, 1968–1973. *Medicine* 1978;57:105–127.

5. Sandre RM, Shafran SD. Infective endocarditis: Review of 135 cases over 9 years. *Clin Infect Dis* 1996;22:276–286.

6. Pelletier LL Jr, Petersdorf RG. Infective endocarditis: A review of 125 cases from the University of Washington Hospitals, 1963–72. *Medicine* 1977;56:287–313.

7. Watanakunakorn C, Burkert T. Infective endocarditis at a large community teaching hospital, 1980–1990. *Medicine* 1993;72:90–102.

8. Terpenning MS, Buggy BP, Kauffman CA. Infective endocarditis: Clinical features in young and elderly patients. *Am J Med* 1987;83:626–634.

9. Lederman MM, Sprague L, Wallis RS, et al. Duration of fever during treatment of infective endocarditis. *Medicine* 1992;71:52–57.

10. Blumberg EA, Robbins N, Adimora A, et al. Persistent fever in association with infective endocarditis. *Clin Infect Dis* 1992;15:983–990.

11. Hutter AM Jr, Moellering RC. Assessment of the patient with suspected endocarditis. *JAMA* 1976;235:1603–1605.

12. Weinstein L, Rubin RH. Infective endocarditis–1973. *Prog Cardiovasc Dis* 1973;16: 239–274.

13. Weinstein L, Brusch JL. *Infective Endocarditis*. New York, NY, Oxford University Press, 1996. pp 165–193.

14. Lerner PI, Weinstein L. Infective endocarditis in the antibiotic era. *N Engl J Med* 1966;274:199–206,259–266,323–331,388–393.

15. Weinstein L, Schlesinger JJ. Pathoanatomic, pathophysiologic and clinical correlations in endocarditis. *N Engl J Med* 1974;291:832–837,1122–1126.

16. Gross NJ, Tall R. Clinical significance of splinter haemorrhages. *Brit Med J* 1963;2:1496–1498.

17. Kilpatrick ZM, Greenberg PA, Sanford JP. Splinter hemorrhages: Their clinical significance. *Arch Intern Med* 1965;115:730–735.

18. Kerr A Jr, Tan JS. Biopsies of the Janeway lesion of infective endocarditis. *J Cutan Pathol* 1979;6:124–129.

19. Yee J, McAllister CK. Osler's nodes and the recognition of infective endocarditis: A lesion of diagnostic importance. *South Med J* 1987;80:753–757.

20. Alpert JS, Krous HF, Dalen JE, et al. Pathogenesis of Osler's nodes. *Ann Intern Med* 1976;85:471–473.

21. Rubenfeld S, Min K-W. Leukocytoclastic angiitis in subacute bacterial endocarditis. *Arch Dermatol* 1977;133:1073–1074.

22. Heffner JE. Extracardiac manifestations of bacterial endocarditis. *West J Med* 1979;131:85–91.

23. Falcone PM, Larrison WI. Roth spots seen on ophthalmoscopy: Diseases with which they may be associated. *Conn Med* 1995;59:271–273.

24. Kim JE, Han DP. Premacular hemorrhage as a sign of subacute bacterial endocarditis. *Am J Ophthalmol* 1995;120:250–251.

25. Beatty S, Harrison RJ, Roche P. Bilateral macular holes resulting from septic embolization. *Am J Ophthalmol* 1997;123:557–558.
26. Churchill MA, Geraci JE, Hunder GG. Musculoskeletal manifestations of bacterial endocarditis. *Ann Intern Med* 1977;87:754–759.
27. Hermans PE. The clinical manifestations of infective endocarditis. *Mayo Clin Proc* 1982;57:15–21.
28. Feinstein EI. Renal complications of bacterial endocarditis. *Am J Nephrol* 1985; 5:457–469.
29. Krause JR, Levison SP. Pathology of infective endocarditis. In Kaye D (ed.) *Infective Endocarditis*. Baltimore, MD, University Park Press, 1976. pp 55–86.
30. Sexauer WP, Quezado Z, Lippman ML, et al. Pleural effusions in right-sided endocarditis: Characteristics and pathophysiology. *South Med J* 1992;85: 1176–1180.
31. Haft JI. Computed tomography of the abdomen in the diagnosis of splenic emboli. *Arch Intern Med* 1988;148:193–197.
32. Ting W, Silverman, NA, Arzouman DA, et al. Splenic septic emboli in endocarditis. *Circulation* 1990;82 (Suppl IV):105–109.
33. Olaison L, Hogevik H, Alestig K. Fever, C-reactive protein, and other acute-phase reactants during treatment of infective endocarditis. *Arch Intern Med* 1997;157:885–892.
34. Sheagren JN, Tuazon CU, Griffin C, et al. Rheumatoid factor in acute bacterial endocarditis. *Arthritis Rheum* 1976;19:887–890.
35. Bayer AS, Theofilopoulos AN, Eisenberg R, et al. Circulating immune complexes in infective endocarditis. *N Engl J Med* 1976;295:1500–1505.
36. Karchmer AW. Infective endocarditis. In Eagle KA, Haber E, DeSanctis RW, et al (eds.) *The Practice of Cardiology*. Boston, MA, Little, Brown & Co., 1980. pp 833–862.
37. Werner AS, Cobbs CG, Kaye D, et al. Studies on the bacteremia of bacterial endocarditis. *JAMA* 1967;202:127–131.
38. Pesanti EL, Smith IM. Infective endocarditis with negative blood cultures: An analysis of 52 cases. *Am J Med* 1979;66:43–50.
39. Pazin GJ, Saul S, Thompson ME. Blood culture positivity: Suppression by outpatient antibiotic therapy in patients with bacterial endocarditis. *Arch Intern Med* 1982;142:263–268.
40. Tunkel AR, Kaye D. Endocarditis with negative blood cultures. *N Engl J Med* 1992;326:1215–1217.
41. O'Keefe JP, Gorbach SL. Laboratory diagnosis of infective endocarditis. In Rahimtoola SH (ed.) *Infective Endocarditis*. New York, NY, Grune and Stratton, 1978. pp 307–325.
42. Van Scoy RE. Culture-negative endocarditis. *Mayo Clin Proc* 1982;57:149–154.
43. Shapiro DS, Kenney SC, Johnson M. Brief report: Chlamydia psittaci endocarditis diagnosed by blood culture. *N Engl J Med* 1992;326:1192–1195.
44. Carpenter JL. Perivalvular extension of infection in patients with infectious endocarditis. *Rev Infect Dis* 1991;13:127–138.
45. Wiseman J, Rouleau J, Rigo P, et al. Gallium-67 myocardial imaging for the detection of bacterial endocarditis. *Radiology* 1976;120:135–138.
46. Morguet AJ, Munz DL, Ivancevic V, et al. Immunoscintigraphy using technetium- 99m-labeled anti-NCA-95 antigranulocyte antibodies as an adjunct to echocardiography in subacute infective endocarditis. *J Am Coll Cardiol* 1994; 23:1171–1178.

47. Sty JR, Boedecker RA. The advantage of 99m-technetium glucoheptonate imaging in acute bacterial endocarditis. *Wisc Med J* 1979;78:32–33.

48. Vagenakis AG, Abreau CM, Braverman LE. Splenic infarction diagnosed by photoscanning. *J Nucl Med* 1972;13:563–564.

49. Cowan JC, Patrick D, Reid DS. Aortic root abscess complicating bacterial endocarditis: Demonstration by computed tomography. *Br Heart J* 1984;52:591–593.

50. Chawla K, Ismailer I, Alexander LL. CT findings in renal ischemia and infarction. *Computerized Radiol* 1984;8:223–227.

51. Friedman SG, Pogo GJ, Moccio CG. Mycotic aneurysm of the superior mesenteric artery. *J Vasc Surg* 1987;6:87–90.

52. Caduff JH, Hernandez RJ, Ludomirsky A. MR visualization of aortic valve vegetations. *J Comput Assist Tomogr* 1996;20:613–615.

53. Akins EW, Slone RM, Wiechmann BN, et al. Perivalvular pseudoaneurysm complicating bacterial endocarditis: MR detection in five cases. *AJR* 1991;156:1155–1158.

54. Hwang SW, Yucel EK, Bernard S. Aortic root abscess with fistula formation. *Chest* 1997;111:1436–1438.

55. Schwartz DR, Belkin RN, Pucillo AL, et al. Aneurysm of the mitral-aortic intervalvular fibrosa complicating infective endocarditis. Preoperative characterization by two-dimensional and color flow Doppler echocardiography, magnetic resonance imaging, and cineangiography. *Am Heart J* 1990;119:196–199.

56. Spyridopoulos I, Helber U, Mewis C, et al. Tricuspid valve endocarditis due to a jet lesion detected by echocardiography in a 27-year-old man with congenital ventricular septal defect. *J Cardiovasc Surg* 1996;37:517–520.

57. Pazin GJ, Peterson KL, Griff FW, et al. Determination of site of infection in endocarditis. *Ann Intern Med* 1975;82:746–750.

58. Hosenpud JD, Greenberg BH. The preoperative evaluation in patients with endocarditis: Is cardiac catheterization necessary? *Chest* 1983;84:690–694.

59. Bennish M, Weinstein RA, Kabins SA, et al. False localization of site of endocarditis by cardiac catheterization with quantitative cultures. *Am J Clin Pathol* 1985;83:130–131.

60. Mills J, Abbott J, Utley JR, et al. Role of cardiac catheterization in infective endocarditis. *Chest* 1977;72:576–582.

61. Welton DE, Young JB, Raizner AE, et al. Value and safety of cardiac catheterization during active endocarditis. *Am J Cardiol* 1979;44:1306–1310.

62. Von Reyn CF, Levy BS, Arbeit RD, et al. Infective endocarditis: An analysis based on strict case definitions. *Ann Intern Med* 1981;94 (Part 1):505–518.

63. Durack DT, Lukes AS, Bright DK, et al. New criteria for diagnosis of infective endocarditis: Utilization of specific echocardiographic findings. *Am J Med* 1994;96:200–209.

64. Bayer AS, Ward JI, Ginzton LE, et al. Evaluation of new clinical criteria for the diagnosis of infective endocarditis. *Am J Med* 1994;96:211–219.

65. Hoen B, Selton-Suty C, Danchin N, et al. Evaluation of the Duke criteria versus the Beth Israel criteria for the diagnosis of infective endocarditis. *Clin Infect Dis* 1995;21: 905–909.

66. Olaison L, Hogevik H. Comparison of the von Reyn and Duke criteria for the diagnosis of infective endocarditis: A critical analysis of 161 episodes. *Scand J Infect Dis* 1996;28:399–406.

67. Hiero M, Nikoskelainen J, Hartiala JJ, et al. Diagnosis of infective endocarditis: Sensitivity of the Duke vs. von Reyn criteria. *Arch Intern Med* 1998;158:18–24.

68. Cecchi E, Parrini I, Chinaglia A, et al. New diagnostic criteria for infective endocarditis: A study of sensitivity and specificity. *Eur Heart J* 1997;18: 1149–1156.

69. Lamas CC, Eykyn SJ. Suggested modifications to the Duke criteria for the clinical diagnosis of native valve and prosthetic valve endocarditis: Analysis of 118 pathologically proven cases. *Clin Infect Dis* 1997;25:713–719.

70. Nettles RE, McCarty DE, Corey GR, et al. An evaluation of the Duke criteria in 25 pathologically confirmed cases of prosthetic valve endocarditis. *Clin Infect Dis* 1997;25: 1401–1403.

71. Del Pont JM, De Cicco LT, Vartalitis C, et al. Infective endocarditis in children: Clinical analyses and evaluation of two diagnostic criteria. *Pediatr Infect Dis J* 1995;14: 1079–1086.

72. Sekeres MA, Abrutyn E, Berlin JA, et al. An assessment of the usefulness of the Duke criteria for diagnosing active infective endocarditis. *Clin Infect Dis* 1997;24:1185–1190.

73. Hoen B, Béguinot I, Rabaud C, et al. The Duke criteria for diagnosing infective endocarditis are specific: Analysis of 100 patients with acute fever or fever of unknown origin. *Clin Infect Dis* 1996;23:298–302.

74. Dodds GA III, Sexton DJ, Durack DT, et al. Negative predictive value of the Duke criteria for infective endocarditis. *Am J Cardiol* 1996;77:403–407.

75. Bayer AS. Editorial: Diagnostic criteria for identifying cases of endocarditis: Revisiting the Duke criteria two years later. *Clin Infect Dis* 1996;23:303–304.

Chapter 6

Echocardiographic Diagnosis and Findings in Infective Endocarditis

David S. Bach, M.D.

Introduction

Echocardiographic imaging has assumed an increasingly important role in the past 2 decades in the assessment and management of patients with known or suspected infective endocarditis (IE). Valvular vegetations associated with infective endocarditis have been described using M-mode and, subsequently, two-dimensional echocardiographic imaging. The enhanced sensitivity of transesophageal echocardiography (TEE) aids detection of vegetations and allows reliable early recognition of complications of endocarditis including paravalvular abscess, aneurysm formation, fistula formation and leaflet destruction or perforation. As such, echocardiographic imaging has assumed a pivotal role in the assessment of the need for and timing of surgical intervention among patients with complications of endocarditis. Finally, accompanying its improved ability to detect and define cardiac pathology, echocardiography has become an important adjunct in the diagnosis of endocarditis, and echocardiographic findings are incorporated in current criteria for the clinical diagnosis of infective endocarditis. The present work describes the echocardiographic findings associated with infective endocarditis and its sequelae, the echocardiographic descriptors that may help define prognosis among patients with infective endocarditis, and the impact of echocardiography on the diagno-

From: Vlessis AA, Bolling S (eds): *Endocarditis: A Multidisciplinary Approach to Modern Treatment.* © Futura Publishing Co., Armonk, NY, 1999.

sis and management of patients with known or suspected infective endocarditis.

Echocardiographic Detection of Vegetations

Infective endocarditis is a disease in which infective organisms invade the endothelial lining of the heart, most commonly affecting the heart valves. On echocardiographic imaging, the pathological hallmark of endocarditis is the presence of one or more vegetations, irregular excrescences formed by the accumulation of infective organisms and surrounding tissue. Echocardiographic imaging is well suited to the interrogation of intracardiac structures, allowing the clinician to "see" vegetations that affect both valvular and nonvalvular structures. Echocardiography is the only noninvasive imaging method that allows the visualization of vegetations associated with endocarditis, and it is useful not only for the detection of vegetations but also for the assessment of the location and extent of infective involvement.

M-mode Echocardiography

Vegetations were first described in 1973 by Dillon using M-mode imaging as thick, shaggy echoes displaying rapid oscillations associated with normally moving valves.[1] This description attempts to differentiate the presence of a vegetation from other causes of valve thickening. Although many disease processes may result in focal or diffuse valvular thickening, the finding of a rapidly oscillating mass associated with an otherwise normal valve has a relatively high specificity for the identification of a vegetation. However, investigators also appreciated that some patients with clinical evidence of endocarditis had other more subtle echocardiographic abnormalities suggestive of valvular involvement that did not meet these criteria as diagnostic of vegetations.

Using M-mode echocardiography, the detection rate for valvular vegetations among patients with clinical evidence of endocarditis has been reported between 12% and 78%.[2-12] Although pathological confirmation of echocardiographically-detected vegetations was not available in many patients included in these studies, there appeared to be acceptably low rates of false positive and false negative echocardiographic findings among patients for whom surgical or autopsy confirmation was available, with high estimates of sensitivity for the detection of vegetations. However, pathological confirmation of the presence of a vegetation requires either surgery or autopsy, defining a group with potentially more fulminant or more advanced disease than in a general population of patients referred for echocardiographic evaluation of possible endocarditis. More extensive valvular involvement among these patients would be more reliably visualized on echocardiography compared with potentially more subtle findings among other patients with less advanced disease. In this regard, the early data supporting a high accuracy of M-mode echocardiography were likely biased toward the detection of vegetations among patients with more aggressive or more advanced forms of endocarditis.

Two-dimensional Imaging

Vegetations were first described on two-dimensional echocardiographic imaging in 1977 by Gilbert,[13] and many others have subsequently reported two-dimensional echocardiographic evidence of vegetations in patients with endocarditis.[3,7,8,10,12,14–16] The frequency with which vegetations were found using two-dimensional and M-mode echocardiographic imaging among patients with clinically suspected endocarditis in reports from the same time period is shown in Table 1. Compared to M-mode echocardiography, two-dimensional imaging has inherently superior spatial resolution. As demonstrated by the comparative studies in Table 1,[7,8,10,12] this results in an increased rate of detection of vegetations among patients with clinically suspected endocarditis. However, caution should again be used in evaluating the reported sensitivities of M-mode and two-dimensional echocardiography for the demonstration of vegetations. Not all patients with clinical endocarditis have discrete vegetations that are visible on echocardiographic imaging. In addition, not all detected vegetations are necessarily indicative of active infection. Because of the lack of pathological confirmation for most reports and the previously noted referral bias inherent to obtaining pathological confirmation, the absolute accuracy of two-dimensional echocardiography for the detection of vegetations is difficult to establish. However, the spatial resolution afforded by two-dimensional imaging clearly allows more thorough assessment of valvular anatomy and function.

On two-dimensional imaging, the echocardiographic characteristics of a vegetation are of a mass of echoes with rapid oscillation attached to or replacing normal valve tissue and with motion independent of other cardiac structures. As was noted in the M-mode echocardiographic description of a vegetation, demonstration of rapid independent oscillatory motion helps to differentiate vegetations from other forms of focal valvular thickening.

Vegetations typically occur on the low pressure aspect of a high veloc-

Table 1
Transthoracic Echocardiographic Detection of Vegetations on M-mode and Two-dimensional Imaging

Author	Year	Number of Patients	M-mode/2D Echo	Vegetations on Echocardiography	Number (%) of Patients Identified
Roy[2]	1976	32	M-mode	25 (7A, 12M, 3A + M)	22 (69%)
Wann[3]	1976	65	M-mode	22 (10A, 9M, 3T)	22 (32%)
Gilbert[13]	1977	7	2D	7 (4A, 1M, 2T)	7 (100%)
Minzt[4]	1979	32	M-mode	12 (12A)	12 (38%)
Wann[5]	1979	23	M-mode & 2D	19 (8A, 7M, 3T, 1Pr)	18 (78%)
Davis[6]	1980	30	M-mode	22 (8A, 4M, 5A + M)	17 (57%)
Martin[7]	1980	43	M-mode	13A, 10M, 7T, 12Pr, 1 other	5 (12%)
			2D		34 (79%)
Stewart[8]	1980	87	M-mode & 2D	51 (18A, 12M, 6T, 8A + M, 2M + T, 1A + M + T)	47 (54%)
Hickey[9]	1981	36	M-mode	24 (18A, 6M)	22 (61%)
Melvin[10]	1981	33	M-mode	16 (1A, 3M, 8T, 2P, 1A + T)	15 (45%)
			2D	28 (4A, 4M, 14T, 2P, 2A + T)	26 (79%)
Come[11]	1982	51	M-mode	23 (8A, 12M, 3T)	19 (37%)
Stafford[14]	1985	62	2D	45 (21A, 20M, 2T, 2 other)	45 (73%)
Buda[15]	1986	50	2D	10A, 8M, 3T	21 (42%)
Lutas[12]	1986	77	M-mode	45 (22A, 17M, 2T, 2A + M);	35 (45%)
			2D	[4Pr nos]	43 (56%)
Jaffe[16]	1990	70	2D	70 (28A, 16M, 16T, 1P, 3A + M, 3 other); [4Pr nos]	54 (76%)

M-mode = M-mode echocardiography; 2D = two-dimensional echocardiography; A = aortic valve; M = mitral valve; T = tricuspid valve; P = pulmonic; Pr = prosthetic valve; other = nonvalvular; nos = not otherwise specified.

ity, turbulent jet. Therefore, vegetations typically are seen on the left atrial aspect of the mitral valve in patients with mitral regurgitation and on the left ventricular aspect of the aortic valve in patients with aortic regurgitation. Similarly, right-sided endocarditis typically involves vegetations on the right atrial aspect of the tricuspid valve, with less common involvement of the pulmonic valve. An example of a tricuspid valve vegetation on two-dimensional echocardiographic imaging is shown in Figure 1. This demonstrates the typical soft tissue density appearance of an active vegetation and a typical location on the low pressure aspect of an atrio-ventricular valve.

Vegetations are not limited to the heart valves, but may occur at any site of intracardiac endothelium. Nonvalvular locations of vegetations typically involve either the low pressure aspect of a shunt or the site of impact of a turbulent or high velocity jet. For example, in a patient with ventricular septal defect and left-to-right shunt, a vegetation may occur on the right ventricular endocardium either adjacent to the septal defect or on the right ventricular free wall at the site of impact of the jet created

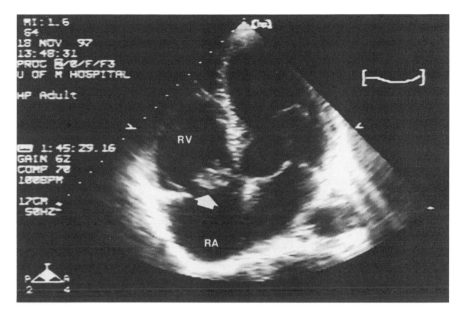

Figure 1. Apical four-chamber view demonstrating large tricuspid valve vegetation. Approximately 1 cm × 2 cm soft-tissue density mass is attached to right atrial aspect of septal leaflet of tricuspid valve (arrow). RA = right atrium; RV = right ventricle.

by the defect. Similarly, the presence of mitral regurgitation creates a high velocity jet that may impact the left atrial wall and create a nidus for vegetation formation. The presence of aortic regurgitation similarly creates a high velocity jet that may impact the endothelium of the left ventricular outflow tract, mitral valve, mitral chordae or papillary muscles, similarly creating sites for potential seeding of infection and growth of vegetations.

In addition to its greater ability to detect vegetations, the superior spatial resolution afforded by two-dimensional echocardiographic imaging offers an improved ability to characterize the size, location and morphology of vegetations. Such characteristics, available only from two-dimensional imaging, may be useful in assessment of prognosis. As will be discussed subsequently, several investigators have described relationships between vegetation size, risk of embolization and need for surgery.

Doppler Imaging

One of the hallmarks of any infective process is tissue destruction. Although different pathological organisms have specific characteristics with respect to rate of growth, vegetation size and accompanying valvular destruction, some amount of tissue destruction typically accompanies IE. Along with advances in the quality and resolution of echocardiographic imaging, modern echocardiographic equipment allows Doppler interrogation for evidence of regurgitation or shunt. Because of a high sensitivity for the detection and characterization of regurgitant lesions, Doppler imaging can provide important information in patients with known or suspected endocarditis.

In some patients, the presence or absence of regurgitation can help in the assessment of a focal valvular excrescence, and specifically helps to determine whether a focal thickening is likely representative of a vegetation. Infective endocarditis resulting in growth of a valvular vegetation typically is accompanied by some amount of tissue destruction and detectable regurgitation. The converse is also true, and the absence of regurgitation in the setting of focal valvular thickening suggests a diagnosis other than active endocarditis.

Imaging constraints may preclude the detection of small vegetations in some patients, particularly on transthoracic imaging. Although small vegetations may not be visible, the presence of regurgitation may suggest tissue destruction and is a sensitive finding for endocarditis.[16] However, regurgitation on echocardiographic Doppler imaging is a common and nonspecific finding. The presence of valvular regurgitation alone does not prove the diagnosis of endocarditis, although the absence of regurgitation makes the diagnosis of endocarditis less likely.

When present, regurgitation can be quantified with respect to severity. In addition, the characteristics of a regurgitant jet can provide ancillary evidence to support a diagnosis of endocarditis. Although not pathognomonic of endocarditis, an eccentric regurgitant jet reflects abnormal underlying anatomy and is suggestive of possible leaflet perforation or paravalvular fistula formation. The presence of a central noneccentric regurgitant jet does not exclude the diagnosis of endocarditis, but the finding of an eccentric regurgitant jet accompanying a focal valvular thickening may help support a diagnosis of IE.

Transesophageal Imaging

Transthoracic echocardiography is limited in its ability to penetrate sufficiently to allow reproducible imaging of posterior cardiac structures and in its ability to resolve fine anatomic detail. Imaging constraints due to poor transmission of ultrasound by lung and bone limit the acoustic windows through which transthoracic echocardiography can be performed to predominantly anterior locations in the parasternal, apical and subcostal regions. In addition, the lower-frequency transducers necessary for ultrasound penetration are limited in resolution and therefore in the ability to distinguish detail. Because of the posterior location of the heart valves, transthoracic imaging has accompanying limitations in its ability to define valvular anatomy and pathology and in detecting valvular vegetations.

Transesophageal echocardiography removes most imaging constraints associated with transthoracic imaging. From within the esophagus, transesophageal imaging is not affected by the poor ultrasound transmission characteristics associated with lung and rib. The position of the ultrasound transducer in close proximity to the posterior cardiac structures obviates the need for deep penetration of ultrasound and permits the use of higher-frequency transducers that allow greater image resolution and therefore superior discrimination of fine detail. For these reasons, transesophageal echocardiography is especially useful in the evaluation of valvular heart disease, including the evaluation of patients with known or suspected endocarditis.

Several reports have described the use of transesophageal echocardiography for the detection of vegetations associated with infective endocarditis.[17-25] A number of early reports in which transesophageal imaging was compared with transthoracic echocardiography for the detection of vegetations are summarized in Table 2. All the investigators concluded that transesophageal echocardiography has a higher test sensitivity for the detection of vegetations, with rates of detection ranging from 48% to 100% for transesophageal echocardiography compared with 18% to 63% for transthoracic imaging.[17-25] Several authors noted that image quality was the greatest factor favoring the detection of vegetations with trans-

Table 2
Transesophageal Versus Transthoracic Echocardiographic Detection of Vegetations

Author	Year	Sensitivity		Specificity	
		TTE (%)	TEE (%)	TTE (%)	TEE (%)
Drexler[17]	1987	27/96 (28%)	46/96 (48%)	n/a	n/a
Daniel[18]	1987	33/82 (40%)*	77/82 (94%)*	n/a	n/a
Erbel[19]	1988	12/19 (63%)	19/19 (100%)	1/1 (100%)	0/1 (0%)
Taams[20]	1990	6/33 (18%)	23/33 (70%)	n/a	n/a
Shively[21]	1991	7/16 (44%)	15/16 (94%)	49/50 (98%)	50/50 (100%)
Birmingham[22]	1992	10/33 (30%)	29/33 (88%)	30/30 (100%)	29/30 (97%)
Daniel[23]	1993	12/33 (36%)	27/33 (82%)	n/a	n/a
Shapiro[24]	1994	18/30 (60%)	26/30 (87%)	31/34 (91%)	31/34 (91%)
Chirillo[25]	1995	48/84 (57%)*	76/84 (90%)*	82/92 (89%)*	70/92 (76%)*

TTE = transthoracic echocardiography; TEE = transesophageal echocardiography; n/a = not available.
* Data reported by valve rather than by patient.

esophageal imaging.[21,22] One investigator noted that the mitral and aortic valves were visualized with average or better than average quality in 100% and 96% of transesophageal echocardiograms, respectively, compared with 89% and 68% of transthoracic echocardiograms.[21] Similarly, another author found that 69% of transthoracic echocardiograms were of good or excellent quality compared with 95% of transesophageal studies, whereas 11% of transthoracic studies were of poor quality compared with no transesophageal studies.[22] Figure 2 demonstrates paired images from

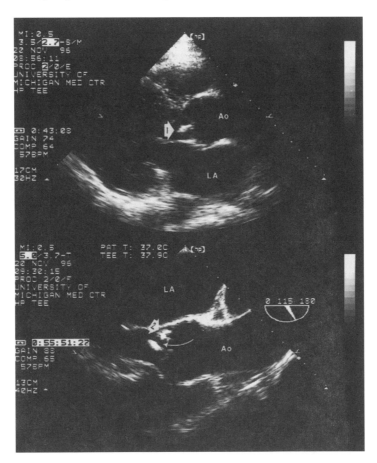

Figure 2. Paired images from transthoracic (top panel) and transesophageal (bottom panel) echocardiograms in patient with aortic valve endocarditis. Vegetation is demonstrated on left ventricular aspect of aortic valve on transthoracic imaging (arrow [1]). Transesophageal imaging demonstrates second, smaller vegetation (arrow [2]) and area of echo dropout suggestive of leaflet perforation (curved arrow) in addition to larger vegetation seen on transthoracic imaging. Ao = ascending aorta; LA = left atrium.

transthoracic and transesophageal echocardiograms in a patient with aortic valve endocarditis. Although a vegetation is visible on transthoracic imaging, a second vegetation and evidence of valve perforation are demonstrated only by transesophageal imaging.

The superior image quality of transesophageal echocardiography is probably responsible for the ability to detect smaller lesions than those detectable by transthoracic echocardiography. In 2 studies, small vegetations were more reliably detected using transesophageal echocardiography than with transthoracic imaging.[17,19] Equal numbers of vegetations greater than 11 mm in size were detected using transesophageal and transthoracic imaging. However, transesophageal imaging was able to demonstrate 24 vegetations less than 5 mm in size whereas transthoracic imaging was able to demonstrate only 6. Similarly, other investigators found that transesophageal echocardiography more reliably allowed detection of vegetations less than 1 cm in size, with only 5 of 12 vegetations less than 1 cm demonstrated using transthoracic imaging.[24] A small mitral valve vegetation on transesophageal imaging is demonstrated in Figure 3. The vegetation, which measures approximately 5 mm $\times$ 8 mm, was not visible on transthoracic imaging.

Vegetation location may also have an impact on the ability to image lesions transesophageally rather than transthoracically. Several investigators found a higher rate of success for detection of vegetations associated with the aortic valve using transesophageal compared with transthoracic imaging.[17,19,21,22] In these studies, rates of detection of aortic valve vegetations with transesophageal imaging ranged from 1.9 to 3.5 times those with transthoracic echocardiography. Similarly, vegetations associated with the mitral valve tended to be more reliably visualized using transesophageal imaging. However, the differences were not as great as those for the aortic valve, with rates of detection with transesophageal echocardiography ranging from 1.3 to 2.0 times those with transthoracic imaging. Investigation of the relative benefits of transesophageal echocardiography for the detection of right-sided vegetations has been limited by a relatively low incidence of tricuspid and pulmonic vegetations in the populations studied.[17,19,21,22,24,26,27] However, most studies found that right-sided lesions were more reliably detected using transesophageal imaging. Indwelling pacemaker catheters and prosthetic heart valves represent special diagnostic challenges for the detection of vegetations. However, transesophageal echocardiography has clear advantages for detection of vegetations associated with such intracardiac devices.[19,20,23] Finally, paravalvular involvement by the infective process can be far more reliably detected using transesophageal imaging.[18,23]

Biplane and multiplane transducers have further enhanced the utility of transesophageal echocardiographic imaging. Several studies have eval-

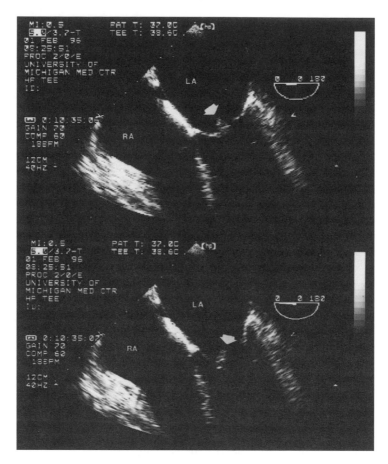

Figure 3. Transesophageal echocardiogram demonstrating small mitral valve vegetation (arrows) in systole (top panel) and diastole (bottom panel). Vegetation measures approximately 5 mm × 8 mm and was not visible on transthoracic imaging. Vegetation demonstrates typical features including soft-tissue density, location on low-pressure (left atrial) aspect of valve and high frequency oscillatory motion evident in real-time imaging. LA = left atrium; RA = right atrium.

uated the use of single plane, biplane and multiplane transesophageal echocardiography in the evaluation of patients with endocarditis.[28–30] Biplane and multiplane imaging were found to be superior to monoplane imaging for the detection of vegetations.[29] In addition, probes using multiple imaging planes were found to allow better definition of vegetation size and characteristics,[28,29] as well as allowing substantially improved description of related tissue destruction and paravalvular complications of infection.[29,30] Finally , there is typically operator preference for the use of biplane and multiplane probes in the evaluation of the complex lesions associated with endocarditis. The complex nature of tissue destruction and alteration of normal tissue planes that may occur with endocarditis are typically more easily interrogated with the additional imaging flexibility afforded by biplane and multiplane probes.

Special Imaging Considerations

Several conditions require special consideration in the use of echocardiography for the detection of vegetations in patients with known or suspected endocarditis. Such conditions include the echocardiographic assessment of prosthetic valve endocarditis, assessment for nonvalvular vegetations, and the recognition of noninfected focal valve lesions.

Prosthetic Valves

Prosthetic valve endocarditis presents a special diagnostic challenge, both because of increased risks for patients and because of limitations in echocardiographic imaging. Patients with prosthetic valves are at increased risk of developing infective endocarditis, and treatment of the infection is more difficult in the presence of prosthetic material. Compared with patients in whom endocarditis affects native valves, patients with prosthetic valve endocarditis are at increased risk of suffering major complications, including the need for surgical intervention and the risk of increased mortality.

Echocardiographic imaging is limited among patients with prosthetic heart valves, and resolution of fine detail of the prosthetic material and the immediately surrounding tissues may be especially challenging. The prosthetic materials associated with valve sewing rings, occluders and struts prohibit penetration of ultrasound, resulting in strong acoustic shadowing which precludes imaging of structures distal to the prosthetic material. In addition, the strong echo- reflectivity of the prosthetic materials results in reverberation artifact, limiting the ability to differentiate small vegetations from normal prosthetic valve echoes. In practical terms, the combination of acoustic shadowing and reverberation artifact results in a limited ability to detect vegetations associated with prosthetic valves and at times to distinguish normal from abnormal paravalvular anatomy.

Superior image resolution with transesophageal echocardiography makes it clearly superior to transthoracic imaging for the detection of vegetations and paravalvular complications associated with prosthetic valve endocarditis.[23,31–33] The greatest difference of transesophageal compared with transthoracic imaging is in the assessment of mechanical valves, including both disk-type and ball and cage prostheses. In one study, investigators demonstrated an increase in sensitivity from 22% to 83% using transesophageal imaging for the detection of vegetations associated with mechanical valve prostheses.[23] Other investigators have confirmed the finding that absence of a visible vegetation associated with a mechanical prosthesis on transthoracic echocardiography has poor predictive power, and that transesophageal echocardiography may allow detection of vegetations despite a normal transthoracic examination.[31–33] Figures 4 and 5 demonstrate examples of endocarditis affecting prosthetic valves. In Figure 4, a vegetation associated with a mechanical mitral valve prosthesis is shown on transesophageal imaging. Figure 5 demonstrates partial dehiscence of a composite aortic valve and aortic root graft due to endocarditis.

In addition to an impaired ability to detect vegetations, transthoracic echocardiography is limited in its ability to demonstrate prosthetic mitral regurgitation in the setting of mechanical prostheses. Because of acoustic shadowing associated with a mechanical prosthesis, the left atrium remains at least partially shielded from view in all transthoracic windows. Although mitral regurgitation may be evident on transthoracic imaging,

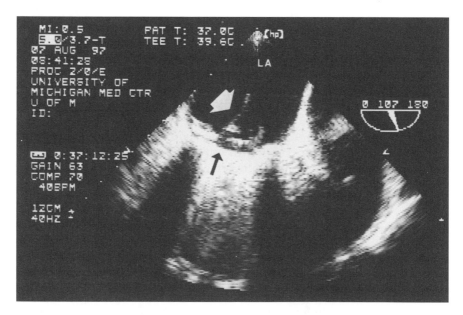

Figure 4. Vegetation (white arrow) on left atrial aspect of mechanical mitral valve prosthesis on transesophageal imaging. Acoustic shadowing from prosthetic disk (black arrow) precluded detection of vegetation on transthoracic echocardiography. LA = left atrium.

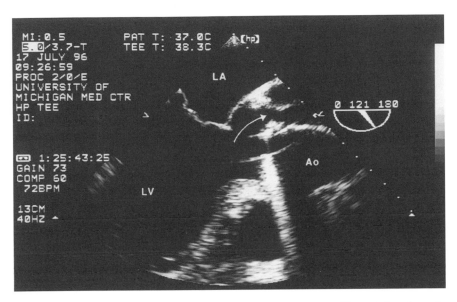

Figure 5. Partial dehiscence (curved arrow) of composite aortic valve and aortic root on transesophageal echocardiography. Although aortic regurgitation was evident on transthoracic echocardiography, transesophageal imaging was necessary to demonstrate anatomy of dehiscence of prosthetic root. Ao = ascending aorta; LA = left atrium; LV = left ventricle.

complete evaluation for mitral regurgitation in a patient with a mechanical mitral prosthesis requires transesophageal imaging.[32,33] In contrast to mitral regurgitation, aortic regurgitation can usually be assessed adequately from transthoracic windows despite the presence of a mechanical prosthesis.[33] In the case of aortic insufficiency, the regurgitant jet enters the left ventricle, which is not shadowed by the prosthetic valve.

Because bioprosthetic valves have less prosthetic material than mechanical valves, there is typically less acoustic shadowing and less reverberation artifact. Although transesophageal echocardiography has a higher sensitivity than transthoracic imaging for the detection of vegetations associated with bioprosthetic aortic and mitral valves, the differences are not as pronounced as with mechanical prostheses.[23,33]

The same problem of acoustic shadowing that affects transthoracic echocardiography similarly affects transesophageal imaging. Although transesophageal echocardiography allows superior image resolution compared to transthoracic imaging, it allows interrogation of only the posterior aspect of mechanical prostheses inasmuch as transthoracic echocardiography allows visualization of only the anterior surfaces. Reliance solely on transesophageal imaging can lead to false negative examinations if vegetations are located on the left ventricular aspect of a mechanical prosthesis.[34] In addition, the most accurate Doppler interrogation of transvalvular gradients is available from transthoracic windows; an otherwise unexplained increase in transvalvular gradients can suggest mechanical valvular obstruction, possibly due to a vegetative mass. Because of these limitations, transthoracic and transesophageal imaging should be viewed as complementary in the interrogation of prosthetic valve anatomy and function. Combined transthoracic and transesophageal examinations should be performed in any patient with a question of prosthetic valve dysfunction, including assessment for possible prosthetic valve endocarditis.

Nonvalvular Vegetations

Infective endocarditis may occur on any endothelial surface, and although valves are the most common site of infection, vegetations may occur in other intracardiac locations. Nonvalvular vegetations are frequently demonstrable on echocardiographic imaging. In patients with known or suspected endocarditis, the echocardiographic examination should not be limited to assessment of valvular anatomy and function, but should also include interrogation for evidence of vegetations involving nonvalvular surfaces including atrial and ventricular endothelium.

Patients with ventricular septal defect are at risk of developing infective endocarditis with nonvalvular vegetations. As with valvular lesions, the low pressure aspect of the ventricular septal defect may serve as a nidus for infection. In addition, damaged endothelium resulting from the impact of a high velocity jet may create a site predisposed to vegetation formation, typically on tricuspid chordae or the right ventricular free wall in the presence of a left-to-right shunt. Echocardiographic imaging is useful for the detection of nonvalvular vegetations, and has been used to describe vegetations located on the right ventricular free wall,[35] the Eustachian valve[36] and the left ventricular endocardium.[37,38]

Noninfective Valve Lesions

Not all mass lesions associated with a heart valve are infective in etiology. Sterile vegetations may be seen in association with the mitral and aortic valves in collagen vascular diseases such as systemic lupus erythematosis or primary antiphospholipid syndrome.[39,40] Nonbacterial thrombotic endocarditis may be seen in patients with underlying malignancy and less often in patients with acute septicemia or burns.[41] In addition, primary cardiac tumors including myxoma, lipoma and papillary fibroelastoma may mimic valvular vegetations.[39] Typically, there are no echocardiographic features of noninfective lesions that can be used to reliably differentiate them from infective vegetations, although the absence of valve destruction may suggest a noninfective process. Clinical history is often the most helpful in differentiating infective from noninfective lesions. The incidental finding of a focal valve mass is not likely to represent an infective lesion in an afebrile patient in whom infective endocarditis was not previously considered.

Improvements in echocardiographic imaging and the use of transesophageal echocardiography have led to an increased ability to detect small focal valve lesions. Often noted as an incidental finding, focal thickening of one or more valves may be seen in a large number of patients, and is neither of presumed infective origin nor indicative of underlying infective endocarditis. However, a similar finding of focal valvular thickening may take on greater significance in patients in whom echocardiography is performed to evaluate for signs of possible endocarditis. It is of obvious importance to distinguish incidental findings of focal valvular thickening from findings suggestive of a vegetation and underlying infective endocarditis. In one study, investigators evaluated the power of 12 diagnostic criteria on transesophageal echocardiography for sensitivity and specificity in the diagnosis of vegetations.[25] Among the criteria tested, chaotic motion was the variable most strongly associated with presence of a vegetation. The coexistence of chaotic motion, size less than 0.5 cm and uneven margins had a sensitivity of 93.3% and a specificity of 83.7% for the detection of vegetations. Other investigators have described a rapid independent oscillatory motion characteristic of infective vegetations.[42] Although focal valve lesions that lack the described rapid oscillatory motion may represent a vegetation, the absence of this finding carries a lower specificity for the diagnosis of infective endocarditis. In general, the diagnosis of a visualized mass as a vegetation will carry a higher specificity if the mass appears to be attached to an endocardial surface, is seen consistently throughout the cardiac cycle, is apparent in multiple views and displays oscillatory motion that is independent of other cardiac structures.[16]

Complications of Endocarditis

Infective endocarditis can result in complications including paravalvular abscess, aneurysm formation, fistula formation between cardiac chambers and advanced tissue destruction or leaflet perforation. Echocardiographic imaging can play a pivotal role in the detection and treatment of complications of endocarditis. Some findings such as paravalvular abscess may dictate the need for surgical intervention. Others, such as fistula formation with shunt or leaflet destruction with valve regurgitation, may have an impact on short-term therapy for hemodynamic support. Early echocardiographic detection of the complications of endocarditis contributes to the ability to individualize therapy, potentially preventing more advanced tissue destruction. Detailed anatomic information afforded by transesophageal imaging allows optimal planning in the surgical correction of mechanical complications of endocarditis.

Paravalvular Abscess

Extension of the infective process into tissues adjacent to an involved valve may result in development of a paravalvular abscess. The limited vascular supply to tissues that form the fibrous skeleton of the heart results in specific locations where an abscess most readily forms. The most frequent locations for abscess formation are in the aortic valve annulus and in the mitral-aortic intervalvular fibrosa, located at the junction of the aortic root and the anterior mitral annulus. In addition, paravalvular abscesses may occur adjacent to the mitral valve, in other paravalvular locations, or, more rarely, within the myocardium. A paravalvular abscess cavity is most often confined to the region immediately adjacent to the valve. However, the abscess cavity may also extend into other cardiac structures. Paravalvular abscesses originating in the aortic root are known to extend into the interventricular septum, the right ventricular outflow tract, the interatrial septum and the anterior mitral valve. Ideally, identification of not only the presence but also the location and extent of a paravalvular abscess can influence surgical intervention.

On echocardiographic imaging, a paravalvular abscess appears as an echo-free space adjacent to an involved valve. The space may appear entirely free of echoes, implying complete liquefaction of the contents, or there may be inhomogeneity within the space, with a faint distribution of echoes indicative of contained necrotic material. In addition to the characteristic echolucency, an abscess cavity is further distinguished by exclusion of flow. Because the abscess represents a closed space, its contents are isolated from the surrounding blood flow and there should be no evidence of pulsatile flow within the cavity. This is best demonstrated on color flow Doppler imaging with Nyquist limits set to relatively low velocities.

Paravalvular abscesses have been described on transthoracic echocardiographic imaging.[43–50] However, both their number and extent are underestimated.[45,47] In one report,[47] only 1 of 22 patients with an abscess identified at surgery was identified using preoperative two-dimensional transthoracic imaging. However, other findings on transthoracic imaging have been found to improve the positive and negative predictive values for the detection of large abscesses. In one such study, investigators found that a rocking motion of a valve prosthesis, presence of a sinus of Valsalva aneurysm, thickening of the anterior or posterior aortic root greater than or equal to 10 mm or a paravalvular echo-density within the interventricular septum that measures greater than or equal to 14 mm are predictors of abscess formation among patients requiring surgery for infective endocarditis.[47] However, it should be noted that predictors such as these may apply selectively to patients who are already candidates for surgery and therefore presumably have advanced infective lesions; the same criteria are not predictive of smaller abscesses occurring in patients with less advanced disease.

Because of the posterior location and potentially small size of abscesses, the sensitivity for detection with transthoracic echocardiography is relatively low.[46,47,51,52] However, the imaging advantages afforded by transesophageal echocardiography dramatically improve diagnostic accuracy. A number of studies have demonstrated the superior diagnostic accuracy of transesophageal imaging for the detection of paravalvular abscesses.[51–53] The advantages of transesophageal imaging are especially important in the evaluation for abscess complicating prosthetic valve endocarditis.[51] Reverberation artifact and acoustic shadowing associated with mechanical prostheses make detection of paraprosthetic abscesses extremely difficult on transthoracic imaging. From a clinical perspective, transthoracic imaging may be useful in the evaluation of paravalvular abscess only if there is demonstration of an abscess cavity. An abscess cannot be safely excluded without transesophageal imaging.

Figures 6, 7, and 8 show 3 examples on transesophageal echocardiography of paravalvular abscesses complicating aortic valve endocarditis. Figure 6 demonstrates a small paravalvular abscess complicating native aortic valve endocarditis. Figure 7 demonstrates a larger abscess complicating prosthetic aortic valve endocarditis. Figure 8 shows an example of atypical extension of the paravalvular abscess into the interventricular septum.

Abscess formation represents one stage in a continuum in which an infective process extends to structures adjacent to an infected valve. In earlier stages, echocardiography may demonstrate only thickening and edema of soft tissue structures in an area of infective involvement, with no discrete central clear space. Following necrosis of tissues in the involved region that may occur over the course of a few days, echocardiography demonstrates the typical findings of an echo-free space that are diagnostic of an abscess. Subsequently, the infective process may lead to perforation of one or more walls of the abscess cavity with formation of an

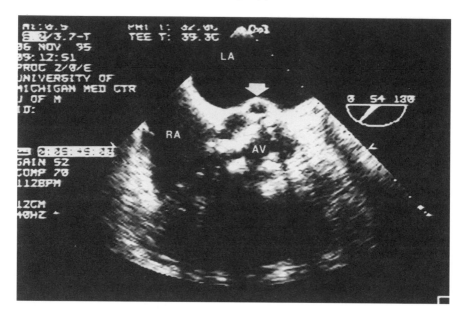

Figure 6. Small paravalvular abscess (arrow) complicating native aortic valve endocarditis on transesophageal echocardiography. Aortic valve is heavily calcified. AV = aortic valve; LA = left atrium; RA = right atrium.

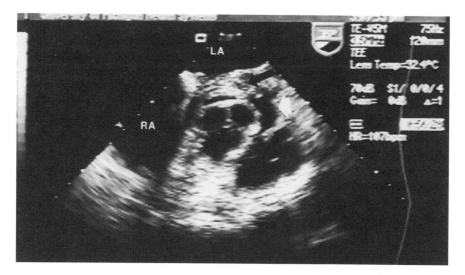

Figure 7. Transesophageal echocardiography demonstrating large paravalvular abscess complicating stentless tissue prosthetic aortic valve endocarditis. In addition to echolucent abscess cavity (white arrow), there is paravalvular soft tissue density (black arrow) representing edema and inflammation prior to necrosis and liquefaction. LA = left atrium; RA = right atrium.

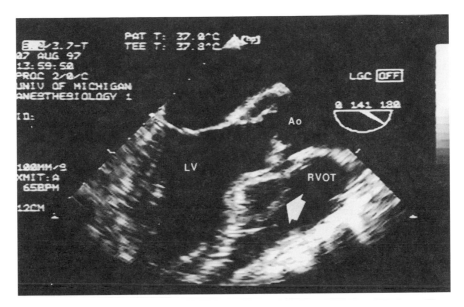

Figure 8. Paravalvular abscess (arrow) extending from aortic valve into interventricular septum on transesophageal echocardiography. Ao = ascending aorta; LV = left ventricle; RVOT — right ventricular outflow tract.

aneurysm or a fistula communicating between adjacent cardiac chambers. Serial echocardiographic studies may be needed to follow the infective process and its response to therapy.

Aneurysm Formation

Infective endocarditis involving the aortic valve can result in secondary involvement of subaortic structures, mediated either by direct extension or by an aortic regurgitation jet seeding secondary sites of impact.[54,55] In either instance, the anterior mitral leaflet or the mitral-aortic intervalvular fibrosa are especially prone to secondary involvement. Once seeding of an area has occurred, there is a continuum of pathological processes that may be observed. The earliest evidence of secondary infection may be vegetation growth or abscess formation. Because of high pulsatile pressures to which an abscess may be exposed, abscesses that occur in proximity to either the left ventricle or the aorta may expand and form an aneurysm or may rupture into an adjacent chamber with subsequent fistula formation.[54–59]

On echocardiography, aneurysm formation of the mitral-aortic intervalvular fibrosa is seen as an echo-free space bounded by thin tissue typically near the base of the anterior mitral leaflet and extending into the left atrium.[54,56,57] Because of the high pulsatile pressures generated by the left ventricle, the aneurysm typically expands into the left atrium during systole with subsequent diastolic collapse.[54] In addition, an aneurysm may occur within the body of the anterior mitral leaflet.[54,58,59] Similar to an aneurysm located in the intervalvular fibrosa, an aneurysm of the mitral leaflet typically demonstrates systolic expansion into the left atrium with subsequent diastolic collapse. It may be difficult to distinguish between an aneurysm that originates from the intervalvular fibrosa and one that originates from the base of the anterior mitral leaflet. Although tissue planes may be distinct on surgical inspection, the two locations are only millimeters apart, and both aneurysms demonstrate pulsatile extension into the left atrium. Aneurysms within the body of the mitral leaflet may be more readily identified by the location farther within the anterior mitral leaflet body and more distant from the intervalvular fibrosa.

In addition to aneurysms of the intervalvular fibrosa and of the anterior mitral valve leaflet, acquired aneurysms of the sinuses of Valsalva may occur as a complication of aortic valve endocarditis. Detectable on echocardiographic imaging, a sinus of Valsalva aneurysm may occur in any of the 3 aortic sinuses.[60] Although most congenital aneurysms of the aortic sinuses tend to extend into the right atrium or right ventricle, acquired sinus of Valsalva aneurysms complicating infective endocarditis may expand and rupture into the right atrium, right ventricle, left atrium, or an extracardiac space.

Leaflet Perforation and Fistula Formation

Tissue destruction associated with infective endocarditis may cause leaflet destruction with perforation or fistula formation. Perforation and fistula formation are presumably mediated by continued weakening of the affected tissues due to the infective process accompanied by continued exposure to high intracardiac pressures, ultimately leading to loss of tissue integrity.

Echocardiography and Doppler imaging are excellent methods of detecting and localizing tissue perforation and fistula formation. Rupture of an aneurysm of the mitral-aortic intervalvular fibrosa into the left atrium can be detected as systolic shunting of blood from the left ventricular outflow tract into the left atrium. Although rupture of an aneurysm of the intervalvular fibrosa results in a clinical picture identical to mitral regurgitation, echocardiographic/Doppler imaging can demonstrate high velocity flow from the left ventricle to the left atrium above the level of the mitral annulus, also termed "supra-annular mitral regurgitation."[54,61]

Similarly, perforation of the anterior mitral leaflet results in a high velocity turbulent systolic jet with flow from the left ventricle to the left atrium.[54,55,58,62–64] Although mitral regurgitation may have many potential etiologies, mitral regurgitation associated with leaflet perforation may be eccentric[54] and typically is characterized by a jet with an atypical origin distinct from the coaptation zone of the mitral leaflets.[62–64] Examples of anterior mitral leaflet perforation are shown in Figures 9 and 10. In Figure 9, a large perforation of the anterior mitral leaflet complicating aortic valve endocarditis is evident on transthoracic imaging. Figure 10 demonstrates a large mitral valve vegetation with leaflet perforation that is evident on color Doppler imaging.

Perforation of an aortic valve cusp can similarly occur as a complication of aortic valve endocarditis. Echocardiographic imaging may demonstrate a partial flail of one or more cusps, and the resulting aortic insufficiency jet tends to be eccentric. Aortic leaflet perforation is also associated with a dense, high frequency pattern of diastolic reverberation noted on continuous wave Doppler through the aortic valve, which is presumably due to vibration of partially destroyed cusp tissue caused by the high velocity diastolic flow of aortic regurgitation. Figure 11 demonstrates tis-

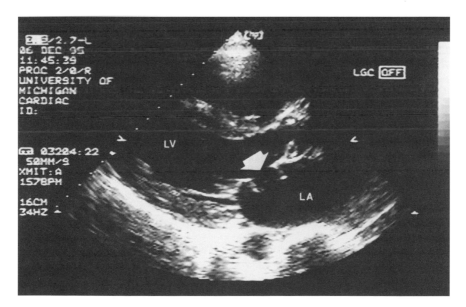

Figure 9. Large perforation of anterior mitral valve leaflet (arrow) complicating aortic valve endocarditis on transthoracic echocardiography. Aortic valve endocarditis led to aortic regurgitation and secondary infection of mitral valve at site of jet impact. LA = left atrium; LV = left ventricle.

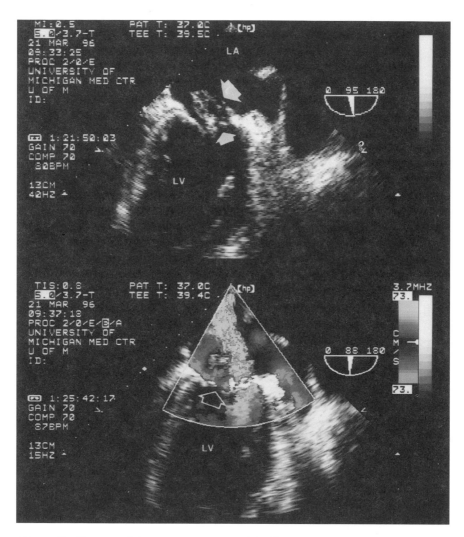

Figure 10. Top panel: Large anterior mitral leaflet vegetation (large arrow) with accompanying perforation (small arrow). Bottom panel: Color flow Doppler demonstrates large regurgitant jet through perforation. Note site of jet origin distinct from point of leaflet coaptation with posterior mitral leaflet (open arrow). LA = left atrium; LV = left ventricle. (See color appendix.)

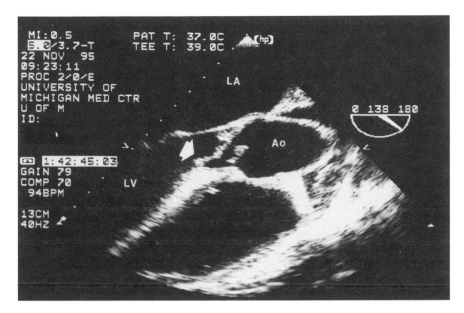

Figure 11. Tissue destruction and flail of aortic valve cusp complicating aortic valve endocarditis on transesophageal echocardiography. Soft tissue densities in left ventricular outflow tract (arrow) comprise vegetative material as well as flail aortic valve cusp. Ao − ascending aorta; LA = left atrium; LV = left ventricle.

sue destruction and flail of an aortic valve cusp complicating aortic valve endocarditis.

As well as seeding the anterior mitral valve leaflet, aortic regurgitation accompanying aortic valve endocarditis can result in secondary seeding of the mitral valve papillary muscles with subsequent papillary muscle rupture and severe valvular mitral regurgitation.[65] Similar to other causes of mitral leaflet flail, the resultant regurgitant jet is markedly eccentric and directed opposite the affected leaflet. Finally, systolic shunting of blood from the left ventricle to the left atrium can be mediated by rupture of an aortic root abscess with fistulous connection between the left ventricle below the level of the aortic valve and the left atrium above.[66] Although the associated jet may appear similar to that accompanying perforation of the basal anterior mitral leaflet or rupture of an intervalvular fibrosa aneurysm, shunting through a fistulous aortic root abscess can be distinguished echocardiographically by the location of the shunt origin and by the observed disruption of the normal continuity between the left ventricular outflow tract and the anterior mitral leaflet.[66]

Because the infective process associated with aortic valve endocarditis may not adhere to normal anatomic tissue planes, perforation and subsequent shunt formation can be observed in several other more unusual locations. Atypical shunts have been described using echocardiographic and Doppler imaging, including communication between the left ventricle and right atrium,[67,68] the left and right ventricles via the membranous interventricular septum[69] and fistulous communication between the left and right atria.[70]

Imaging Modality and Complications of Endocarditis

It is important to note that many of the complications of endocarditis may be preferentially demonstrated by Doppler evidence of pathological regurgitation or shunt.[54,55,58-70] Although echocardiographic imaging may provide important anatomic detail and more definitive diagnostic information, image resolution on transthoracic imaging is often limited and may not establish a firm diagnosis.

As expected, transesophageal echocardiography has substantial advantages over transthoracic imaging for the detection of complications of endocarditis including paravalvular abscess or aneurysm formation, leaflet or aneurysm perforation, and fistula formation between cardiac chambers.[54,59,61,63-65,67,69-71] Transesophageal echocardiography should be considered the imaging modality of choice for the assessment of paravalvular abscess because of the posterior location, the potentially small size of abscesses and no associated abnormal flow in the absence of perforation or fistulization. Transthoracic echocardiography cannot be used reliably to evaluate for paravalvular abscess complicating infective endocarditis. Although transthoracic echocardiography and Doppler imaging may frequently demonstrate evidence of regurgitation[59,65] or shunt,[61,63,67,69,70] transesophageal echocardiography provides significantly improved imaging resolution which in turn permits accurate preoperative diagnosis of abscess, aneurysm, perforation and fistula formation.[54,59,61,63-65,67,69-71] As previously noted, the advantages of transesophageal imaging are even more pronounced in the setting of complications of prosthetic valve endocarditis.[23,31-33]

Prognostic Implications of Echocardiographic Findings

Many investigators have sought to define whether the presence or morphologic characteristics of vegetations on echocardiographic imaging are predictive of clinical outcome among patients with known or suspected infective endocarditis.[2-6,8,9,11,12,14-16,19,72-77] In general, investigations have sought to define whether echocardiographic features can predict complications of endocarditis such as embolic phenomena, congestive heart failure, subsequent need for surgical intervention or mortality. There is a general although not unanimous consensus that the echocardiographic detection of vegetations in patients with infective endocarditis may suggest an increased risk.

Echocardiographic Detection of Vegetations

Data compiled from a variety of investigations that describe the respective incidences of congestive heart failure, embolic complications, need for surgery and patient mortality based on the presence or absence of vegetations on echocardiographic imaging are shown in Table 3. Early studies using M-mode echocardiography relied on the simple detection of vegetations as a risk for subsequent events.[2–4,6,9,11] As was the case with data derived for estimation of the sensitivity of echocardiography for the detection of vegetations, studies were retrospective analyses and may have been biased to include patients with more advanced disease. In addition, sample sizes tended to be relatively small, precluding most observed differences from reaching statistical significance. However, there was fairly good agreement that the detection of vegetations on M-mode echocardiography suggests a worse prognosis among patients with known or suspected endocarditis, with higher observed rates of congestive heart failure,[3,6,9,11] embolization,[2–4,6,9,11] need for surgery[2,3,6, 9,11] and death.[3,9,11]

Investigators subsequently used two-dimensional echocardiography for the similar assessment of prognosis among patients with known or suspected endocarditis. Although most investigators found that risk was increased in the setting of vegetations evident on echocardiographic imaging,[5,8,14–16,74] not all studies were able to confirm these observations.[12,73, 75,76] Some of the populations studied may have included patients with more aggressive or more advanced disease, leading to nonuniformity in findings. Further, because most of the studies were retrospective analyses, it is difficult to determine whether knowledge of echocardiographic findings may have affected subsequent patient management. Finally, most of the study populations were small and, as was the case with studies using M-mode echocardiography, observed trends often failed to reach statistical significance.

Vegetation Size, Mobility and Location

The additional spatial resolution afforded by two-dimensional echocardiography allows morphologic characterization of vegetations with respect

Table 3

Incidence of Complications of Endocarditis and Mortality Associated with Echocardiographic Evidence of Vegetation

Authors	Year	Modality	n	Vegetation Visualized on Echo					No Vegetation Visualized on Echo					Corr.
				n	CHF	Embolus	Surgery	Death	n	CHF	Embolus	Surgery	Death	
Roy[2]	1976	M-mode	32	22	n/a	55%	n/a	n/a	10	n/a	20%	n/a	n/a	yes
Wann[3]	1976	M-mode	65	22	100%	18%	82%	9%	43	28%	0	0	0	yes
Mintz[4]	1979	M-mode	32	12	n/a	75%	n/a	n/a	20	n/a	15%	n/a	n/a	yes
Davis[6]	1980	M-mode	30	17	82%	47%	100%	35%	13	46%	15%	15%	23%	yes
Hickey[9]	1981	M-mode	36	22	82%	50%	64%	36%	14	29%	36%	21%	14%	ns
Come[11]	1982	M-mode	51	24	58%	25%	29%	33%	27	19%	7%	4%	4%	ns
Wann[5]	1979	2D	23	19%	63%	37%	63%	5%	4	0%	0%	0%	0%	ns
Stewart[8]	1980	2D	87	47	32%	30%	26%	11%	40	3%	10%	5%	5%	yes
Stafford[14]	1985	2D	62	45	58%	47%	53%	27%	17	53%	12%	53%	0%	yes
Lutas[12]	1986	2D	77	43	53%	26%	12%	7%	34	35%	18%	21%	12%	no
Buda[15]	1986	2D	50	21	38%	48%	43%	24%	29	21%	14%	17%	7%	yes
Jaffe[16]	1990	2D	70	43	n/a	40%	n/a	n/a	15	n/a	40%	n/a	n/a	ns
Steckelberg[73]	1991	2D	207	79	n/a	14%	39%	n/a	82	n/a	11%	11%	n/a	no
Sanfilippo[74]	1991	2D	148	98	21%	41%	24%	11%	26	0%	31%	0	8%	yes
Heinle[75]	1994	2D	41	30	n/a	47%	n/a	n/a	11	n/a	30%	n/a	n/a	no
Erbel[19]	1988	TEE	96	46	n/a	24%	n/a	n/a	50	n/a	6%	n/a	n/a	yes
Mügge[71]	1989	TEE	105	96	22%	31%	n/a	15%	9	33%	33%	n/a	44%	yes
De Castro[76]	1997	TEE	57	54	n/a	44%	n/a	n/a	3	n/a	33%	n/a	n/a	no

Corr. = correlation between echocardiographic presence of vegetation and complications; n/a = not available; ns = not significant; 2D = two-dimensional echocardiography; TEE = transesophageal echocardiography; CHF = congestive heart failure.

to size, shape and mobility. Many investigators have sought to define whether characteristics of vegetations are useful in predicting prognosis.[5,8,12,14–16,19,72–77] The most widely investigated and perhaps the most controversial question has been whether vegetation size is an independent risk for subsequent embolization. Published data addressing the impact of vegetation size on embolic risk are summarized in Table 4. These reports demonstrate a division between investigators who concluded that vegetation size is a predictor of embolic events[14,16,72,74,77] and those who concluded that it is not.[5,12,15,19,73,75,76] As noted previously, many studies included small numbers of patients, and sometimes strong trends toward difference did not reach criteria for statistical significance.[5,12,14,16] However, one investigator demonstrated statistical significance for vegetation size greater than 10 mm as an embolic risk after pooling findings with data from 4 previously published reports.[16] Another investigator made the same conclusion after performing a meta-analysis using data from 10 previously published reports including a total of 415 patients.[77]

One investigator described an observable decrease in vegetation size on serial echocardiograms performed on patients before and after clinical embolic events, including one patient who suffered a stroke and 2 who experienced peripheral arterial embolic events.[5] Later, others observed that excluding from analysis those patients who had experienced embolic events prior to echocardiographic imaging resulted in a stronger observed relationship between vegetation size and embolic risk.[16,72] The implication of these findings is that larger vegetations may present a risk of subse-

Table 4
Reported Embolization Rates as a Function of Vegetation Size

Author	Year	N	Size	Embolization Rate		p	Correlation
				Larger	Smaller		
Wann[5]	1979	7	qualitative	57%	27%	0.33*	n/a
Stafford[14]	1985	21	>6 mm	51%	0%	0.11*	yes
Lutas[12]	1986	11	>10 mm	35%	12%	0.16*	no
Buda[15]	1986	10	>10 mm	55%	57%	1.0*	no
Erbel[19]	1988	11	>11 mm	21%	22%	1.0*	no
Mügge[71]	1989	33	>10 mm	47%	19%	<0.01	yes
Jaffe[16]	1990	10†	>10 mm	26%	11%	0.19	yes (ns)
Steckelberg[73]	1991	27	>10 mm	hazard ratio 1.4	>0.2	no
Sanfilippo[74]	1991	48	maximum	n/a	n/a	0.03‡	yes
Heinle[75]	1994	20	>10 mm	50%	42%	0.5	no
De Castro[76]	1997	25	>10 mm	42%	47%§	0.78*	no

N = number of patients with embolic events; 'Size' = size threshold between large and small vegetations; n/a = not available; ns = not significant.
* p value calculated from provided data using Fisher exact test; † limited to left-sided endocarditis; ‡ based on multiple stepwise logistic regression analysis; § includes vegetations <10 mm and no visible vegetation.

quent embolization, but that imaging after an embolic event fails to correlate with prior events. Performance of echocardiograms among patients with antecedent embolic events will not reveal the size of vegetations that have already embolized, and the correlation between vegetation size and embolic risk may be underestimated.

Other investigators have separately addressed the question of whether vegetation size is related to prognosis for vegetations found exclusively associated with right-sided endocarditis.[78,79] Both groups of investigators noted the generally benign course of right-sided endocarditis. One investigator found that the echocardiographic documentation of vegetations greater than 1.0 cm was associated with a lower rate of response to appropriate medical therapy and an increased need for surgical intervention.[78] Similarly, after studying a large population of intravenous drug users with right-sided endocarditis, another investigator concluded that despite a generally favorable prognosis, the presence of larger vegetations on echocardiographic imaging was associated with significantly higher mortality.[79]

In addition to vegetation size, investigators have used the spatial resolution afforded by two-dimensional echocardiography to further characterize other morphologic features of vegetations. Vegetations that appear to have increased mobility on echocardiographic imaging have been found to pose an increased risk of embolization compared to sessile vegetations.[72] However, vegetation mobility appears to be strongly related to vegetation size,[16,72] and it may not be possible to adequately separate vegetation mobility from vegetation size as a risk of embolization. A semiquantitative echocardiographic scheme has been devised to further characterize the morphologic characteristics of vegetations.[74] The analyzed features included vegetation size (in 2 dimensions), vegetation mobility (graded as fixed, mobile edge, pedunculated or prolapsing), vegetation extent (graded as single, multiple on one valve or on multiple valves) and vegetation consistency (graded as completely calcified, partially calcified, denser than myocardial echoes or equal to myocardial echoes). With this scheme, vegetation mobility, extent and size appeared to be independent predictors of combined risk in endocarditis.

Finally, investigators have evaluated whether echocardiographic determination of vegetation location predicts subsequent prognosis. Here again not all investigators are in agreement,[73,75] but several investigators have demonstrated an increased risk of systemic embolization if vegetations are located on the mitral valve as opposed to the aortic valve.[16,72, 74,80]

The prognostic value of morphologic features of vegetations on echocardiography may be due to a single factor or a combination of 2 factors. Failure of host defense mechanisms or inadequate treatment may result in vegetations of larger size which are more readily detectable on echocardiographic imaging. In this case, morphologic features of vegetations may serve strictly as a marker of response to therapy. Alternatively, larger vegetations may present a risk simply by virtue of their physical characteristics, with increased risks of valve destruction, obstruction or embolization. As noted above, there is no consensus as to whether vegetation size, mobility or other echocardiographic characteristics portend an increased risk for subsequent morbid events. In addition, there are no prospective studies that test whether surgery decreases overall risk among patients with large or mobile vegetations. Given these uncertainties, surgical intervention is not presently recommended based solely on echocardiographic evidence of large or mobile vegetations.

The Negative Echocardiographic Examination

There is important prognostic information associated with an echocardiographic examination that reveals neither vegetations nor other evidence of infective endocarditis.[81–83] Inasmuch as early literature suggested a relatively high sensitivity for the echocardiographic detection of vegetations in patients with endocarditis,[2–16] some studies revealed significant rates of false negative examinations.[3,4,8,9,11,12,15] However, improved imaging quality and in particular the use of transesophageal echocardiography have increased the sensitivity for detection of abnormalities in patients with endocarditis. High imaging sensitivity and the presumption that undetected vegetations are small and without significant associated tissue destruction imply that a normal echocardiographic study of good quality carries a favorable prognosis and, depending on other clinical factors, a significant likelihood that the patient may not have infective endocarditis.

In one study, investigators followed patients with possible endocarditis who had neither vegetations nor evidence of abscess on monoplane transesophageal echocardiography.[81] Of these 65 patients, 56 (86%) did not have endocarditis and other diagnoses were subsequently established. Four patients were treated for endocarditis based on clinical history and equivocal echocardiographic findings. The remaining 5 patients, representing 8% of the total group, were subsequently found to have endocarditis based on clinical course, pathological examination or follow-up transesophageal echocardiography. These authors concluded that, although a negative monoplane transesophageal echocardiogram cannot definitively exclude endocarditis, it reduces the probability of the diagnosis. However, follow-up imaging may be warranted if another diagnosis is not established. These findings were confirmed by other investigators, who followed 93 patients without discrete vegetations on monoplane or biplane transesophageal echocardiography.[82] These investigators found a 100% negative predictive value for excluding the diagnosis of infective endocarditis among patients with native valves and a 90% negative predictive value among patients with prosthetic valves. Both of these studies used absence of vegetations as criteria for a negative echocardiographic examination. However, some patients had abnormal valvular findings that indicated valvular pathology but did not meet strict diagnostic criteria for vegetations. The negative predictive value for infective endocarditis of a completely normal transesophageal echocardiogram is presumably even higher. Finally, although not independently addressed, the improved imaging capabilities associated with multiplane transesophageal echocardiography may further strengthen the power of a negative examination.

Transesophageal imaging may not always be necessary to exclude the diagnosis of endocarditis. In one study, only 2 of 46 patients (4%) with no vegetations on transthoracic echocardiography of good quality were found to have vegetations on transesophageal imaging, whereas 17 of 47 patients (36%) with nondiagnostic transthoracic studies had evidence of vegetations on transesophageal imaging.[83] Based on these findings, a negative transthoracic study appears to reduce the likelihood but cannot exclude the diagnosis of endocarditis. As previously noted, transesophageal imaging appears to have incremental diagnostic value in the detection of vegetations, and clearly incremental value in the detection of paravalvular abscess.[17–25] The decision regarding the use of transesophageal imaging should be influenced by the pre-test likelihood for the diagnosis of endocarditis.

Echocardiographic Evaluation of Patients

Echocardiography is frequently used among patients with known or suspected endocarditis to search for and characterize vegetations, paravalvular abscess and valvular or other tissue destruction. Although the diagnosis of infective endocarditis remains a clinical one and must take into account the presence of an infective illness and evidence of bacteremia, the use of echocardiography has gained importance in helping to establish a diagnosis as well as in evaluating patients with known endocarditis.

Diagnosis of Endocarditis

Echocardiographic imaging is useful in the evaluation of patients with a clinical suspicion of endocarditis and in patients with unexplained bacteremia. Modern criteria for establishing the diagnosis of endocarditis rely heavily on echocardiographic data. The Duke criteria for endocarditis require 2 major, one major and 3 minor, or 5 minor criteria to establish a diagnosis of endocarditis.[42] Major criteria comprise only blood culture evidence of endocarditis and evidence of endocardial involvement by echocardiography, including evidence of a discrete vegetation, abscess, partial prosthetic valve dehiscence or new valvular regurgitation. The designation of vegetation on echocardiography requires the demonstration of an oscillating intracardiac mass in a typical location including valvular, in the path of a regurgitant jet or on implanted material. Other echocardiographic evidence consistent with endocarditis but not meeting the major criteria is considered a minor criterion. The Duke criteria for endocarditis therefore weigh echocardiographic evidence of endocarditis equally with blood culture data, in contrast to the previously accepted von Reyn criteria which did not use echocardiographic data in establishing a diagnosis of endocarditis.[84] The Duke criteria appear to have high diagnostic accuracy for both the detection[42,85] and the exclusion of endocarditis.[86]

The relative impact of transthoracic and transesophageal echocardiography has been evaluated among patients with suspected endocarditis.[87,88] Among a general population referred for echocardiographic evaluation in the setting of possible endocarditis, transthoracic echocardiography appears to categorize adequately most patients as to the likelihood of disease.[87] In general, technically adequate transthoracic imaging can usually exclude the diagnosis of endocarditis when the pretest likelihood of disease is moderate or low. However, transesophageal imaging should be routinely used for patients with prosthetic valves,[89] and should be considered for those in whom transthoracic imaging is either technically inadequate or indicative of an intermediate probability of disease, as well as for patients with a higher pre-test likelihood of endocarditis. Among patients with a higher pre-test likelihood of endocarditis, transesophageal echocardiography has been found to have a significant impact on diagnosis.[88] As a general recommendation, echocardiography should be performed on all patients in whom a diagnosis of infective endocarditis is considered. Transthoracic imaging should be the initial imaging modality among patients with native valves and lower pre-test probability of disease. Patients with prosthetic valves and those with a higher likelihood of endocarditis should undergo evaluation that includes transesophageal imaging.

Evaluation of Patients with Known Endocarditis

All patients with an established diagnosis of endocarditis should undergo echocardiographic imaging.[90] Echocardiography is useful in the detection and characterization of the pathological and hemodynamic consequences of infection, including vegetations, regurgitant lesions and assessment of ventricular function.[89] Furthermore, echocardiography can provide important prognostic information and help in the assessment of sequelae of endocarditis that may influence management of the disease, including the detection of paravalvular abscess, leaflet perforation, ruptured chordae and shunt.

Transthoracic echocardiography appears to be adequate for the initial evaluation of hemodynamically uncompromised patients with native valve endocarditis.[89] If imaging is technically adequate, transthoracic echocardiography can provide confirmation of the presence and location of vegetations and assessment of valvular regurgitation. Repeated imaging can help assure adequate response to therapy. Transesophageal imaging should be considered for all patients with prosthetic valves, for patients in whom transthoracic imaging provides suboptimal characterization of valvular anatomy or function, for patients who have hemodynamically significant sequelae of infection and for those who fail to respond to adequate therapy.[89] Arguably, it is reasonable for all patients diagnosed with endocarditis to undergo transesophageal echocardiography during treatment to screen for abscess formation or other sequelae that could alter management.[90] In addition, transesophageal echocardiography should be performed in all patients who require surgical intervention for endocarditis in order to optimally define cardiac and particularly valvular anatomy and function including assessment for secondary lesions that may have an impact on the surgical procedure.

An echocardiographic view of vegetation size and consistency can provide additional information reflecting response to therapy. Vegetations may resolve during therapy.[91] Alternatively, successful therapy can be accompanied by a decrease in size[91-93] and increase in echogenicity of vegetations,[91,92] changes that can be monitored during treatment. Evidence of progressive valvular dysfunction or failure of anticipated changes in the appearance of vegetations on echocardiographic imaging may suggest a delayed or incomplete response to therapy. Because vegetations that do not decrease in size during therapy appear to be associated with a higher incidence of complications and greater requirement for valve replacement,[93] echocardiographic monitoring during treatment may allow reassessment of prognosis and potentially even allow alteration in therapy prior to the development of complications. Figure 12 demonstrates the bright, echo-dense appearance of a vegetation that is inactive and healed, distinguished from the soft tissue density associated with active vegetations shown in other figures.

Finally, echocardiography during therapy may be useful in the conservative management of some patients. Although patients with pros-

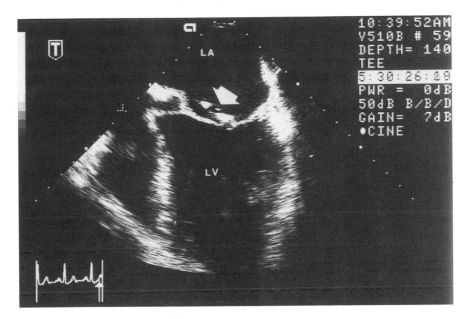

Figure 12. Bright, echo-dense appearance of mitral valve vegetation (arrow) on transesophageal echocardiography suggests vegetation that is inactive and healed. Bright appearance is distinguished from soft tissue density associated with active vegetations. LA = left atrium; LV = left ventricle.

thetic valve endocarditis often require surgical valve replacement, there are reports of conservative medical management using transesophageal echocardiography to follow vegetation size and morphology for adequacy of response to therapy.[94] With this strategy, the echocardiographic demonstration of vegetation resolution may help support the clinical decision to treat with antibiotics rather than repeated valve replacement. Although echocardiographically monitored conservative therapy may be appropriate for some patients, this strategy has not been prospectively tested.

Echocardiography and Surgical Intervention

Therapy for infective endocarditis typically involves prolonged treatment with antibiotics. However, surgical intervention is required in a subset of patients. Surgery may be required early in the course of disease if there is hemodynamic compromise due to regurgitation or shunt, for evidence of failure of antibiotic therapy or for abscess formation. In addition, surgery may be required later during treatment for the repair of valvular regurgitation, fistula formation or shunt occurring as sequelae of infection.

In general, echocardiography may affect surgical intervention for endocarditis in 3 ways, which are explained below.

Detection of Complications

The presence of paravalvular abscess complicating endocarditis predicts that infection will not be eradicated by medical therapy alone, and surgical intervention is usually necessary. As previously noted, echocardiographic imaging is an accurate means to detect paravalvular abscess.[45–47,49,51–53,95–97] Although abscesses have been described using transthoracic imaging, the sensitivity for detection is clearly superior using transesophageal echocardiography.[51–53] If transesophageal echocardiography is not routinely performed in all patients treated for endocarditis, it should be performed to evaluate for abscess in any patient with persistent or recurrent fevers or other evidence of incomplete response to therapy. Similarly, echocardiography should be performed to evaluate for leaflet perforation or fistula formation if there is a new murmur, a change in murmur or a change in hemodynamic status during therapy for endocarditis.

Preoperative Assessment

Patients with endocarditis are at risk for secondary sites of infection and for other sequelae of infection that may affect surgical planning. Although a patient may require surgery due to abscess formation, valvular tissue destruction resulting in significant regurgitation may require intervention during the same procedure. Similarly, patients referred for surgical repair of valvular perforation, regurgitation or shunt may have additional hemodynamically important sequelae of infection that may require intervention. Because abscess formation or secondary sites of tissue destruction may affect the timing and extent of surgery, preoperative transesophageal echocardiography should be considered in all patients who require surgical intervention for infective endocarditis.

Intraoperative Echocardiography

Intraoperative echocardiography allows the assessment and potential revision of reparative cardiac surgical procedures before the patient leaves the operating room. Either transesophageal or epicardial echocardiography is commonly used following mitral valve reconstruction to interrogate for residual mitral insufficiency, and for aortic leaflet mobility and presence of aortic insufficiency following aortic allograft valve replacement. In addition, closure of leaflet perforation or repair of fistulae complicating endocarditis can be interrogated for presence of residual regurgitation or shunt. The intraoperative determination of the adequacy of surgical intervention allows any necessary revisions to be performed during the same procedure, and serves as a baseline measure of cardiac anatomy and function against which any future changes can be measured.

Summary

Echocardiography plays a pivotal role in the diagnosis and treatment of infective endocarditis. Two-dimensional transthoracic imaging can provide important information regarding the presence of endocarditis and of associated complications. Transesophageal echocardiography has improved the ability to identify vegetations accurately and to identify and characterize complications of endocarditis including paravalvular abscess, aneurysm formation, leaflet perforation or destruction and fistula formation. Echocardiographic imaging provides important prognostic as well as diagnostic information, and plays an important role in monitoring therapy and in defining the need for, as well as assessing, the results of surgical intervention for endocarditis.

References

1. Dillon JC, Feigenbaum H, Konecke LL, et al. Echocardiographic manifestations of valvular vegetations. *Am Heart J* 1973;86:698–704.
2. Roy P, Tajik AJ, Giuliani ER, et al. Spectrum of echocardiographic findings in bacterial endocarditis. *Circulation* 1976;53:474–482.
3. Wann LS, Dillon JC, Weyman AE, et al. Echocardiography in bacterial endocarditis. *N Engl J Med* 1976;295:135–139.
4. Mintz GS, Kotler MN, Segal BL, et al. Survival of patients with aortic valve endocarditis: Prognostic implications of the echocardiogram. *Arch Intern Med* 1979;139:862–866.
5. Wann LS, Hallam CC, Dillon JC, et al. Comparison of M-mode and cross-sectional echocardiography in infective endocarditis. *Circulation* 1979;60:728–736.
6. Davis RS, Strom JA, Frishman W, et al. The demonstration of vegetations by echocardiography in bacterial endocarditis; An indication for early surgical intervention. *Am J Med* 1980;69:57–63.
7. Martin RP, Meltzer RS, Chia BL, et al. Clinical utility of two-dimensional echocardiography in infective endocarditis. *Am J Cardiol* 1980;46:379–385.
8. Stewart JA, Silimperi D, Harris P, et al. Echocardiographic documentation of vegetative lesions in infective endocarditis: Clinical implications. *Circulation* 1988;61:374–380.

9. Hickey AJ, Wolfers J, Wilcken DEL. Reliability and clinical relevance of detection of vegetations by echocardiography in bacterial endocarditis. *Br Heart J* 1981;46:624–628.

10. Melvin ET, Berger M, Lutzker LG, et al. Noninvasive methods for detection of valve vegetations in infective endocarditis. *Am J Cardiol* 1981;47:271–278.

11. Come PC, Isaacs RE, Riley MF. Diagnostic accuracy of M-mode echocardiography in active infective endocarditis and prognostic implications of ultrasound-detectable vegetations. *Am Heart J* 1982;103:839–847.

12. Lutas EM, Roberts RB, Devereux RB, et al. Relation between the presence of echocardiographic vegetations and the complication rate in infective endocarditis. *Am Heart J* 1986;112:107–113.

13. Gilbert BW, Haney RS, Crawford F, et al. Two-dimensional echocardiographic assessment of vegetative endocarditis. *Circulation* 1977;55:346–353.

14. Stafford WJ, Petch J, Radford DJ. Vegetations in infective endocarditis: Clinical relevance and diagnosis by cross sectional echocardiography. *Br Heart J* 1985; 53:310–313.

15. Buda AJ, Zotz RJ, LeMire MS, et al. Prognostic significance of vegetations detected by two- dimensional echocardiography in infective endocarditis. *Am Heart J* 1986;112:1291–1296.

16. Jaffe WM, Morgan DE, Pearlman AS, et al. Infective endocarditis, 1983–1988: Echocardiographic findings and factors influencing morbidity and mortality. *J Am Coll Cardiol* 1990;15:1227–1237.

17. Drexler M, Erbel R, Rohmann S, et al. Diagnostic value of two-dimensional transoesophageal versus transthoracic echocardiography in patients with infective endocarditis. *Eur Heart J* 1987;8:303–306.

18. Daniel WG, Schroder E, Nonnast-Daniel B, et al. Conventional and transoesophageal echocardiography in the diagnosis of infective endocarditis. *Eur Heart J* 1987;8:287–292.

19. Erbel R, Rohmann S, Drexler M, et al. Improved diagnostic value of echocardiography in patients with infective endocarditis by transoesophageal approach: A prospective study. *Eur Heart J* 1988;9:43–53.

20. Taams MA, Gussenhoven EJ, Bos E, et al. Enhanced morphological diagnosis in infective endocarditis by transoesophageal echocardiography. *Br Heart J* 1990;63:109–113.

21. Shively BK, Gurule FT, Roldan CA, et al. Diagnostic value of transesophageal compared with transthoracic echocardiography in infective endocarditis. *J Am Coll Cardiol* 1991;18:391–397.

22. Birmingham GD, Rahko PS, Ballantyne F III. Improved detection of infective endocarditis with transesophageal echocardiography. *Am Heart J* 1992;123: 774–781.

23. Daniel GD, Mügge A, Grote J, et al. Comparison of transthoracic and transesophageal echocardiography for detection of abnormalities of prosthetic and bioprosthetic valves in the mitral and aortic positions. *Am J Cardiol* 1993;71: 210–215.

24. Shapiro SM, Young E, De Guzman S, et al. Transesophageal echocardiography in diagnosis of infective endocarditis. *Chest* 1994;105:377–382.

25. Chirillo F, Bruni A, Giujusa T, et al. Echocardiography in infective endocarditis: Reassessment of the diagnostic criteria of vegetation as evaluated from the precordial and transesophageal approach. *Am J Card Imaging* 1995;9:174–179.

26. Herrera CJ, Mehlman DJ, Hartz RS, et al. Comparison of transesophageal and

transthoracic echocardiography for diagnosis of right-sided cardiac lesions. *Am J Cardiol* 1992;70:964–966.

27. San Román JA, Vilacosta I, Zamorano JL, et al. Transesophageal echocardiography in right- sided endocarditis. *J Am Coll Cardiol* 1993;21:1226–1230.

28. Tardif JC, Schwartz SL, Vannan MA, et al. Clinical usefulness of multiplane transesophageal echocardiography: Comparison to biplanar imaging. *Am Heart J* 1994;128:156–166.

29. Job FP, Franke S, Lethen H, et al. Incremental value of biplane and multiplane transesophageal echocardiography for the assessment active infective endocarditis. *Am J Cardiol* 1995;75:1033–1037.

30. Daniel WG, Mügge A, Grote J, et al. Evaluation of endocarditis and its complications by biplane and multiplane transesophageal echocardiography. *Am J Card Imaging* 1995;9:100–105.

31. Khandheria BK, Seward JB, Oh JK, et al. Value and limitations of transesophageal echocardiography in assessment of mitral valve prostheses. *Circulation* 1991;83:1956–1968.

32. Alton ME, Pasierski TJ, Orsinelli DA, et al. Comparison of transthoracic and transesophageal echocardiography in evaluation of 47 Starr-Edwards prosthetic valves. *J Am Coll Cardiol* 1992;20:1503–1511.

33. Alam M, Rosman HS, Sun I. Transesophageal echocardiographic evaluation of St. Jude Medical and bioprosthetic valve endocarditis. *Am Heart J* 1992;123: 236–239.

34. Tenenbaum A, Fisman EZ, Vered Z, et al. Failure of transesophageal echocardiography to visualize a large mitral prosthesis vegetation detected solely by transthoracic echocardiography. *J Am Soc Echocardiogr* 1995;8:944–946.

35. Zijlstra F, Fioretti P, Roelandt JRTC. Echocardiographic demonstration of free wall vegetative endocarditis complicated by a pulmonary embolism in a patient with ventricular septal defect. *Br Heart J* 1986;55:497–499.

36. Vilacosta I, San Roman JA, Roca V. Eustachian valve endocarditis. *Br Heart J* 1990;64:340–341.

37. Shenoy MM, Kalakota M, Uddin M, et al. Left ventricular mural bacterial endocarditis: Diagnosis by transesophageal echocardiography. *Can J Cardiol* 1992;8:57–59.

38. Shirani J, Keffler K, Gerszten E, et al. Primary left ventricular mural endocarditis diagnosed by transesophageal echocardiography. *J Am Soc Echocardiogr* 1995;8:554–556.

39. Joffe II, Jacobs LE, Owen AN, et al. Noninfective valvular masses: Review of the literature with emphasis on imaging techniques and management. *Am Heart J* 1996;131:1175–1183.

40. Galve E, Candell-Riera J, Pigrau C, et al. Prevalence, morphologic types and evolution of cardiac valvular disease in systemic lupus erythematosus. *N Engl J Med* 1988;319:817–823.

41. Blanchard DG, Ross RS, Dittrich HC. Nonbacterial thrombotic endocarditis: Assessment by transesophageal echocardiography. *Chest* 1992;102:954–956.

42. Durack DT, Lukes AS, Bright DK. New criteria for diagnosis of infective endocarditis: Utilization of specific echocardiographic findings. *Am J Med* 1994;96: 200–209.

43. Mardelli TJ, Ogawa S, Hubbard FE, et al. Cross-sectional echocardiographic detection of aortic ring abscess in bacterial endocarditis. *Chest* 1978;74:576–578.

44. Scanlan JG, Seward JB, Tajik AJ. Valve ring abscess in infective endocarditis:

Visualization with wide angle two-dimensional echocardiography. *Am J Cardiol* 1982;49:1794–1800.

45. Nakamura K, Suzuki S, Satomi G, et al. Detection of mitral ring abscess by two-dimensional echocardiography. *Circulation* 1982;65:816–819.

46. Neimann JL, Danchin N, Godenier JP, et al. Two-dimensional echocardiographic recognition of aortic valve ring abscess. *Eur Heart J* 1984;5:59–65.

47. Ellis SG, Goldstein J, Popp RL. Detection of endocarditis-associated perivalvular abscesses by two-dimensional echocardiography. *J Am Coll Cardiol* 1985; 5:647–653.

48. Pollak, SJ, Felner JM. Echocardiographic identification of an aortic valve ring abscess. *J Am Coll Cardiol* 1986;7:1167–1173.

49. Saner HE, Asinger RW, Homans DC, et al. Two-dimensional echocardiographic identification of complicated aortic root endocarditis: Implications for surgery. *J Am Coll Cardiol* 1987;10:859–868.

50. Aguado JM, González-Vílchez F, Martin-Durén R, et al. Perivalvular abscesses associated with endocarditis: Clinical features and diagnostic accuracy of two-dimensional echocardiography. *Chest* 1993;104:88 93.

51. Daniel WG, Mügge A, Martin RP, et al. Improvement in the diagnosis of abscesses associated with endocarditis by transesophageal echocardiography. *N Engl J Med* 1991;324:795–800.

52. Blumberg EA, Karalis DA, Chandrasekaran K, et al. Endocarditis-associated paravalvular abscesses. Do clinical parameters predict the presence of abscess? *Chest* 1995;107:898–903.

53. Rohmann S, Erbel R, Mohr-Kahaly S, et al. Use of transoesophageal echocardiography in the diagnosis of abscess in infective endocarditis. *Eur Heart J* 1995; 16 (Suppl B):54–62.

54. Karalis DG, Bansal RC, Hauck AJ, et al. Transesophageal echocardiographic recognition of subaortic complications in aortic valve endocarditis: Clinical and surgical implications. *Circulation* 1992;86:353–362.

55. Harpaz D, Shah P, Hicks G, et al. Transesophageal echocardiographic recognition of an unusual complication of aortic valve endocarditis. *J Am Soc Echocardiogr* 1994;7:72–78.

56. Vandenbossche JL, Hartenberg K, Leclerc JL. Mitral valve aneurysm formation documented by cross-sectional echocardiography. *Eur Heart J* 1986;7:171–175.

57. Polak PE, Gussenhoven WJ, Roelandt JRTC. Transoesophageal cross-sectional echocardiographic recognition of an aortic valve ring abscess and a subannular mycotic aneurysm. *Eur Heart J* 1987;8:664–666.

58. Decroly PH, Vandenbossche JL, Englert M. Anterior mitral valve aneurysm perforation secondary to aortic valve endocarditis detected by Doppler colour flow mapping. *Eur Heart J* 1989;10:186–189.

59. Karalis DG, Chandrasekaran K, Wahl JM, et al. Transesophageal echocardiographic recognition of mitral valve abnormalities associated with aortic valve endocarditis. *Am Heart J* 1990;119:1209–1211.

60. Ryan T, Markel ML, Waller BF, et al. Doppler echocardiographic detection of a ruptured acquired aneurysm of the sinus of Valsalva: Clinical-morphologic correlations. *Chest* 1987;91:626–629.

61. Bansal RC, Graham BM, Jutzy KR, et al. Left ventricular outflow tract to left atrial communication secondary to rupture of mitral-aortic intervalvular fibrosa in infective endocarditis: Diagnosis by transesophageal echocardiography and color flow imaging. *J Am Coll Cardiol* 1990;15:499–504.

62. Miyatake K, Yamamoto K, Park YD, et al. Diagnosis of mitral valve perforation by real-time two-dimensional Doppler flow imaging technique. *J Am Coll Cardiol* 1986;8:1235–1239.

63. Nomeir AM, Downes TR, Cordell AR. Perforation of the anterior mitral leaflet caused by aortic valve endocarditis: Diagnosis by two-dimensional, transesophageal echocardiography and color flow Doppler. *J Am Soc Echocardiogr* 1992;5:195–198.

64. De Castro S, d'Amati G, Cartoni D, et al. Valvular perforation in left-sided infective endocarditis: A prospective echocardiographic evaluation and clinical outcome. *Am Heart J* 1997;134:656–664.

65. Habib G, Guidon C, Tricoire E, et al. Papillary muscle rupture caused by bacterial endocarditis: Role of transesophageal echocardiography. *J Am Soc Echocardiogr* 1994;7:79–81.

66. Fisher EA, Estioko MR, Stern EH, et al. Left ventricular to left atrial communication secondary to a para-aortic abscess: Color flow Doppler documentation. *J Am Coll Cardiol* 1987;10:222–224.

67. Elian D, Di Segni E, Kaplinsky E, et al. Acquired left ventricular-right atrial communication caused by infective endocarditis detected by transesophageal echocardiography: Case report and review of the literature. *J Am Soc Echocardiogr* 1995;8:108–110.

68. Trehan N, Goldfarb A, Gindea AJ, et al. Echocardiographic diagnosis of atrioventricular septal perforation caused by an aortic valve vegetation. *J Am Soc Echocardiogr* 1988;1:150–151.

69. Winslow TM, Friar DA, Larson AW, et al. A rare complication of aortic valve endocarditis: Diagnosis with transesophageal echocardiography. *J Am Soc Echocardiogr* 1995;8:546–550.

70. Sheppard RC, Chandrasekaran K, Ross J, et al. An acquired interatrial fistula secondary to para-aortic abscess documented by transesophageal echocardiography. *J Am Soc Echocardiogr* 1991;4:271–276.

71. Kan MN, Chen YT, Lee AYS. Comparison of transesophageal to transthoracic color Doppler echocardiography in the identification of intracardiac mycotic aneurysms in infective endocarditis. *Echocardiography* 1991;8:643–648.

72. Mügge A, Daniel WG, Frank G, et al. Echocardiography in infective endocarditis: Reassessment of prognostic implications of vegetation size determined by the transthoracic and the transesophageal approach. *J Am Coll Cardiol* 1989;14:631–638.

73. Steckelberg JM, Murphy JG, Ballard D, et al. Emboli in infective endocarditis: The prognostic value of echocardiography. *Ann Intern Med* 1991;114:635–640.

74. Sanfilippo AJ, Picard MH, Newell JB, et al. Echocardiographic assessment of patients with infectious endocarditis: Prediction of risk for complications. *J Am Coll Cardiol* 1991;18:1191–1199.

75. Heinle S, Wilderman N, Harrison JK, et al. Value of transthoracic echocardiography in predicting embolic events in active infective endocarditis. *Am J Cardiol* 1994;74:799–801.

76. De Castro S, Magni G, Beni S, et al. Role of transthoracic and transesophageal echocardiography in predicting embolic events in patients with active infective endocarditis involving native cardiac valves. *Am J Cardiol* 1997;80:1030–1034.

77. Tischler MD, Vaitkus PT. The ability of vegetation size on echocardiography to predict complications: A meta-analysis. *J Am Soc Echocardiogr* 1997;10:562–568.

78. Robbins MJ, Frater RWM, Soeiro R, et al. Influence of vegetation size on clinical outcome of right-sided infective endocarditis. *Am J Med* 1986;80:165–171.

79. Hecht SR, Berger M. Right-sided endocarditis in intravenous drug users: Prognostic features in 102 episodes. *Ann Intern Med* 1992;117:560–566.

80. Rohmann S, Erbel R, Gorge G, et al. Clinical relevance of vegetation localization by transoesophageal echocardiography in infective endocarditis. *Eur Heart J* 1992;13(4):446–452.

81. Sochowski RA, Chan KL. Implication of negative results on a monoplane transesophageal echocardiographic study in patients with suspected infective endocarditis. *J Am Coll Cardiol* 1993;21:216–221.

82. Lowry RW, Zoghbi WA, Baker WB, et al. Clinical impact of transesophageal echocardiography in the diagnosis and management of infective endocarditis. *Am J Cardiol* 1994;73:1089–1091.

83. Irani WN, Grayburn PA, Afridi I. A negative transthoracic echocardiogram obviates the need for transesophageal echocardiography in patients with suspected native valve active infective endocarditis. *Am J Cardiol* 1996;78:101–103.

84. Von Reyn CF, Levy BS, Arbeit RD, et al. Infective endocarditis: An analysis based on strict case definitions. *Ann Intern Med* 1981;94:505–518.

85. Bayer AS, Ward JI, Ginzton LE, et al. Evaluations of new clinical criteria for the diagnosis of infective endocarditis. *Am J Med* 1994;96:211–219.

86. Dodds GA III, Sexton DJ, Durack DT, et al. Negative predictive value of the Duke criteria for infective endocarditis. *Am J Cardiol* 1996;77:403–407.

87. Lindner JR, Case RA, Dent JM, et al. Diagnostic value of echocardiography in suspected endocarditis: An evaluation based on the pretest probability of disease. *Circulation* 1996;93:730–736.

88. Fowler VG Jr, Li J, Corey GR, et al. Role of echocardiography in evaluation of patients with Staphylococcus aureus bacteremia: Experience in 103 patients. *J Am Coll Cardiol* 1997;30:1072–1078.

89. Cheitlin MD, Alpert JS, Armstrong WF, et al. ACC/AHA guidelines for the clinical application of echocardiography: Executive summary. A report of the American College of Cardiology/American Heart Association Task Force on Practice Guidelines (Committee on Clinical Application of Echocardiography). *J Am Coll Cardiol* 1997;29:862–879.

90. Khandheria BK. Suspected bacterial endocarditis: To TEE or not to TEE (editorial). *J Am Coll Cardiol* 1993;21:222–224.

91. Vuille C, Nidorf M, Weyman AE, et al. Natural history of vegetations during successful medical treatment of endocarditis. *Am Heart J* 1994;128:1200–1209.

92. Tak T, Rahimtoola SH, Kumar A, et al. Value of digital image processing of two-dimensional echocardiograms in differentiating active from chronic vegetations of infective endocarditis. *Circulation* 1988;78:116–123.

93. Rohmann S, Erbel R, Darius H, et al. Prediction of rapid versus prolonged healing of infective endocarditis by monitoring vegetation size. *J Am Soc Echocardiogr* 1991;4:465–474.

94. Bruss J, Jacobs LE, Kotler MN, et al. Utility of transesophageal echocardiography in the conservative management of prosthetic valve endocarditis. *Chest* 1992;102:1886–1888.

95. Rohmann S, Seifert T, Erbel R, et al. Identification of abscess formation in

native-valve infective endocarditis using transesophageal echocardiography: Implications for surgical treatment. *Thorac Cardiovasc Surg* 1991;39:273–280.

96. Cormier B, Vahanian A. Echocardiography and indications for surgery. *Eur Heart J* 1995;16 (Suppl B):68–71.

97. Brecker SJD, Jin XY, Yacoub MH. Anatomical definition of aortic root abscesses by transesophageal echocardiography: Planning a surgical strategy using homograft valves. *Clin Cardiol* 1995;18:353–359.

Chapter 7

Neurological Complications of Infective Endocarditis

Amy A. Pruitt, M.D.

Introduction

In the century since William Osler's description of the neurological complications of infective endocarditis (IE), retrospective reviews have appeared regularly.[1] The largest series consistently report similar distributions of neurological problems, and all concur that embolic stroke is the most frequent neurological complication. The author's 2 series, separated by 17 years, as well as other reports spanning 6 decades, agree that neurological complications occur in about 30% of patients with IE, about half of whom present with the neurological event.[2-15] In most series, patients with neurological complications have a mortality rate between 1.5 and 3 times that of patients without such complications, though in this author's more recent series, mortality of patients with neurological complications was 45% less than that in the earlier series.[11,15] Table 1 details the percentage of neurological complications and mortality in 879 patients from 5 recent series published during the last 16 years with patient accrual over a 30-year period.

These stable incidence and mortality rates mask an evolving spectrum of conditions predisposing to IE, causative organisms, and diagnostic and therapeutic techniques. The advent of magnetic resonance imaging (MRI) has clarified our understanding of the pathogenesis of many of the neurological complications of endocarditis, and transesophageal echocardiography has permitted better visualization of valvular vegetations. However,

From: Vlessis AA, Bolling S (eds): *Endocarditis: A Multidisciplinary Approach to Modern Treatment.* © Futura Publishing Co., Armonk, NY, 1999.

Table 1

Neurological Complications of Infective Endocarditis

Author/Ref. No/Yr	No. Patients	%Neurological Complication	%Stroke†	Mortality Neuro	
				+	−
Pruitt (11)(1978)	216	39	17	58	20
Salgado (12)(1989)	175	36.5	17	20.6	14.6
Gransden (13)(1989)	178*	33	7		
Kanter (4)(1991)	166*	35	20	35	19
Pruitt (15)(1995)	144	29	18	32	13

* Series included only native valve endocarditis
† Ischemic and hemorrhagic strokes are grouped together

these technical advances have not resolved several major clinical controversies. Disagreement continues about the significance of distribution and size of valvular vegetations and risk of embolic stroke, as does the clinical management controversy with respect to systemic anticoagulation in patients with endocarditis who have suffered an embolic stroke. Optimal timing for cardiac surgery and the degree of risk for further cerebral injury

Table 2

Major Issues in the Management of Patients with Infective Endocarditis and Neurological Involvement

1. **ANTICOAGULATION**
   * What are the risks and benefits of anticoagulation during an episode of endocarditis?
   * Is there a role for heparin or antiplatelet agents?
   * After an embolic stroke, when can anticoagulation be reinstituted safely in patients receiving antibiotics for endocarditis?
   * Should anticoagulation be discontinued when patients with prosthetic valves develop endocarditis?
2. **CARDIAC SURGERY**
   * What is the risk of neurological deterioration if a patient with a stroke requires emergent valve replacement?
   * Should a single cerebral embolus be an indication for valve replacement?
   * Is there an echocardiographically-defined group of patients who will benefit from valve repair surgery and avoid prosthetic valves?
3. **INFECTIOUS INTRACRANIAL (MYCOTIC) ANEURYSMS**
   * Should a search for infectious intracranial aneurysms be undertaken in every endocarditis patient?
   * What is the role of magnetic resonance angiography in the detection and follow-up of infectious intracranial aneurysms?
   * What is the proper management of infectious intracranial aneurysms?

during valve replacement remains under discussion. This chapter will address these and other major clinical management controversies summarized in Table 2.

Epidemiology

The risk of nervous system involvement in endocarditis depends on the conditions predisposing to IE, which have changed greatly in the last 4 decades. In the preantibiotic era, rheumatic heart disease accounted for 39% to 76% of cases.[2,16,17] In more recent series, the declining frequency of rheumatic heart disease and the rising percentage of IE cases for which no underlying cardiac condition is apparent are clear. Among identifiable predisposing conditions, mitral valve prolapse and degenerative changes such as calcific aortic stenosis greatly outweigh congenital heart disease and rheumatic heart disease.[18,19] Along with the altered spectrum of underlying cardiac conditions, the age distribution of the affected population is changing. At this author's institution, the mean ages of patients with and without neurological complications were similar (48 and 53), but the range was larger than in earlier series (18 to 97 years) and there was a "missing middle" with patients clustering in the over age 60 or under age 40 groups. Other institutions report a higher mean age, probably reflecting a lower incidence of intravenous drug abuse and local referral patterns.[14,18,19] Men outnumber women in most series.

Risk factors for IE may be related to underlying cardiac abnormalities, patient behavior and medical or surgical therapies of other conditions. Intravenous drug abuse accounts for an increasing percentage of community-acquired IE and stroke (with or without IE) among young adults.[20-22] Mathew's recent series from Cook County Hospital, in Chicago, identifies several salient features of drug abuse-related IE relevant to neurological morbidity and overall mortality. Right and left heart valves were affected roughly equally; these authors demonstrated tricupsid valve involvement in 46% of patients, mitral valve in 32%, and aortic valve in 9%. *Staphylococcus aureus* was the causative organism in two thirds of these patients.[23] In contrast, 10% to 20% of IE cases in patients over age 60 may be hospital-acquired.[24] Iatrogenic risk factors, including invasive instrumentation of the gastrointestinal or genitourinary tracts and indwelling devices such as arterioarterial fistulas, pacemakers, intra-aortic balloon pumps and central intravenous catheters, play a causative role in these cases. The increasing population with prosthetic valve endocarditis (PVE) poses special diagnostic and management issues discussed later in this chapter.

With these demographic variables, the spectrum of causative organisms has shifted in a pattern predictive of a trend toward increasing IE cases with nervous system involvement from virulent organisms in populations at risk for a variety of often multiple antibiotic-resistant organisms due to concurrent disease such as systemic neoplasia and multiple organ failure. The distribution of causative organisms varies somewhat among institutions due to disparate referral patterns and nosocomial issues, but the decline of streptococci as causative organisms from 90% in the preantibiotic era to less than 50% is a uniform observation.[15,16] Of particular neurological relevance are two streptococci: Group D, of which *Enterococcus fecalis* is the most common, is problematic because it is often antibiotic-resistant, and *S. bovis*, observed in association with digestive tract malignancy, has been the source of late cerebral emboli.

S. aureus now accounts for up to 40% of IE cases in some institutions, and represented 32% of IE cases in the author's recent series.[15,25] Valves with no apparent cardiac lesions are affected in up to 30% of *S. aureus* cases. Staphylococcal species account for nearly one half of PVE pathogens.[12] A wider range of pathogens afflicts elderly patients with multiple system disease and immunocompromised patients. These organisms include the HACEK bacteria group (*Hemophilus, Actinobacillus, Cardiobacterium, Eikenella,* and *Kingella*) and fungal organisms. In these often heavily-pretreated patients, blood cultures are persistently negative, though even in untreated patients, culture-negative endocarditis appears to be increasingly frequent.[26]

In contrast to the above data from the United States, IE in developing countries has a different patient base and bacteriologic spectrum. A review of 110 patients from a southern Indian referral hospital between 1977 and 1994 determined that rheumatic heart disease remained the most frequent underlying cardiac lesion in endocarditis patients with a mean age of 24. However, neurological complications were frequent (52.7%) and mortality higher in the group with neurological complications possibly because delay in diagnosis of IE was more common in the group with neurological complications.[27] As international travel increases the likelihood that patients from developing countries will be seen by US-trained neurologists and emergency personnel, the varying demographics of IE must be known in order to maintain an appropriate index of suspicion when a young patient presents with a stroke.

From the neurologist's perspective, it is the increasing incidence of *S. aureus* IE coupled with the older age range of the population that alters the pace and severity of neurological problems. Table 3 highlights features of neurological relevance in *S. aureus* endocarditis. Though intravenous drug abuse is a major risk factor, the behavior of this virulent organism does not depend on the predisposing factor. A recent Danish series of 250 patients with *S. aureus* endocarditis but no history of intravenous drug abuse reports figures very similar to those in series of intravenous drug

Table 3

Major Clinical Features of *Staphylococcus aureus* Endocarditis

1. **INCIDENCE:** up to 40% of infective endocarditis patients in recent series
2. **RISK FACTORS:** 60% of patients are intravenous drug abusers
   * 50% of intravenous drug abusers had *S. aureus* as pathogen
   * 50% of patients with prosthetic valve endocarditis had *S. aureus* as pathogen
3. **MORTALITY:** 32% *S. aureus* patients vs. 11.2% patients with other pathogens
   * Congestive heart failure, conduction disturbances, and neurological problems explained the excess mortality
4. **NEUROLOGIC COMPLICATIONS:** 39% to 50% of *S. aureus* group vs. 25% others
   * Early cerebral embolism, septic arteritis, purulent meningitis, and mycotic aneurysm are major issues
   * 54% to 66% of *S. aureus* neurological complications occurred at presentation of infective endocarditis vs. 19% for streptococcal cases

Data from references 12–15,23,25,47,48.

abuse-associated IE. In the group with neurological complications, 35% experienced neurological problems, and mortality was higher.[28]

Nervous System Involvement in Infective Endocarditis

In this author's recent University of Pennsylvania series, 29% of IE episodes had neurological complications.[15] Patients with neurological complications differ from those without such problems in several important respects. *S. aureus* is overrepresented as the causative organism, and intravenous drug abuse is disproportionately represented as a risk factor. Vegetations are more frequently detected by echocardiography in the group with neurological complications, but no particular cardiac valve or valves were consistently more affected in the neurological group. These findings differ from the author's earlier series, but concur with several other retrospective series in which the mitral valve was the most frequently affected valve in patients with cerebral embolism, but this frequency did not differ statistically from other valves. The mortality rate in the group with neurological complications was twice that of other patients with IE, and about one half of the mortality could be ascribed directly to the neurological problem. Table 4 compares patients with IE at the University of Pennsylvania with and without neurological involvement on several non-neurological parameters, including demographic characteristics, valve site, predisposing conditions, microbiology and clinical outcome. These data largely concur with those of Salgado, who found that age, duration of prodrome,

Table 4
Comparison of Endocarditis Cases With and Without
Neurological Complications

	Patients With Complications (Total 42)		Patients Without Complications (Total 102)	
	N	%	N	%
Age (mean)	48		53	
Sex				
Male	25	70	70	71
Female	12	30	28	29
Type of valve				
Native	37	88	93	91
Prosthetic	5	12	9	9
Valve affected				
Mitral	21	50	37	37
Aortic	11	26	20	20
Mitral and Aortic	3	7	12	11.7
Tricuspid	2	4.7	9	8.8
Anticoagulation	2	4.7	10	10
Vegetations by echo	22/39	59*	35/84	40.6
Organism				
S. aureus	18	43*	28	28
S. viridans	6	14	25	24
Enterococcus	4	9.6	18	17
S. epidermidis	2	4.8	12	11.7
Culture negative	1	2.4	7	6.8
Other	11	26*	12	11.7
Risk factor				
Intravenous drug use	18	50*	28	28
Rheumatic heart disease	4	11	6	6.1
Nosocomial	5	14	14	14
None identifiable	2	5.4	9	9
Outcome				
Improved without surgery	16	40	65	64
Improved, valve replaced	11	27.5	24	23.5
Death	13	32*	13	12.7
due to neurological complication	6	14	0	0

* $p < 0.05$.
Reprinted, with permission, from reference 15.

anticoagulation at onset and atrial fibrillation were of no predictive value for the development of neurological complications.[12]

Pathophysiology

The major neurological manifestations of endocarditis reflect focal, multifocal, or generalized brain dysfunction and include both ischemic and hemorrhagic stroke, encephalopathy and CNS infection (meningitis, abscess). Three overlapping mechanisms are responsible for these diverse complications: embolization to large and small arteries, infection of brain and meninges, and toxic or immune-mediated injury.

It is postulated that the antithrombotic properties of the cardiac endothelial surface are lost during infective endocarditis. Animal models suggest that bacteria can adhere to damaged endothelium and colonize cardiac tissue with subsequent platelet-fibrin deposition. Colonization with a virulent bacterial species results in further endocardial surface damage and growth of a soft, friable vegetation with a propensity for embolization. Embolism of infected thrombi can result in bland infarction, micro- or macroabscess formation, septic vasculitis or mycotic aneurysm. These events constitute a continuum, the outcome of which depends on host defenses, pathogen virulence and timing of antibiotic therapy. Continuous bacteremia can produce fever with delirium or can result in metastatic infection of the brain or meninges. Therefore, encephalopathy, the presenting symptom in 27% of elderly patients in one series, can be a nonspecific finding or can represent direct brain infection. The differential diagnosis of encephalopathy in IE includes multiple microabscesses, meningitis, toxic reaction to drugs, metabolic derangement and a low flow state based on cardiac compromise in the form of congestive heart failure, perivalvular abscesses and arrhythmias.

A final mechanism of neurological compromise in IE is the formation of circulating immune complexes such as glomerulonephritis that may play a role in systemic dysfunction, in clinical signs such as petechiae, Osler's nodes, and Janeway's lesions, and in several infrequent neurological sequelae, including late aneurysmal rupture and mononeuropathies.[29,30] Alajouanine and colleagues described late focal neurological deficits due to a "proliferative endarteritis" with thrombotic occlusion, and Venger described late, recurrent aneurysmal hemorrhage.[31,32]

Incidence and Type of Neurological Complications

A neurological problem complicated 42 of 144 episodes of IE, or 29%, in the recent University of Pennsylvania series, whose results are quite representative of other institutional experience and so will be reviewed in detail here. Cerebral embolism was the most common neurological complication, occurring in 20 of 144 patients (14%). Sudden focal neurological episodes were all investigated with computed tomography (CT) and in many instances with magnetic resonance imaging (MRI). Cerebral embolism was apparently single in 9 cases and multiple in 11 by neuroimaging studies. Conversion to hemorrhagic infarction occurred spontaneously in 3 patients and in one patient while on heparin.

Primary intracranial hemorrhage was a significantly less common stroke mechanism, occurring in 4.1% of 144 episodes. Demonstrable mycotic aneurysms were found in only 2 of these patients, septic arteritis was believed to account for 3 others, and subdural hematoma and hemorrhage following embolic infarction complicated a third case. CNS infection was demonstrated in the form of brain abscess in 2% of patients and CSF pleocytosis was present in 4.1%, only one third of whom had culture-positive purulent meningitis. Only 18 lumbar punctures were performed to investigate the 144 episodes, 2 of which were done in the group without proven neurological complications.

Seizures complicated 6 courses of IE. Paraspinal abscess occurred in 2 patients. The two mononeuropathies documented were not clearly due to vasculitis and may have been caused by local compression in patients at prolonged bed rest. Visual obscurations, headache and elevated erythrocyte sedimentation rate led to the initial erroneous diagnosis of temporal arteritis in one elderly patient. Table 5 summarizes the distribution and timing of neurologic complications in this series.[15]

Of prime concern to the neurological consultant are those CNS manifestations that precede or coincide with the diagnosis of IE. Early neurological involvement is most characteristic of *S. aureus* endocarditis. Fifty-four percent of neurological events associated with this organism occurred at presentation, whereas only 19% of streptococcal cases presented with a neurological problem.[13] Salgado and others report that 16% to 23% of all types of neurological complications occur at presentation and that another 30% evolve within the first 48 hours after initiation of antibiotic therapy.[12] In the series described above, 13 of 20 embolic strokes (65%) occurred within 48 hours of admission. Of 144 IE episodes, nearly one fifth (19%) presented with a neurological problem, only 3 of which, however, had no other evidence of IE.

Differential Diagnosis

Because IE has protean initial manifestations, the neurologist must consider the possibility of IE in many different types of patients. The readily

Table 5

Neurological Complications in 42 Episodes of Infective Endocarditis

	N	% of Total	% at Presentation
I. *Stroke**			
Cerebral embolism	20	14	7
Single	9		
Multiple	11		
Hemorrhagic	3		
Hemorrhagic on warfarin	1		
Intracranial hemorrhage	6	4.1	2.8
Mycotic aneurysm	2		
Septic arteritis (?)	3		
Subdural hematoma and hemorrhagic infarction	1		
II. *CNS Infection*			
Brain abscess	3		
Meningitis	4		
Aseptic	2		
Purulent	2		
III. *Miscellaneous*			
Seizures	6	4.1	1.3
Paraspinal abscess	2	1.3	1.3
Visual obscurations	1		
Peroneal palsy	1		
Radial palsy	1		
Postoperative lower brachial plexopathy	1		
Delirium	2		
H. zoster	1		
Opiates	1		

* 13 of 20 emboli occurred within 48 hours of presentation at a time of uncontrolled infection (65%).
Reprinted, with permission, from reference 15.

recognizable situation of a febrile patient with focal neurological deficit and changing heart murmur represents the minority of case presentations. The diagnosis of IE should be considered in any febrile patient with a focal neurological deficit or headache, or with an intracranial hemorrhage in a clinical setting devoid of conventional risk factors for cerebral hemorrhage. Patients whose underlying heart condition dictates antimicrobial prophylaxis for various dental or surgical procedures should be questioned about compliance with the regimens outlined by Dajani and colleagues.[33]

Unfortunately, the constellation of focal neurological deficit, fever, elevated erythrocyte sedimentation rate and evidence of CNS infarction can be seen with numerous conditions other than IE, including atrial myxoma, vasculitis and nonbacterial thrombotic endocarditis. In many of these situations, prior diagnosis of vasculitis or neoplasia is absent. Fever, one of the cardinal signs of IE, can be obscured in many hosts, particularly those taking corticosteroids, while in others fever will ultimately be related to some process other than IE. Appropriate blood cultures are therefore essential, and recommendations are outlined in Chapter 2.

Diagnostic Procedures

Although the diagnosis of IE continues to rest on microbiological confirmation, echocardiography plays an important role in early evaluation (see Chapter 6.) Transesophageal echocardiography has proven superior to standard two-dimensional echocardiography for detection of valvular abscesses and for evaluation of PVE. Echocardiographic data contribute to the inclusionary criteria for endocarditis in recent series. Thus, a patient with a febrile illness and new vegetations on echocardiogram, may be classified and treated as a case of IE, even with negative blood cultures. Such a patient would not have been included in series of IE prior to the 1970s, so direct comparison of earlier series of IE to current study populations may not be valid.

This section will address the major controversy surrounding the association between demonstrable valvular vegetations and risk for subsequent embolism as well as increased likelihood of valve replacement for congestive heart failure. Several studies have claimed a positive correlation for embolism and valve replacement outcome criteria.[34-37] However, in 3 series, vegetations did not correlate with embolism risk and were equally common in groups with and without neurological complications.[12,28,38] In the study by Roder, 35% of patients with vegetations experienced embolic stroke versus 26% of those without vegetations (p = 0.38). However, the authors concede that these conclusions are based on the results of transthoracic echocardiograms performed in only half the patients.[28]

Roder's data show that 74% of patients with cerebral emboli had demonstrable valvular vegetations versus 50.6% of patients with all types of neurological complications versus 40.6% of those without any neurological involvement. In 3 cases, transesophageal echocardiography demonstrated vegetations where prior two-dimensional echocardiography studies failed to do so. These figures agree with 2 meta-analyses. Lutas' composite report of 11 studies found an embolic rate of 26% in patients with demonstrable vegetations and 15% in those with normal echocardiograms.[39] Vegetations larger than 10 mm were generally associated with a higher incidence of emboli than smaller lesions (47% versus 19%). These data may be complicated by the fact that early embolization due to pathogens like *S. aureus* may reduce the size of echocardiographically visible lesions. Clinically, repeat embolization is uncommon, and most emboli occur early in the course of the illness. A second meta-analysis by Tischler surveyed 738 patients in 10 studies. Tischler concluded that echocardiographically detected left-sided heart valve vegetations greater than 10 mm increase the risk of systemic embolization and eventual necessity of surgical valve replacement by an odds ratio of 2.8 and 2.95 respectively.[40]

As further data from transesophageal echocardiography become available, management decisions may eventually be based on the presence and size of cardiac vegetations. The presence of vegetations greater than 10 mm and clinical evidence of embolism leads to consideration of valve replacement. In the absence of clinical cerebral embolism, but with large vegetations, the neurological consultant cannot yet justify prophylactic valve replacement as healing of such lesions has been clearly demonstrated. An exception to this policy is the demonstration of large vegetations in fungal endocarditis and certain PVE cases that may be considered for preemptive cardiac valve surgery because of the very high risk for cerebral and systemic embolism.

Specific Management Issues

Cerebral Embolism

Cerebral embolism is the most common complication of IE, occurring in 14% to 20% of patients and being the presenting symptom in about half of those cases. This complication is rare in tricuspid valve endocarditis. Some authors report a slight association of mitral valve infection with an increased risk of cerebral embolism.[11,12] Others do not find this association.[15,38] There is a much stronger association of cerebral ischemia with causative organism. Infection with *S. aureus* has been associated with roughly double the frequency of cerebral embolism compared with that of streptococcal IE cases.[12,14,15]

The advent of CT scanning has brought an increase in detection of multiple emboli (18% in pre-CT era versus 50% post-CT).[1,10,41] CT, which can differentiate bland from hemorrhagic infarctions, is the diagnostic procedure of choice for the emergent investigation of sudden focal neurological deficit in IE. MRI, which demonstrates well the evolution of neuropathological processes from cerebral emboli to cerebritis to microabscess and aneurysm or abscess formation, is more useful in follow-up of cerebral

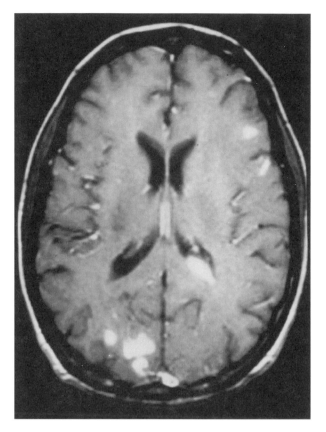

Figure 1. MRI of the brain after gadolinium administration in a patient with *S. aureus* endocarditis involving the mitral valve shows multiple bilateral enhancing lesions consistent with embolic infarctions, some of which were hemorrhagic on unenhanced short TR images (not shown). This patient also had meningitis, whose pathogenesis is suggested by the enhancing choroidal lesion with ependymal extension.

emboli. (Figure 1). Follow-up MRI, if clinically feasible, is done at 1- to 2-week intervals to ensure resolution of microabscesses or cerebritis.

Emboli cluster at presentation or during uncontrolled infection and are accompanied by systemic emboli in nearly half of all cases.[11] Only 3 of 20 emboli (15%) in the recent series by this author occurred more than 2 weeks after initiation of antibiotic therapy. One further case occurred after completion of an appropriate antibiotic course, and one patient suffered an embolic stroke after cardiac valve replacement and well after bacteriologic cure of IE. Similarly, Salgado reported that fewer than 3% of all patients with IE had cerebral emboli after infection was controlled.[12]

Patients with cerebral emboli tend to be sicker than those without such neurological problems. Valve replacement ultimately became necessary in 45% of embolic stroke patients versus 23.5% of patients without neurological complications at this author's institution. Of the 8 cerebral embolism patients who underwent lumbar puncture, 5 (62.5%) had concomitant CSF pleocytosis. Thus, multiple neurological complications of IE in a single patient are quite common.

Despite the early morbidity and mortality from cerebral embolism, a case of cured native valve endocarditis (NVE) does not change future stroke risk in patients with valvular heart disease. Salgado followed a group of 140 patients for 22 months after bacteriologic cure. Of these patients, 15 developed stroke, 14 of whom had received prosthetic valves.[12] In most longitudinal studies, stroke subsequent to cured IE was explained readily by atherosclerotic risk factors, new IE, prosthetic valves or inappropriate intensity of anticoagulation.

Anticoagulation

The above data suggest that anticoagulation is not indicated to prevent recurrent emboli in cured NVE. A more pressing question for the neurological consultant is the role of anticoagulation during an episode of IE. Over 50 years ago, it was taught that anticoagulation would improve antibiotic penetration and prevent thrombus propagation.[6] More recently, Weinstein has argued that there is no role for anticoagulation in IE because valvular vegetations are not primarily platelet/fibrin propagating thrombi and can break off regardless of anticoagulation with subsequent risk for cerebral hemorrhage.[42] Experimental evidence suggests that the risk of hemorrhage while anticoagulated may be particularly pronounced when cerebral emboli are septic.[43] Clinical series have produced worrisome statistics, such as the 1978 observation that one-half of cerebral hemorrhages occurred in the 3% of patients anticoagulated at the time of embolism.[11]

Such observations have resulted in a confusing set of recommendations about 1) instituting anticoagulation after cerebral emboli; 2) withholding and reinstituting anticoagulation during the course of treatment of IE in patients for whom chronic anticoagulation is otherwise indicated; and 3) withholding anticoagulation in PVE. The advent of CT and MRI has given us a better understanding of the rate of transformation of bland to hemorrhagic infarction and the time course of resolution of blood. In this context, the issues of anticoagulation in NVE and PVE will be addressed separately.

In NVE, the embolic recurrence rate is low after infection is controlled. Because most emboli occur within the first 48 hours, anticoagulation is of no benefit in preventing recurrent embolic stroke. If recurrent emboli develop, vigorous effort to control infection should be made, including consideration of cardiac surgery for patients with large or growing vegetations (greater than 10 mm). The neurologist should counsel withholding of anticoagulation for at least 48 hours in cardiac situations for which it is otherwise indicated to minimize risk of bleeding into infarcted cerebrum. If emboli develop in an anticoagulated patient, the neurologist should advise cessation of anticoagulation for at least 48 hours for similar reasons, with a follow-up CT before reinstitution of anticoagulation to insure that there has been no hemorrhagic transformation. On the other hand, the uncomplicated development of NVE or PVE without emboli does not dictate cessation of otherwise indicated anticoagulation therapy.[44,45] Aspirin and other antiplatelet drugs have been evaluated in several small studies. In the study by Taha, the incidence of stroke on CT was prospectively compared in patients with IE randomized to low-dose (75 mg) aspirin or no aspirin for 38 days. One patient in the nontreated group developed a cerebral infarction.[46] A larger trial is needed to establish the efficacy of aspirin prophylaxis for embolic infarction in IE. Consideration is being given to a trial of low molecular weight heparin therapy (enoxaparin) in this setting as well.

Prosthetic Valve Endocarditis: Special Considerations

Patients with bioprosthetic or mechanical cardiac valves have a 1% to 4% incidence of IE, conventionally divided into "late" (more than 60 days postoperatively) and "early" (less than 60 days postoperatively). Overall, the incidence of cerebral embolism is about equal in NVE and PVE. Although the percentage of PVE cases in various series reflects hospital referral patterns, aggregate analysis of more than 200 patients in the literature suggests that inadequately anticoagulated patients with mechanical valves are at greatest risk for embolism during IE.[16,47,48] Thus, anticoagulation should be continued at the onset of PVE in a high-risk mechanical valve. However, the occurrence of a hemorrhage after embolization in an anticoagulated patient is associated with a mortality rate in excess of 80%. A recent study by Leport suggests that heparin may be safer than warfarin in the high-risk population of patients with mechanical prosthetic valves. Fifteen of 16 such patients treated with heparin were embolism-free.[49] If embolism occurs in an anticoagulated patient, anticoagulation should be discontinued for 48 hours with repeat CT scanning before reinstitution of heparin. For the highest-risk mechanical valves such as those manufactured by St. Jude Medical (St. Paul, MN) or Bjork-Shiley (Irvine, CA), modification of this procedure may be necessary, with careful monitoring of ongoing

Table 6
Summary of Recommendations for Anticoagulation
in Infective Endocarditis

1. The development of native valve or prosthetic valve infective bacterial endocarditis does not dictate automatic cessation of otherwise indicated warfarin theapy.
2. Anticoagulation is not indicated for the prevention of recurrent embolic stroke in native valve endocarditis.
3. Anticoagulation should be withheld for 48 hours in patients suffering a cerebral embolism while receiving anticoagulation. CT should be obtained prior to reinstitution of anticoagulation.
4. If fungal prosthetic valve endocarditis is present, consider discontinuation of anticoagulation in all but the highest risk prostheses.
5. Routine initiation of anticoagulants to prevent stroke in bioprosthetic valve endocarditis is not justified.
6. Follow-up MRI, if clinically feasible, should be done in 1–2 weeks following cerebral embolism to allow documentation of resolution of cerebritis and/or microabscesses.

heparinization. Table 6 summarizes anticoagulation recommendations for NVE and PVE. Areas of future study include the role of antiplatelet agents in prevention of embolism, confirmation of the encouraging reports of heparin safety in PVE and refinement of echocardiographic data about vegetations and the indication for cardiac surgery. The role of valve repair surgery, which may avert the long-term risk of prosthetic valves, must be clarified for patients with large vegetations at high embolic risk.

Cardiac Surgery

Patients with IE come to cardiac surgery for a combination of indications including, at times, the neurological situation. The occurrence of cerebral emboli may contribute to the decision about timing of valve replacement. The neurologist is frequently asked to comment about the risk of bleeding into an ischemic stroke during cardiac bypass or about the effect of nonpulsatile blood flow or hypotension on a recent cerebral infarction. What appears clear from various series, including this author's, is that cardiac valve replacement is not mandatory for patients with an epdisode of cerebral embolism in the absence of other cardiac indications. If emergent cardiac surgery is required for hemodynamic reasons, several studies have suggested that patients operated on within a few days of stroke may suffer further neurological deterioration.[50,51] The neurological complication rate of cardiac surgery in the author's series was 30% for patients who required valve replacement within 2 weeks of a stroke. In a recent Japanese study

---

Table 7
Indications for Cardiac Surgery in Endocarditis[1]

ABSOLUTE
  * Refractory congestive heart failure
  * Myocardial or perivalvular abscess
  * Repeated relapses of infective endocarditis despite antibiotic therapy
  * Unstable prostheses
  * Fungal endocarditis
RELATIVE
  * *Multiple cerebral embolic episodes*[2]
UNCERTAIN
  * *Single cerebral embolic episode*
  * *>10 mm cardiac valve vegetation by echocardiography*

---

[1] Indications based on neurologic issues are highlighted by italics.
[2] Multiple cerebral infarctions should be assessed by magnetic resonance imaging (see Figure 1 in this chapter).

---

of 181 patients with cerebral emboli among 2523 surgical cases of IE, a significant correlation was found between the interval from stroke and risk of exacerbation of cerebral symptoms. Of these patients, 30% had worsening neurological deficit (mechanism not defined) if operated on within one week of embolism, 16% within 2 weeks, and 10% after 2 weeks.[52] A contrary point of view is offered by Zisbrod, who suggests that emergent valve replacement confers no increased risk.[53] The consensus in the literature, and in this author's opinion, however, is that if one has the luxury one should wait until cerebral edema has subsided—at least one week and preferably more than 2. Table 7 summarizes the indications for cardiac surgery with emphasis on the role of neurological complications.

Intracranial Hemorrhage

Intracranial hemorrhage occurs in 3% to 6% of patients with IE.[11,12,14,15] Four mechanisms have been identified: rupture of mycotic aneurysm, septic arteritis, hemorrhagic transformation of initially bland embolic infarction and (rarely) immune complex injury to vasculature resulting in aneurysm formation months to years after the episode of IE.[32,54] Hemorrhagic transformation of cerebral infarction and the role of anticoagulation in IE is dealt with in this chapter under cerebral embolism. Septic arteritis produces acute pyogenic necrosis of the vasculature, and occurs early in the course of IE caused by virulent pathogens, primarily *S. aureus*. It may be more common when there is purulent meningeal inflammation.[32,55]

Mycotic Aneurysms

Infectious intracranial aneurysms, more commonly known by the slightly misleading Oslerian term "mycotic aneurysms," are recognized in 1% to 5% of IE cases and represent 2.5% to 5% of all intracranial aneurysms.[56] The true incidence almost certainly exceeds the reported one, since many aneurysms may heal after antibiotic therapy. Aneurysms associated with IE are typically found at sites where septic emboli are likely to lodge and tend to be more peripheral than those associated with extravascular infectious sources. Three quarters of mycotic aneurysms involve branches of the middle cerebral artery, and at least 20% are multiple.[11] Fungal IE is associated with large proximal aneurysms. Figure 2 shows a distal middle cerebral artery aneurysm in a patient with *S. bovis* endocarditis who was

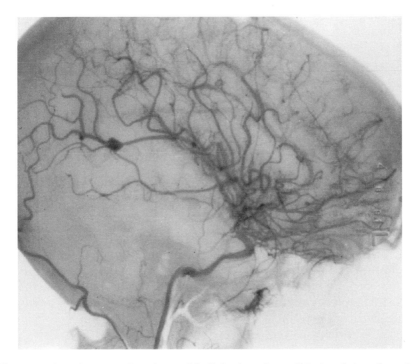

Figure 2. Arteriogram of patient with *S. bovis* endocarditis involving the mitral valve reveals an 8 mm aneurysm at the junction of the posterior temporal and angular branches of the middle cerebral artery in the posterior sylvian region. Three small aneurysms (not shown) were seen in distal branches of the calcarine artery and all resolved with medical treatment. Despite large vegetations seen by echocardiography on this patient's mitral valve, cardiac surgery was delayed for 6 weeks to allow healing of the mycotic aneurysms, and she received a mechanical prosthesis.

treated successfully with medical therapy and later with mitral valve replacement. Rarely, mycotic aneurysms can occur in the extracranial carotid artery.[57]

Mycotic aneurysms sometimes arise by superinfection of congenital aneurysms, but neuropathological study of most mycotic aneurysms confirms Molinari's original concept of pathogenesis. His dog studies demonstrated that aneurysm development depends on embolic site, host defenses, and efficacy and timing of antimicrobial therapy. Untreated animals developed mycotic aneurysm within 3 days, whereas antibiotics delayed the formation of aneurysms by 7 to 10 days or resulted in the formation of brain abscess. Invasion of the vessel wall occurred from the vasa vasorum of the adventitia with weakening and subsequent rupture.[58]

Few debates in neurological management have thrived as long as the controversy about detection and therapy of mycotic aneurysms in IE. That there is a divergence of opinion is not surprising given the conflicting outcomes of medical treatment reported in large series. In Ojemann's study of 27 aneurysms followed with angiography during antibiotic treatment, only 8 disappeared, 5 decreased in size, 4 were unchanged, 6 enlarged, and in 4 cases new aneurysms formed.[59] Schold has reported cerebral hemorrhage from mycotic aneurysms late during appropriate antibiotic treatment.[60] Bamford and Venger report new aneurysm development after bacteriologic cure, perhaps due to damage to cerebral vessels by circulating immune complexes.[61,32]

Adding 28 of their own cases to these cautionary reports, Brust and colleagues have become the major advocates for early aggressive search for mycotic aneurysms in all cases of IE. They emphasize that initial neurological symptoms were attributable to aneurysm in the minority of these patients. Four aneurysms ruptured during appropriate antibiotic treatment and a fifth patient suffered hemorrhage after completion of therapy.[62] Brust emphasizes the high morbidity and mortality from aneurysmal rupture and concludes that all patients with IE should undergo CT and lumbar puncture. Those with neurological abnormalities, including isolated CSF pleocytosis, should undergo four-vessel cerebral angiography. Brust recommends that single accessible mycotic aneurysms in medically stable patients be promptly excised.

Opposing this view are Hart, Kanter and others who emphasize the rarity of mycotic aneurysms, their symptomatic clustering in the early stages of infection, and the extremely low incidence of later rupture after bacteriologic cure.[54,63-65] Healing of mycotic aneurysms during antibiotic therapy has been documented in numerous reports.[65-69] Stilhart's systematic study correlated CT and four-vessel angiography and found a high frequency of multiple aneurysms (in 5 of 11 patients) and a high incidence of aneurysms in patients with focal neurological signs (11 of 35). However, there were no mycotic aneurysms in patients with normal CT scans, and Stilhart concluded that CT is a practical screen for aneurysm.[70] Stilhart's data must be confirmed and do not agree with those of Salgado, who found no incidental unruptured aneurysm among 24 patients who underwent angiography or autopsy.[65] Corr's recent longitudinal study of 14 patients with mycotic aneurysms on antibiotic treatment found that no new aneurysms developed during treatment.[71] There have been no longitudinal studies of the sensitivity of magnetic resonance angiography (MRA) compared with four-vessel angiography for the detection and follow-up of mycotic aneurysms, though current consensus is that MRA would miss small, distal aneurysms (which, nevertheless, might be those least likely to hemorrhage during appropriate antibiotic therapy).[72]

This author interprets the above data to justify a more conservative approach to the management of mycotic aneurysm than that suggested by Brust. The prevalence of unruptured mycotic aneurysms in patients with IE is unknown, so that for the 1% to 2% of patients who experience rupture of mycotic aneurysm after hospital admission, there is no accurate denominator for the frequency of unruptured mycotic aneurysm to determine risk. Recognizing that rupture will occasionally occur at presentation or too early for meaningful intervention, current management at the author's institution includes emergent CT for patients with neurological symptoms. The presence of blood on CT dictates four-vessel angiography, and decisions about emergent surgery will depend on the patient's medical condition and the location and integrity of the aneurysm or aneurysms. In most situations excision of mycotic aneurysms still requires ligation of the affected vessel and the likelihood of severe neurological deficit should be weighed in the management decision. Surgical techniques for mycotic aneurysm have evolved in the past 5 years, however. CT now allows localized stereotactic craniotomy with laser-guided localization and excision of distal arterial branches with infectious intracranial aneurysms.[73,74]

Though this author's policy is not to commit all IE patients to cerebral angiography, several important clinical symptoms should not be ignored even when the neurological examination and CT are normal. Severe persistent headache or "sentinel" transient embolic symptoms with normal CT scan findings dictate lumbar puncture. Because minimal aneurysm leakage can result in a focal meningeal reaction, CSF pleocytosis would sway the decision in favor of four-vessel angiography. Still to be gathered are prospective data on several high-risk groups. As the incidence rises of S. aureus as the causative organism, it can be expected that early aneurysm formation may increase. Serial prospective CT and MRA/angiography correlation would allow definitive demonstration of the true incidence and clinical consequences of mycotic aneurysms. It is possible that because one of the mechanisms of aneurysm formation is adventitial invasion,

Table 8
Summary of Management Recommendations for Infectious Intracranial (Mycotic) Aneurysms

1. Routine angiography for all patients with endocarditis and cerebral embolism is not justified. CT-documented blood should prompt four-vessel arteriography as should persistent focal headache with cerebrospinal fluid pleocytosis.
2. The indications for neurosurgical repair of aneurysm must be individualized by organism, location, number, and size, and the patient's medical condition.
3. Serial arteriography is indicated for intracranial aneurysms that are being treated medically.
4. Arteriography to detect asymptomatic aneurysms is not required prior to anticoagulation of all patients requiring emergent valve replacement. However, those who have documented aneurysms should have cardiac surgery delayed, if possible, to allow healing of aneurysms.
5. Magnetic resonance angiography (MRA) screening is not a substitute for four-vessel arteriography in high-risk situations.

clinicians should consider those patients with *S. aureus* meningitis at particular risk and deserving of preemptive angiography.

Another high-risk group consists of patients requiring acute valve replacement and short- or long-term anticoagulation. Some authorities have recommended angiography in all such patients preoperatively. While perioperative aneurysm rupture has been reported, and while the often young patients involved may receive lifelong anticoagulation with mechanical prostheses, it remains this author's opinion that available information on the low incidence of later hemorrhage, even in these groups, does not justify routine angiography.[65,75] Table 8 summarizes recommendations for the diagnosis and management of mycotic aneurysms in IE.

Brain Abscess

There is a continuum between ischemic/hemorrhagic cerebrovascular disease in IE and CNS infection, the outcome of which depends on the interplay of host factors, organism, and antibiotic therapy. MRI has proved to be a sensitive tool for the demonstration of cerebritis and microabscess formation (see Figure 1).[76] However, the incidence of macroscopic brain abscess has remained low in series that predate and those that postdate CT and MRI imaging.[11,12,77,78] In the author's recent series, three macroscopic brain abscesses developed on antibiotic therapy and resolved without surgical intervention. CT-guided needle aspiration proved useful in the management of one of these cases.

A recent clinical-pathological conference discussed by Logigian raises a cautionary tale about superinfection of cerebral embolic infarctions in the setting of central venous line-induced septicemia. A presumably initially bland cerebral infarction may have been seeded by *S. aureus* and resulted in the development of brain abscesses months after completion of a 17-day course of antibiotics.[79] Patients with "uncomplicated" septicemia and recent cerebral infarction may deserve a full IE antibiotic course, and transesophageal echocardiography may disclose vegetations and lead to reassignment of some patients with bacteremia to a longer course of antimicrobial therapy.

Miscellaneous Neurological Complications

Ocular Symptoms and Signs

Ocular manifestations of IE may be the presenting symptoms or may be asymptomatic clues to the presence of IE, particularly in fungal IE.[80] Mechanisms common to the other neurological manifestations of IE explain eye symptoms. Emboli account for central retinal artery occlusion and retinal hemorrhages, although Roth spots (retinal hemorrhages with a small white center) are believed to be due to immunologic mechanisms.[16] The unusual presentation of IE as macular holes from ocular emboli has been described recently.[81] Increased intracranial pressure from meningitis, multiple cerebral emboli or hemorrhage can produce papilledema.

Cranial and Peripheral Neuropathies

Acute cranial and peripheral mononeuropathies have been reported largely with *S. viridans* IE. Such lesions are often multiple, and, in a detailed report of 5 such cases by Jones, were the initial manifestation of IE in 4.[82] Cutaneous emboli and splinter hemorrhages corresponded to the affected peripheral nerve and embolic occlusion of the vaso vasorum seemed a more likely mechanism in this acute phase of the illness than did early immune-mediated injury in both the Jones cases and in a more recent report by Andreas.[83] Multiple nerves were involved simultaneously in several cases, making IE a consideration in the differential diagnosis of mononeuritis multiplex.[10,11] Multiple nerve root involvement also could cause diagnostic confusion with critical illness polyneuropathy.

Musculoskeletal and Spinal Complications

Back pain is a frequent symptom in patients with bacteremia. Epidural abscess, however, is extremely uncommon and no cases of IE were among those reported in a large series by Baker.[84] Three cases were seen in the author's recent series, probably reflecting a trend due to the high frequency of *S. aureus* IE. No emboli to the spinal cord were seen in this author's series or in any of the other large reports of IE. Though the syndrome of epidural abscess is familiar to most clinicians, less familiar is the clinical presentation of sepsis with pyomyositis, the infection being most often due to *S. aureus* and most frequently involving the calf, gluteal and thigh areas. Though HIV patients are most commonly affected, severe leg muscle pain as a presenting symptom of sepsis has been described in patients with organ transplantation, diabetes, neutropenia and intravenous drug use with consequent IE.[85,86]

Neurological Toxicities of Antimicrobial Agents

When a patient who has been promptly and appropriately treated for IE develops new neurological abnormalities during the treatment course, the differential diagnosis includes mycotic aneurysm development, recurrent or resistant infection, simultaneous infection with another microorganism, metabolic derangement, low flow state due to cardiac failure, seizure and coagulopathy such as dissemminated intravascular coagulation or sinus thrombosis. However, the clinician should also consider the possibility that the patient's new symptoms are due to potential toxicities of antimicrobial agents. These range from potentiation of neuromuscular blockade and peripheral neuropathy to pseudotumor cerebri, delirium and seizures. Indeed, it is those IE patients with meningeal inflammation and thus blood-brain barrier disruption who are most at risk for seizures from penicillin in the high doses necessary to treat their infection. Potential neurological toxicities of antimicrobial agents are summarized in Table 9.

Summary

Despite earlier detection, better neuro-imaging and better antibiotic therapy, the frequency of neurological complications of IE remains high in a broadening group of at-risk patients.[87] Patients with neurological complications are distinguished from those without such problems by more frequent echocardiographically demonstrable vegetations, a higher frequency of *S. aureus* IE, a rising rate of intravenous drug abuse as the underlying risk factor, and an increased mortality rate. Approximately half the mortality is due directly to the neurological complication and the balance to cardiac compromise.

The advent of MRI has altered our classification of neurological com-

Table 9
Neurologic Toxicities of Antimicrobial Agents

Neurologic Problem	Potential Causative Drugs
Seizures	Penicillin G[1], Imipenem, Aztreonam Gentamicin, Ciprofloxacin, Ofloxacin Metronidazole, Amphotericin B Acyclovir[2], Foscarnet, Praziquantel
Potentiation of Neuromuscular Blockade	Aminoglycosides, Cephalosporins
Pseudotumor cerebri	Minocycline, Tetracycline
Ototoxicity	Vancomycin, Aminoglycosides, Erythromycin
Delirium	Ciprofloxacin, Ofloxacin, Metronidazole, Foscarnet, Praziquantel, Amphotericin B[3]
Headache	Ciprofloxacin, Ofloxacin, Bactrim, Fluconazole, Itraconazole, Foscarnet, Praziquantel
Dizziness	Aminoglycosides, Minocycline, Isoniazid, Fluconazole, Itraconazole
Chemical Meningitis	Bactrim
Optic Neuropathy	Ethambutol
Tremor	Acyclovir, Cephalosporins
Peripheral Neuropathy	Metronidazole, Isoniazid, Zalcitabine (ddC), Stavudine (d4T)
Myopathy	Zidovudine

1 = high dose (e.g. for endocarditis) in patients with impaired renal function
2 = intravenous
3 = leukoencephalopathy
Reprinted with permission, from Pruitt AA: Infections of the nervous system. Neurol Clin N Amer 1998;16:440.

plications of IE, making distinction among syndromes more of a pathophysiologic continuum. An increased frequency of MRI-diagnosable cerebritis and microabscesses now explains diffuse encephalopathy in some patients with IE.

Major management controversies continue to plague clinicians who try to provide the best therapy for IE patients. The algorithm in Figure 3 summarizes the author's approach to the management of a patient with known or suspected IE and a neurological abnormality in accordance with the following clinical series-based conclusions.

1) Anticoagulation is not indicated to prevent recurrent cerebral emboli in NVE. Anticoagulants should not be discontinued because of the development of uncomplicated IE in patients with mechanical valves,

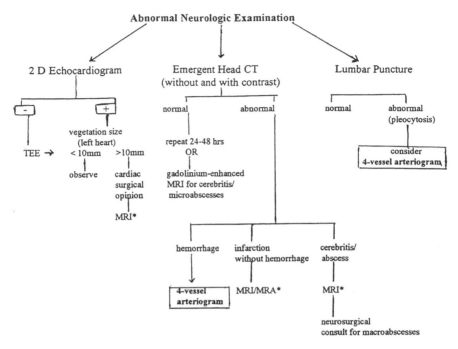

Figure 3. Management algorithm: the patient with known or suspected endocarditis and neurological abnormalities. In this management algorithm, MRI helps to define the multiplicity of cerebral emboli, thus enabling the clinician to determine the urgency of cardiac valvular replacement. It is also a better tool than CT to follow the resolution of cerebritis and abscesses. Pathways leading to 4-vessel arteriography include CT-demonstrated hemorrhage and purulent meningitis even with a normal CT, both situations being associated with a significant risk for infectious intracranial aneurysm. Arteriography is not mandatory for all patients with cerebral embolism requiring urgent cardiac valve replacement. TEE = transesophageal echocardiography; MRI/MRA = magnetic resonance imaging/angiography.

and anticoagulation should be withheld for 48 hours after a cerebral embolus to minimize the risk of hemorrhage.

2) If emergent valve replacement is necessary in an IE patient with a recent cerebral infarction, the risk of neurological deterioration remains high through the first 2 weeks after the cerebral event. If possible, surgery should be delayed for at least 2 weeks after stroke in the setting of IE.

3) Routine search for mycotic aneurysm in all IE patients is not justified. Medical treatment may suffice for many aneurysms. Advances in surgical technique may decrease the morbidity of vessel ligation, and each

Table 10

Evolving Neurological Management Issues in Infective Endocarditis

1. **Transesophageal echocardiography (TEE):** The role of TEE in defining patients who can receive a shorter course of antibiotics and in committing certain patients to valve replacement or repair must be developed further.
2. **Anticoagulation:** The role of heparin in preventing embolism in prosthetic valve endocarditis must be confirmed. The possible role of antiplatelet agents or low molecular weight heparinoids in reducing the risk of cerebral embolism is worthy of further study.
3. **Magnetic resonance angiography (MRA):** The sensitivity of MRA/MRI for detection of unruptured infectious intracranial aneurysms must be correlated with conventional arteriography. The issue of whether MRA/MRI will give sufficient follow-up information about reduction in aneurysm size, thereby avoiding repeat arteriography, is unresolved.
4. **Infectious intracranial (mycotic) aneuryms:** To resolve the controversy about aneurysm incidence, consequences, and management, a subgroup of patients at great risk for cerebral embolism (those with *S. aureus* endocarditis) should be studied prospectively with CT, MRI/MRA, and arteriography.

case should be considered on the basis of multiplicity of aneurysms, their location and the patient's medical condition.

The major challenge in the diagnosis of IE is to keep abreast of the evolving spectrum of host factors and organisms, and the major challenge in management of such patients is the establishment of criteria for identifying the few patients for whom early surgical intervention can minimize neurological morbidity. Table 10 summarizes the diagnostic and therapeutic issues for which clinicians must look to future clinical investigations for definitive answers.

References

1. Osler W. Gulstonian lectures on malignant endocarditis. *Lancet* 1885;1: 415–508.
2. Rabinovich S, Evans J, Smith IM, et al. A long-term view of bacterial endocarditis. 337 cases 1924–1963. *Ann Intern Med* 1965;63:185–198.
3. Lerner PI, Weinstein L. Infective endocarditis in the antibiotic era. Parts 1 and 2. *N Engl J Med* 1996;274:199–266.
4. Harrison MJG, Hampton JR. Neurological presentation of bacterial endocarditis. *Br Med J* 1967;2:148–151.
5. Winkelman NW, Eckel JL. The brain in bacterial endocarditis. *Arch Neurol Psychiatry* 1930;23:1161–1182.

6. Kernohan JW, Woltman HW, Barnes AR. Involvement of the nervous system associated with endocarditis. *Arch Neurol Psychiatry* 1939;42:789–809.

7. Toone EC. Cerebral manifestations of bacterial endocarditis. *Ann Intern Med* 1941;12:1551–1573.

8. Krinsky CM, Merritt HH. Neurological manifestations of subacute bacterial endocarditis. *N Engl J Med* 1938;218:563–566.

9. Ziment I. Nervous system complications of bacterial endocarditis. *Am J Med* 1969;47:593–607.

10. Jones HR, Siekert RG, Geraci JE. Neurologic manifestations of bacterial endocarditis. *Ann Intern Med* 1969;71:21–28.

11. Pruitt AA, Rubin RH, Karchmer AW, et al. Neurologic complications of bacterial endocarditis. *Medicine* 1978;57:329–343.

12. Salgado AV, Furlan AJ, Keyes TF, et al. Neurologic complications of endocarditis: A 12-year experience. *Neurology* 1989;39:173–178.

13. Gransden WR, Eykyn SJ, Leach RM. Neurological presentations of native valve endocarditis. *QJM* 1989;73(272):1135–1142.

14. Kanter MC, Hart RG. Neurologic complications of infective endocarditis. *Neurology* 1991;41:1015–1020.

15. Pruitt AA. Neurologic complications of infective endocarditis: A review of an evolving disease and its management issues in the 1990s. *Neurologist* 1995;1: 20–34.

16. Francioli PB. Central nervous system complications of infective endocarditis. In Scheld WM, Whitley RJ, Durack DT (eds.) *Infections of the Central Nervous System.* New York, NY. Raven Press, 1991.

17. Cherubin CE, Neu HC. Infective endocarditis at the Presbyterian Hospital in New York City from 1938–1967. *Am J Med* 1971;51:83–95.

18. Terpenning MS, Buggy BP, Kaufmann CA. Infective endocarditis: Clinical features in young and elderly patients. *Am J Med* 1987;83:626–634.

19. McKinsey DS, Ratts TE, Bisno AL. Underlying cardiac lesions in adults with infective endocarditis: The changing spectrum. *Am J Med* 1987;82:681–688.

20. Bevan H, Sharma K, Bradley W. Stroke in young adults. *Stroke* 1990;21: 382–386.

21. Kaku DA, Lowenstein DH. Emergence of recreational drug abuse as a major risk factor for stroke in young adults. *Ann Intern Med* 1990;113:821–827.

22. Sloan MA, Kittner SJ, Feeser BR, et al. Illicit drug-associated ischemic stroke in the Washington Young Stroke Study. *Neurology* 1998;19:1688–1693.

23. Mathew J, Addai T, Anand A, et al. Clinical features, site of involvement, bacteriologic findings, and outcome of infective endocarditis in intravenous drug users. *Arch Intern Med* 1995;155:1641–1648.

24. Aragon T, Sande MA. Infective endocarditis. In Stein JH (ed.) *Internal Medicine.* 4th ed. St Louis, MO. Mosby-Year Book, 1994. p 190.

25. Sanabria TJ, Alpert JS, Goldberg R, et al. Increasing frequency of staphylococcal infective endocarditis: Experience at a university hospital, 1981–1988. *Arch Intern Med* 1990;150:1305–1309.

26. Tunkel AR, Kaye DL. Endocarditis with negative blood cultures. *N Engl J Med* 1992;326:1215–1217.

27. Santoshkumar B, Radhakrishnan K, Balakrishnan KG, et al. Neurologic complications of infective endocarditis observed in a south Indian referral hospital. *J Neurol Sci* 1996;137:139–144.

28. Roder BL, Wandall DA, Espersen F, et al. Neurologic manifestations in Staphylococcus aureus endocarditis: A review of 260 bacteremic cases in nondrug addicts. *Am J Med* 1997;102:379–386.
29. Rubenfield S, Min KW. Leukoclastic angiitis in subacute bacterial endocarditis. *Arch Dermatol* 1977;113:1073.
30. Kauffmann RH, Thompson J, Valentijn M, et al. The clinical implications and the pathogenetic significance of circulating immune complexes in infective endocarditis. *Am J Med* 1981;71:17.
31. Alajouanine T, Castaigne P, Lhermitte F, et al. L'arterite cerebrale de la maladie d'Osler: Ses complications tardives. *Sem Hop Paris* 1959;35:1160.
32. Venger GH, Aldama AE: Mycotic vasculitis with repeated intracranial aneurysmal hemorrhage. *J Neurosurg* 1988;69:775–779.
33. Durack DT. Prevention of infective endocarditis. *N Engl J Med* 1995;32:38–41.
34. Buda AJ, Zota RJ, LeMire MS, et al. Prognostic significance of vegetations detected by two-dimensional echocardiography in infective endocarditis. *Am Heart J* 1986;112:1291–1296.
35. Mügge A, Daniel WG, Frank G, et al. Echocardiography in infective endocarditis: Reassessment of prognostic implications of vegetation size determined by the transthoracic and transesophageal approach. *J Am Coll Cardiol* 1989;14: 631–638.
36. Jaffe WM, Morgan DE, Pearlman AS, et al. Infective endocarditis, 1983–1988: Echocardiographic findings and factors influencing morbidity and mortality. *J Am Coll Cardiol* 1990;15:1227–1233.
37. Shapiro SM, Bayer AS. Transesophageal and Doppler echocardiography in the diagnosis and management of infective endocarditis. *Chest* 1991;100: 1125–1130.
38. Hart RG, Foster JW, Luther MF, et al. Stroke in infective endocarditis. *Stroke* 1990,21.695–700.
39. Lutas EM, Roberts RB, Devereux RB, et al. Relation between the presence of echocardiographic vegetations and the complication rate in infective endocarditis. *Am Heart J* 1986;112:107–113.
40. Tischler MD, Vaitkus PT. The ability of vegetation size on echocardiography to predict clinical complications: A meta-analysis. *J Am Soc Echocardiogr* 1997; 10:562–568.
41. Le Cam B, Guivarch G, Boles JM, et al. Neurologic complications in a group of 86 bacterial endocarditis cases. *Eur Heart J* 1984;5 (Suppl C):97–100.
42. Weinstein L. Life-threatening complications of infective endocarditis and their management. *Arch Intern Med* 1986;146:953–957.
43. Foote RA, Reagan TJ, Sandok BA. Effects of anticoagulants in an animal model of septic cerebral embolization. *Stroke* 1978;9:573–579.
44. Paschalis C, Pugsley W, John R, et al. Rate of cerebral embolic events in relation to antibiotic and anticoagulant therapy in patients with bacterial endocarditis. *Eur Neurol* 1990;30:87.
45. Delahaye JP, Poncet PH, Malquarti V. Cerebrovascular accidents in infective endocarditis: Role of anticoagulation. *Eur Heart J* 1990;11:1074–1078.
46. Taha TH, Durrant SS, Mazeika PK, et al. Aspirin to prevent growth of vegetations and cerebral emboli in infective endocarditis. *J Intern Med* 1992;231: 543–546.
47. Davenport J, Hart RG. Prosthetic valve endocarditis 1976–1987: Antibiotics, anticoagulation and stroke. *Stroke* 1990;21:993–999.

48. Keyser DL, Biller J, Coffman TT, et al. Neurologic complications of late prosthetic valve endocarditis. *Stroke* 1990;21:472–475.

49. Leport C, Vilde JL, Bricaire F, et al. Fifty cases of late prosthetic valve endocarditis: Improvement in prognosis over a 15-year period. *Br Heart J* 1987;58:66–71.

50. Maruyama M, Kuriyama Y, Sawada T, et al. Brain damage after open heart surgery in patients with acute cardioembolic stroke. *Stroke* 1989;20:1305–1310.

51. Ting W, Silverman N, Levitsky S. Valve replacement in patients with endocarditis and cerebral septic emboli. *Ann Thorac Surg* 1991;51:18–22.

52. Eishi K, Kawazoe K, Kuriyama Y, et al. Surgical management of infective endocarditis associated with cerebral complications: Multi-center retrospective study in Japan. *J Thorac Cardiovasc Surg* 1995;110:1745–1755.

53. Zisbrod Z, Rose DM, Jacobowitz IJ, et al. Results of open heart surgery in patients with recent cardiogenic embolic stroke and CNS dysfunction. *Circulation* 1987;76 (Suppl V) V109–V112.

54. Hart RG, Kagan-Hallet K, Joerns SE. Mechanisms of intracranial hemorrhage in infective endocarditis. *Stroke* 1987;18:1948–1956.

55. Perry JR, Bilbao JM, Gray T. Fatal basilar vasculopathy complicating bacterial meningitis. *Stroke* 1992;23:1175–1178.

56. Barrow DL, Prats AR. Infectious intracranial aneurysms: Comparison of groups with and without endocarditis. *Neurosurgery* 1990;27:562–573.

57. Hubaut JJ, Albait B, Fropier JM, et al. Mycotic aneurysm of the extracranial carotid artery: An uncommon complication of bacterial endocarditis. *Ann Vasc Surg* 1997;11:634–636.

58. Molinari GH, Smith L, Goldstein MN, et al. Pathogenesis of cerebral mycotic aneurysms. *Neurology* 1973;23:325–332.

59. Ojemann RG, Heros RC, Crowell RH. Infectious intracranial aneurysms. In Ojemann RG (ed.) *Surgical Management of Cerebrovascular Disease*. 2nd ed. New York, NY. Williams & Wilkins, 1988. p 337–346.

60. Schold C, Earnest MP. Cerebral hemorrhage from a mycotic aneurysm developing during appropriate antibiotic therapy. *Stroke* 1978;9:267–268.

61. Bamford J, Hodges J, Warlow C. Late rupture of a mycotic aneurysm after cure of bacterial endocarditis. *J Neurol* 1986;233:51–53.

62. Brust JCM, Dickinson PCT, Hughes JED, et al. The diagnosis and treatment of cerebral mycotic aneurysms. *Ann Neurol* 1990;27:238–246.

63. Kanter MC, Hart RG. Cerebral mycotic aneurysms are rare in infective endocarditis. *Ann Neurol* 1990;28:590–591.

64. Kanter MC, Webb RM, Hart RG, et al. Management of acute stroke in infective endocarditis. *Neurology* 1990;40 (Suppl 1):S417.

65. Salgado AV, Furlan AJ, Keys TF. Mycotic aneurysm, subarachnoid hemorrhage and indications for cerebral angiography in infective endocarditis. *Stroke* 1987;18:1057.

66. Cantu RC, LeMay M, Wilkinson HA. The importance of repeated angiography in the treatment of mycotic-embolic intracranial aneurysm. *J Neurosurg* 1966;25:189–193.

67. Morawetz RW, Karp RB. Evolution and resolution of intracranial bacterial (mycotic) aneurysms. *Neurosurgery* 1984;15:43–49.

68. Meyer YJ, Batjer HH. Resolution of a recurrent/residual bacterial aneurysm during antibiotic therapy. *Neurosurgery* 1990;26:537–539.

69. Frazee JG, Cahan LD, Winter J. Bacterial intracranial aneurysms. *Neurosurgery* 1986;233:51–53.
70. Stilhart B, Aboulker J, Khouadja F, et al. Should the aneurysms of Osler's disease be investigated and operated on prior to hemorrhage? *Neurochirurgie* 1986;32:410–417.
71. Corr P, Wright M, Handler LC. Endocarditis-related cerebral aneurysms: Radiologic changes with treatment. *AJNR* 1995;16:745–748.
72. Hackney D, personal communication.
73. Elowiz EH, Johnson WD, Milhorat TH. CT-localized stereotactic craniotomy for excision of a bacterial intracranial aneurysm. *Surg Neurol* 1995;44:265–269.
74. Malik LM, Kamiryo T, Goble J, et al. Stereotactic laser-guided approach to distal middle cerebral artery aneurysm. *Acta Neurochir Wien* 1995;132:138–144.
75. Bullock R, VanDellen JR. Rupture of bacterial intracranial aneurysms following replacement of cardiac valves. *Surg Neurol* 1982;17:9–11.
76. Bertorini TE, Lasater RE, Thompson BR, et al. Magnetic resonance imaging of the brain in bacterial endocarditis. *Arch Intern Med* 1989;149:815–817.
77. Chun CH, Johnson JD, Hofstetter M, et al. Brain abscess: A study of 45 consecutive cases. *Medicine* 1986;65:415–431.
78. Mampalam TJ, Rosenblum ML. Trends in the management of bacterial brain abscesses: A review of 102 cases over 17 years. *Neurosurgery* 1988;23:451–458.
79. Case records of the Massachusetts General Hospital: Case 31-1991. *N Engl J Med* 1991;321:341–350.
80. Edwards JE, Roos RY, Montgomerie JZ, et al. Ocular manifestations of Candida septicemia: Review of seventy-six cases of hematogenous Candida endophthalmitis. *Medicine* 1974;53:47–75.
81. Beatty S, Harnson RJ, Roche P. Bilateral macular holes resulting from septic embolization. *Am J Ophthalmol* 1997;123:557–559.
82. Jones HR, Siekert RG. Embolic mononeuropathy and bacterial endocarditis. *Arch Neurol* 1968;19:535–537.
83. Andreas S, Tebbe U, Holzgraef M, et al. Embolic mononeuropathy in subacute bacterial endocarditis. *Clin Cardiol* 1990;13:666.
84. Baker AS, Ojemann RG, Schwartz MN. Spinal epidural abscess. *N Engl J Med* 1975;293:463–467.
85. Bofill L, Gunnarsson G, Lewis WD, et al. Staphylococcal pyomyositis in liver transplantation: Case report and review. *Infect Dis Clin Prac* 1996;4:60.
86. Christin L, Sarosi GA. Pyomyositis in North America: Case reports and review. *Clin Infect Dis* 1992;15:668.
87. Jones HR, Siekert RG. Neurological manifestations of infective endocarditis. Review of clinical and therapeutic challenges. *Brain* 1989;112:1295–1315.

III

Management

Chapter 8

Medical Treatment and Prevention of Infective Endocarditis

N. Cary Engleberg, M.D.

Introduction

The antimicrobial therapy of endocarditis presents certain difficulties that are novel compared to the treatment of most other serious infections. In endocarditis, organisms are usually concentrated at very high density within a cardiac vegetation. Vegetations may contain as many as 10^9 or 10^{10} organisms per gram of tissue. At this high density, microorganisms grow very slowly and metabolize at a very slow rate. As a consequence, they are also killed very slowly by most antimicrobial agents and long durations of therapy are required.[1] In most infections, antimicrobial therapy that stops the growth of the infecting agent is sufficient to reverse the course of the disease. This is because the host immune system is able to clear disabled pathogens from tissues. In endocarditis, the vegetation with its layers of fibrin and platelets is a relatively privileged site. The elements of the host immune system that would normally clear these infectious agents (e.g. phagocytic cells) are unable to penetrate and to accumulate at the site of infection. As a result, spontaneous cures of endocarditis are virtually unheard of. In addition, therapy is effective only when the antimicrobial agents are able to permeate the vegetation, kill the infecting agent, and sterilize the valve.

This chapter will describe how the novel pathological features of en-

From: Vlessis AA, Bolling S (eds): *Endocarditis: A Multidisciplinary Approach to Modern Treatment.* © Futura Publishing Co., Armonk, NY, 1999.

docarditis dictate the choice and duration of medical therapy. Successful regimens for the most common etiologic agents of infective endocarditis will be discussed, and recent efforts to simplify and to shorten these therapies will be evaluated. The less stringent therapeutic requirements for the prevention of endocarditis will also be outlined.

Treatment of Endocarditis

General Principles

All patients with endocarditis should be hospitalized at bed rest and monitored carefully for signs of changing murmurs, hemodynamic compromise, evidence of embolization, signs of myocardial abscess, or extracardial infection (e.g. metastatic infection, mycotic aneurysm). At least 3 sets of blood cultures (with at least 10 ml of blood per bottle) should be obtained within the first 24 hours. Since bacteremia is continuous in endocarditis, most etiologic agents are recovered with very high probability with 2 or more blood culture sets. More than 3 cultures may be necessary if the patient has been previously treated with antibiotics. The importance of isolating the infecting agent in order to rationally guide therapy cannot be underestimated.

Because of the pathological processes described above, the successful treatment of endocarditis requires bactericidal antimicrobial therapy to be sustained for a prolonged period of time. Although antibiotics which are inhibitory but not bactericidal (i.e. bacteriostatic antibiotics) may produce a clinical response, relapse is very likely after discontinuation of therapy. The more bactericidal a drug or drug regimen is, the sooner that sterilization of the valve will be achieved. As a result, synergistic combinations of drugs that generate more serumcidal activity than single agents may improve the response to therapy, decrease the rate of relapse, or permit a shorter total duration of therapy.

In general, oral therapy has been discouraged for treating endocarditis because of the potential for erratic gastrointestinal absorption and unpredictable serum bactericidal levels. This approach is being reconsidered in certain situations now that oral antimicrobials with high bioavailability are available.[2–4]

Not all antimicrobials diffuse equally into an established vegetation. Studies with radiolabeled drugs show that some agents (e.g. teichoplanin) fail to penetrate into the center of a vegetation, others (e.g. ceftriaxone, penicillin) generate a concentration gradient with decreasing levels toward the center of the vegetation, and still others (e.g. fluoroquinolones, tobramycin) permeate the entire vegetation homogeneously.[5] Although it is tempting to assume that the penetration of these antimicrobials into the vegetation will be predictive of their efficacy, there are still no data that actually support this notion.

The effectiveness of antimicrobial therapy appears to be the product of bactericidal levels and the time over which these levels are sustained. However, intermittent dosing of antibiotics that generate very high peak levels and low trough levels is likely to be less effective than sustained levels that continuously exceed the minimal bactericidal concentration. Therefore, the object of therapy should be to achieve bactericidal levels within the vegetation and to maintain those levels continuously until valvar sterilization is achieved. All of the recommended courses of therapy described below meet these conditions.

Streptococcal Endocarditis

Most subacute bacterial endocarditis is caused by streptococci, either the viridans streptococci or the nonhemolytic, nonenterococcal group D streptococci (i.e., *Streptococcus bovis*). With a few exceptions, these organisms are usually very sensitive to penicillin G, with 80% to 85% inhibited by 0.2 μg/L or less.

The choice of therapy depends on the sensitivity of the infecting strain. To select therapy with confidence, the streptococcal isolate should be tested to confirm its sensitivity to penicillin G, including a determination of the minimum inhibitory concentration (MIC). Some streptococci manifest drug tolerance. Tolerance is said to occur when the level of antibiotic required to kill the organism in vitro (the minimum bactericidal concentration or MBC) is several dilutions higher than the MIC. The significance of this in vitro phenomenon has never been established, and there are no special treatment recommendations based on the finding of tolerance.

Infections with organisms that are inhibited by penicillin at low concentrations (less than 0.1 μg/mL) can be treated with either penicillin G or ceftriaxone for a total of 4 weeks (Table 1). Therapy with either drug typically results in a cure rate of ~98%.[6,7] For patients who are allergic to beta-lactam antibiotics, a 4-week course of vancomycin is regarded as the best alternative.[8]

In cases of penicillin-sensitive viridans streptococci or *S. bovis* endocarditis without complications or undue risk of aminoglycoside toxicity, the duration of therapy can be reduced by the addition of an aminoglycoside. In a 1981 study, the combination of penicillin G and streptomycin given for 2 weeks was as effective as 4 weeks of therapy with a beta-lactam antibiotic alone.[9] Today, gentamicin is usually substituted for

Table 1
Drug Therapy for Streptococcal Endocarditis (adapted from reference 44)

Drug	Duration
Penicillin-sensitive streptococcal endocarditis	
penicillin G[a]	4 weeks
ceftriaxone[b]	4 weeks
vancomycin[c]	4 weeks
penicillin G[a]	2 weeks
PLUS	
gentamicin[d] OR streptomycin[e]	2 weeks
Relatively resistant streptococcal endocarditis†	
Penicillin G[a] (18 million units per day)	4 weeks
PLUS	
gentamicin[d] OR streptomycin[e]	first 2 weeks
vancomycin[c]	4 weeks
Penicillin-resistant streptococcal or enterococcal endocarditis§	
penicillin G[f] OR ampicillin[i] OR vancomycin[c]	4–6 weeks
PLUS	
gentamicin[d]	4–6 weeks
Streptococcal prosthetic valve endocarditis	
For penicillin-susceptible strains:	
penicillin G[f] OR vancomycin[g] OR a cephalosporin[h]	4–6 weeks
PLUS	
gentamicin[d]	first 2 weeks
For penicillin-resistant strains:	
penicillin G[f] OR ampicillin[i] OR vancomycin[g]	6–8 weeks
PLUS	
gentamicin[d]	6–8 weeks

Antibiotic doses (assuming normal renal function):

[a] Penicillin G 12–18 million units IV daily (given q4h or by continuous infusion)

[b] Ceftriaxone 2 gms IV or IM qd

[c] Vancomycin 15 mg/kg q 12 h (adjust dose so that peak levels 1 hour after infusion are 30–45 μg/ml)

[d] Gentamicin 1 mg/kg q8h (adjust dose so that peak levels are 3 μg/ml and through levels are <1 μg/ml)

[e] Streptomycin 7.5 mg/kg q12h

[f] Penicillin G 18–30 million units IV daily (given q4h or by continuous infusion)

[g] Vancomycin 0.5 gm IV q6h

[h] Cephalothin 2 gms IV q4h, cefazolin 2 gms IV q8h, or the maximal dose of another active cephalosporin

[i] Ampicillin 12 gms IV daily (given q4h or by continuous infusion)

* Once-daily aminoglycoside therapy is not known to be therapeutically equivalent to divided doses in endocarditis and is therefore not recommended.

† MIC >0.1 μg/ml and <0.5 μg/ml

§ includes all enterococci that are susceptible to beta-lactams and gentamicin, viridans streptococci with MIC $\geq$ 1.0 μg/ml, and nutritionally-deficient streptococci streptomycin, since gentamicin therapy is better tolerated and more easily monitored, and the 2 aminoglycosides are considered therapeutically equivalent in this setting. Similarly, a 14-day course of therapy with once-daily ceftriaxone (2 gm intravenously) in combination with another aminoglycoside, netilmicin, also performed favorably in a recent multicenter trial.[10] For convenience of administration and monitoring drug levels, ceftriaxone can be combined with gentamicin, instead of netilmicin, to achieve the same result. To avoid nephrotoxicity and ototoxicity in elderly patients, it may be preferable to avoid aminoglycosides altogether and rely on longer duration beta-lactam therapy when possible.

Intensive therapy is recommended when any streptococcal isolate is more resistant to penicillin, i.e., MIC greater than 0.1 μg/mL, but less than 0.5 μg/mL (Table 1). Although there is limited formal evaluation of treatment regimens for these infections, beta-lactam therapy is usually given for 4 weeks with gentamicin added for the first 2 weeks. When vancomycin must be used instead, gentamicin is not considered necessary. Some authorities suggest that other complicated cases of endocarditis should be treated in this manner also.[11] Cases that require this intensive therapy include those with symptoms lasting for more than 3 months or those complicated by extracardial infections such as mycotic aneurysm.

When viridans streptococci are highly resistant to penicillin (MIC greater than 0.5 μg/mL), the optimal therapy is the same as that recommended for treating penicillin-sensitive enterococcal endocarditis (see Table 1). In these cases, a beta-lactam or vancomycin is given for 4 to 6 weeks and combined with gentamicin for the entire duration of therapy. Intensive regimens are also recommended for treating nutritionally-deficient streptococci. These fastidious organisms grow in culture only in the presence of special additives, such as vitamin B6 or cysteine. As a result, in vitro susceptibility tests with these organisms may be misleading. Clinical experience suggests that these infections are difficult to cure with standard courses of treatment.

Endocarditis with other streptococci, such as group A, B, C and G streptococci and *S. pneumoniae*, is sufficiently rare that direct comparative studies of therapeutic options have not been performed. Group A streptococci continue to be uniformly sensitive to penicillin G. Therefore, treatment of the rare endocarditis cases with penicillin or a first-generation cephalosporin is usually sufficient. In contrast, group B, C or G streptococci may be relatively resistant to penicillin. Many would recommend 4 weeks of beta-lactam therapy with gentamicin for the first 2 weeks in these cases. Although penicillin-sensitive *S. pneumoniae* endocarditis can be treated in the same manner as other sensitive viridans streptococci, i.e., with penicillin G, the emergence of penicillin-resistant *S. pneumoniae* during recent years makes careful in vitro susceptibility testing essential when selecting effective therapy.

Enterococcal Endocarditis

The enterococci share many morphological features with the streptococci but are now recognized as a separate genus. From a therapeutic perspective, the distinction is apropos, since the problems of intrinsic and acquired drug resistance among the enterococci are not encountered among their streptococcal cousins. Both of the dominant enterococcal species, *E. fecalis* and *E. fecium*, are resistant to very high concentrations of cephalosporins and relatively resistant to penicillin and other beta-lactam antibiotics. The penicillins (and vancomycin) may inhibit enterococci at low concentrations, but they are poorly bactericidal at clinically achievable levels for many strains. As explained above, the poor bactericidal activity with these single agents results in unacceptable cure rates for endocarditis. A 1954 Mayo Clinic review reported that only 39% of patients were cured with penicillin alone, although half were cured with daily doses exceeding 6 million units a day.[12] This relative resistance to killing by beta-lactams and vancomycin is an intrinsic property of entercocci that must be assumed even when in vitro testing indicates that a strain is susceptible to penicillin, ampicillin, or vancomycin.

Similarly, the enterococci are also intrinsically resistant to gentamicin and cannot be inhibited by clinically-achievable doses of the drug in vivo. Gentamicin is ineffective because the drug cannot penetrate through the enterococcal cell wall to reach its intracellular target, the ribosome. Fortunately, the combination of a penicillin (or vancomycin) with gentamicin produces a bactericidal combination, and is therefore a classic example of antimicrobial synergy. Theoretically, this synergy occurs because the beta-lactam disrupts the enterococcal cell wall enough to permit the penetration of gentamicin. Since bactericidal activity occurs with neither drug alone but with both together, it is necessary to continue both drugs throughout the entire course of therapy for endocarditis.

The typical therapeutic regimen for endocarditis due to enterococci with intrinsic resistance, but no acquired resistances, is shown in Table 1. High-dose beta-lactam therapy with gentamicin is the combination of choice. Vancomycin can be substituted in patients who are beta-lactam sensitive; however, the combination of vancomycin and gentamicin should not be used routinely, since there is less clinical experience with this combination and since this combination is more likely to be nephrotoxic. Uncomplicated cases should be treated for a minimum of 4 weeks. It is preferable to extend therapy to 6 weeks in established cases with symptoms for more than 3 months.

In recent years, enterococci with acquired resistance to all of these agents have appeared and have occasionally been isolated from patients with endocarditis. Resistance to penicillins, gentamicin and vancomycin have all been introduced into enterococci by transfer of genes from related organisms.

Acquired gentamicin resistance is due to the acquisition of an enzyme that modifies and inactivates the drug. An enterococcal strain carrying such an enzyme is resistant to more than 500 μg/mL of gentamicin in vitro. This level is only slightly less than the concentration of drug in the piggyback bag before it is infused into the patient! With this high level of resistance, gentamicin is of no therapeutic value, even in combination with penicillin or vancomycin. Some gentamicin-resistant strains may be sensitive to streptomycin (i.e. inhibited by less than 2000 μg/mL). Enterococci with this resistance pattern can be treated with streptomycin; however, many high-level gentamicin-resistant strains also have high-level resistance to streptomycin (MIC greater than 2000 μg/mL). For gentamicin and streptomycin, in vitro testing for aminoglycoside susceptibility predicts whether in vivo synergistic killing will occur. This is not necessarily so for other aminoglycosides. For example, E. fecium carries a chromosomal gene which prevents synergistic killing by tobramycin, kanamycin and netilmicin, even in the absence of high-level resistance by in vitro testing. Clinical failure of the combination of penicillin and tobramycin for treatment of E. fecium has been documented.[13]

Similarly, in vitro testing may not predict whether amikacin will fail to produce synergistic killing. As a result, aminoglycosides other than gentamicin and streptomycin should generally be avoided in treating enterococcal endocarditis.

Due to the lack of proven therapy and the paucity of effective antibiotics, there are currently no guidelines for treating aminoglycoside-resistant enterococcal endocarditis. However, a reasonable approach is to use high ampicillin alone for a total of 8 weeks. The expected cure rate will be 50%. Patients who relapse should undergo valve replacement surgery followed by additional monotherapy.[14,15] Alternative approaches offer little or no additional benefit and may be antagonistic.

The combination of vancomycin and ampicillin actually reduces bactericidal effect in vitro, and rifampin is either neutral or antagonistic to other drugs in vitro and has not been shown to add efficacy in standard animal models. Likewise, it is not clear whether the addition of a fluoroquinolone is beneficial.

To compound the problem in recent years, enterococcal strains have acquired resistance to penicillins and vancomycin. Such strains usually also carry high-level resistance to aminoglycosides, leaving few proven therapeutic options. There are a few caveats, however. The beta-lactam resistance of some *E. fecalis* strains depends on the production of a beta-lactamase that can be detected using a nitrocephin disk on agar plates. Although these isolates are resistant to ampicillin in vivo, they are usually sensitive to ampicillin-sulbactam (Unasyn, Pfizer, Inc., New York, NY). Similarly, there are 2 prominent phenotypes of vancomycin resistance in enterococci: The VanA strain is resistant to both vancomycin and the investigational glycopeptide teichoplanin; whereas VanB are sensitive to teichoplanin. Treatment of VanB isolates with teichoplanin has been effective in animals and may be effective in human cases[16] even though this agent penetrates poorly into infected vegetations.

Strains of vancomycin-resistant *E. fecium* (VREF) exist that are resistant to both teichoplanin and ampicillin-sulbactam and are a growing problem in many hospitals. Reports of successful treatment of endocarditis with such strains using nonconventional combinations is anecdotal at best.[17] An investigational agent, Synercid (RhPne-Poulenc Rorer Pharmaceuticals, Courbevoie, France), is a combination of two streptogramin antibiotics (quinupristin and dalfopristin) that has activity against most VREF in vitro. Unfortunately, this agent is usually bacteriostatic at clinically-achievable levels. In addition, emergence of resistant strains has been documented in patients receiving the drug.[18] In the next few years, several pharmaceutical companies plan to launch new products that may have superior activity against resistant enterococci; however, there is presently no therapy that is reliably effective.

Staphylococcal Endocarditis

Acute bacterial endocarditis with methicillin-sensitive strains of *Staphylococcus aureus* (MSSA) should be treated with semisynthetic penicillins or first-generation cephalosporins (Table 2). In the unusual case of a penicillin-susceptible *S. aureus* endocarditis, penicillin G is still the drug of choice and should be used preferentially at a daily dose of 18 million units or more. Since penicillin-sensitive *S. aureus* strains are now a rarity, opportunities to use penicillin G for treatment are infrequent. Most cases of *S. aureus* endocarditis are treated with a semisynthetic, antistaphylococcal penicillin such as oxacillin or nafcillin 2 gm every 4 hours.

The addition of gentamicin to these regimens does not appear to affect the duration of fever or mortality; however, there is evidence that the duration of bacteremia is significantly reduced when gentamicin is given in combination.[19,20] Since the potential benefit of this added therapy is marginal, gentamicin should be reserved for patients at low risk of nephrotoxicity or ototoxicity, and then only until blood cultures turn negative.

Table 2
Drug Therapy for Staphylococcal Endocarditis (adapted from reference 44)

Drug	Duration
Methicillin-sensitive staphylococcal endocarditis	
Semisynthetic antistaphylococcal penicillin[a]	4–6 weeks
+/=	
Gentamicin[b]	3–5 days
Cefazolin[c]	4–6 weeks
+/=	
Gentamicin[b]	3–5 days
Vancomycin[d]	4–6 weeks
Methicillin-sensitive staphylococcal endocarditis (selected cases)*	
Nafcillin[a]	2 weeks
PLUS	
Gentamicin[b]	2 days
Methicillin-resistant staphylococcal endocarditis	
Vancomycin[d]	4–6 weeks
Staphylococcal prosthetic valve endocarditis	
For methicillin-sensitive strains:	
Nafcillin[a]	6–8 weeks
PLUS rifampin[e]	6–8 weeks
PLUS gentamicin[b]	2 weeks
For methicillin-resistant and coagulase-negative strains:	
Vancomycin[d]	6–8 weeks
PLUS rifampin[e]	6–8 weeks
PLUS gentamicin[b]	2 weeks

Antibiotic doses (assuming normal renal function):

[a] Nafcillin 2 gms IV q4h or 12 gms/day by continuous infusion

[b] Gentamicin 1 mg/kg q8h (adjust dose so that peak levels are 3 μg/ml and trough levels are <1 μg/ml)

[c] Cefazolin 2 gms IV q4h

[d] Vancomycin 0.5 gm IV q6h

[e] Rifampin 300 mg po q8h

* Reserved for intravenous drug users whose cases meet the following criteria:[15,45]

1. Endocarditis is due to a methicillin- and gentamicin-sensitive strain of *S. aureus*.
2. Infection is shown, by transesophageal echocardiography, to involve only the tricuspid valve, and the vegetation is <2 cm.
3. Clinical and bacteriologic response occurs within 96 hours of initiating therapy.
4. There is no evidence of emboli, metastatic infection, hemodynamic compromise, or renal failure.

Although there may be a temptation to use vancomycin as the first line of therapy because of the more convenient dosing intervals, there is evidence that suggests vancomycin is inferior to antistaphylococcal penicillin therapy in terms of clinical response and, possibly, cure rate.[21,22] Vancomycin should be reserved for patients with beta-lactam allergy or cases associated with methicillin-resistant *S. aureus* (MRSA) strains.

A subset of patients with uncomplicated staphylococcal endocarditis can be treated successfully with an abbreviated course of therapy. Short-course therapy has been used for intravenous drug users with MSSA endocarditis restricted to the tricuspid valve (Table 2). If the vegetation is less than 2 cm and there is no evidence of extracardial complications, these patients can be treated with a 2-week course of an antistaphylococcal penicillin plus an aminoglycoside.[22-25] One study, with small numbers of patients, raises the question of whether the gentamicin is even necessary.[23] In these cases, short-course therapy with vancomycin cannot be regarded as a substitute for the penicillin, since relapses occur at an unacceptable rate after only 2 weeks of therapy.[22]

Intravenous drug users are difficult to treat with intravenous therapy either in hospital or as outpatients. Because right-sided endocarditis is amenable to treatment with less stringent regimens than other forms of endocarditis, there has been interest in the possibility of oral antibiotic treatment in this group of patients. The fluoroquinolones are a good choice for this type of therapy because of their excellent oral bioavailability. In a 1989 study, the combination of ciprofloxacin and rifampin cured 10 of 10 patients who completed therapy.[26] In this study, ciprofloxacin was given intravenously initially at a dose of 300 mg with oral rifampin 300 mg every 12 hours. The ciprofloxacin was switched to 750 mg every 12 hours with rifampin after no more than 7 days and continued for a total of 28 days. In a direct comparative study, patients were randomized to receive either the oral ciprofloxacin and rifampin regimen described above or conventional parenteral therapy (as described in Table 2). There was no significance between the cure rate in the 2 groups; however, the high dropout rates resulted in relatively small groups of patients who completed therapy and could be analyzed.[2] Experimental evidence suggests that later generation quinolones may be superior in efficacy to ciprofloxacin for endocarditis therapy and are less likely to select for quinolone resistant strains.[27] Nevertheless, the existing high frequency of staphylococcal resistance to quinolones dictates that these agents will not be adequate for empirical therapy, but only when the susceptibility of the infecting strain to the quinolone is already known.

Patients with MRSA endocarditis should be treated with vancomycin (Table 2). Cephalosporins are ineffective and should not be used against these organisms, even if they appear susceptible by in vitro testing. Early reports suggested that the addition of rifampin might be of some benefit in staphylococcal endocarditis; however, a comparative study of patients with MRSA endocarditis treated with either vancomycin or vancomycin plus rifampin showed no advantage to the combination.[28] Rifampin does have a role in staphylococcal prosthetic valve endocarditis (see below).

Gram-negative Endocarditis

Of endocarditis cases not associated with intravenous drug use, 5% to 10% are associated with the HACEK group of microorganisms. This acronym stands for the 5 genera in the group: *Hemophilus parainfluenzae* and *H. aphrophilus*, *Actinobacillus actinomycetemcomitans*, *Cardiobacterium hominis*, *Eikenella corrodens*, and *Kingella kingae*. These organisms are fastidious and may require 2 weeks or more to grow in culture. Occasionally, blood cultures are negative in patients with these types of bacterial endocarditis. HACEK organisms are therefore one possible cause of culture-negative endocarditis In the past, HACEK organisms were uniformly sensitive to ampicillin. Recently, strains producing beta-lactamase have emerged, and monotherapy with ampicillin is no longer recommended.[8] Instead, treatment with a third-generation cephalosporin (e.g. ceftriaxone 2 gm intravenously or intramuscularly.) Therapy is continued for 4 weeks.

A small proportion of endocarditis is due to Enterobacteriaceae or *Pseudomonas* species. This form of endocarditis is seen in hospitalized patients and in intravenous drug users; it is very rare in previously healthy individuals. In general, these infections require synergistic combinations of antibiotics for treatment and may require surgical resection even when the organisms are apparently sensitive, especially when the infection involves the left side of the heart. Sensitive gram-negative organisms such as *E. coli* and *Proteus mirabilis* can be treated with ampicillin 2 gms intravenously every 4 hours and an aminoglycoside at high dose to maintain peak serum levels of 8 to 10 μg/mL. Other gram-negatives should be treated with combinations based on in vitro susceptibility testing.

Pseudomonas endocarditis is treated with ceftazidime or an extended spectrum penicillin and tobramycin, according to in vitro suceptibility. The aminoglycoside should be dosed to achieve peak levels of 15–20 μg/mL and trough levels of 2 μg/mL or less. Both drugs should be continued for a total of 6 weeks. Recent evidence suggests that aminoglycosides may induce "adaptive resistance" in *Ps. aeruginosa* which increases resistance to this class of antibiotics for up to 24 hours. As a consequence, single daily dose therapy in experimental *Pseudomonas* endocarditis appears to sterilize valves more efficiently than twice daily dosing of aminoglycosides.[29]

Fungal Endocarditis

Endocarditis due to *Candida* species has become increasingly common, especially among patients receiving intensive care with broad-spectrum antibiotics and prolonged use of central intravenous catheters. Endocarditis caused by *Candida* is rarely cured by medical therapy alone, and most authorities recommend a combination of medical and surgical treatment. The drug of choice remains amphotericin B, which appears to be superior to fluconazole in experimental endocarditis models. In patients who develop nephrotoxicity associated with amphotericin, a lipid-associated form of the drug should be tried, such as Abelcet (The Liposome Company, Princeton, NJ), Amphotec (Sequus Pharmaceuticals, Menlo Park, NJ), or Ambisome (Fujisawa USA, Deerfield, IL). Although there are no comparative data in humans, experimental animal studies show no evidence of improved valve sterilization when 5-flucytosine or rifampin are given with amphotericin.[30]

In preparation for valve surgery, amphotericin should be administered for 1–2 weeks, when possible. Postoperative therapy should be continued for 6 to 8 weeks. In patients who have absolute contraindications for surgery, amphotericin therapy should be given as recommended above and followed by long-term treatment with oral fluconazole (e.g. 400 mg to 800 mg per day for 6 months or longer).

There are occasional reports of "cure" of candidal endocarditis with long-term oral fluconazole therapy, particularly with right-sided disease.[31,32] However, most experience suggests that patients treated in this way will ultimately relapse. Oral fluconazole may be useful for ongoing suppressive therapy in patients who cannot undergo surgery, but more clinical experience will be needed to know when such an approach may be feasible and safe.

Endocarditis cases involving other fungi are less common. See chapter 15 for further explanation.

Culture-negative Endocarditis

Culture-negative endocarditis is diagnosed when the classic symptoms and clinical manifestations of endocarditis are present, but the blood cultures are repeatedly negative. There are a variety of reasons for negative blood culture, including partial antimicrobial treatment, extended course of illness (especially with right-sided disease), mural endocarditis (e.g. infected ventricular septal defect), infection with a fastidious microorganism (e.g. the HACEK organisms, nutritionally deficient streptococci, *Neisseria* species, *Brucella* species), or infection with an obligate intracellular pathogen (e.g. *Chlamydia*, *Coxiella*, *Histoplasma*) that cannot grow in blood culture.

The choice of empirical therapy should reflect the clinical presentation.[33] Subacute, native valve, culture-negative endocarditis should be treated to cover all streptococci and the HACEK organisms. Ceftriaxone plus gentamicin is a suitable choice for this purpose (see Table 1). If there is a clinical response, then the ceftriaxone should be continued for 4 to 6 weeks. Gentamicin can be discontinued after 2 weeks in patients who respond promptly.

Acute native valve culture-negative endocarditis should be treated to cover *Staphylococcus aureus*, enterococci, *Neisseria* species, and the HACEK organisms. Empirical therapy requires ampicillin for coverage of the enterococci and an antistaphylococcal penicillin or vancomycin to cover possible *S. aureus*. When there is a prosthetic valve involved, then vancomycin is the preferred choice, because of the possibility of coagulase-negative staphylococci or diphtheroid infection. Oral rifampin may be added as well (see Table 2).

Patients with culture-negative endocarditis who defervesce within 7 days of therapy have a favorable prognosis, with 92% survival. However, fever beyond 7 days is associated with a mortality of 50%, with deaths usually due to complications that would be amenable to early valve replacement (e.g. congestive failure, major emboli).[33]

Prosthetic Valve Endocarditis

The general principles of treatment of prosthetic valve endocarditis (PVE) are the same as for native valve infection discussed above. However, the presence of foreign material makes the clearance of these infections much more difficult. Mechanical and bioprosthetic valves have comparable rates of medical cure and mortality and should be treated comparably.[34] In general, standard treatment regimens involve the same antibiotics as those which are recommended for native valve endocarditis, but at higher doses and for longer durations.

Streptococcal PVE requires a minimum of 4 to 6 weeks of therapy with the addition of gentamicin for the first 2 weeks (Table 1). When relatively resistant strains or enterococci are isolated the combination should be continued for 6 to 8 weeks. Treatment of resistant enterococcal PVE is problematic at best. There is one report of cure with quinupristin-dalfopristin (Synercid).[17]

In the past, *S. aureus* PVE was treated with a combination of antistaphylococcal penicillin and gentamicin, or vancomycin (for methicillin-resistant strains). However, experience with PVE due to coagulase-negative staphylococci in humans suggests that gentamicin is an important adjunct to therapy,[35] and there is an important role for rifampin in the regimen when prosthetic materials are present. Coagulase-negative staphylococcal PVE is usually due to methicillin-resistant strains, and is therefore best treated with the combination of intravenous vancomycin and oral rifampin for 6 to 8 weeks plus intravenous gentamicin for the first 2 weeks of therapy.[36] By analogy rather than direct comparative analysis, the American Heart Association Expert Committee now recommends a similar 3-drug regimen for all staphylococcal PVE (Table 2).[8] When the staphylococci are methicillin-sensitive, antistaphylococcal penicillin should be used in place of vancomycin. Clinicians must remember that the use of rifampin will usually require upward adjustment of the warfarin dose.

Gram-negative PVE with Enterobacteriaceae or *Pseudomonas* should be treated with a synergistic beta-lactam and aminoglycoside combination for 6 to 8 weeks. Medical treatment is often insufficient, and surgery is then required. For patients with pseudomonal endocarditis who are refractory to standard therapy and are not surgical candidates, there are a few reports suggesting that oral ciprofloxacin can effectively suppress bacteremia for long periods of time.[37,38]

Candidal PVE carries a significant mortality, especially when complicated by congestive failure or persistent fungemia. Combined surgical and medical therapy should involve intensive preoperative amphotericin B administration, wide debridement of infected tissues, replacement with biological prostheses when possible, and extended postoperative antifungal therapy (e.g. 6 to 8 weeks of amphotericin B, followed by oral fluconazole for several months). Such an approach resulted in a 4-year survival in 8 of 12 patients (67%) with fungal PVE.[39] In support of an alternative approach to therapy, a 1996 case review suggests that the mortality of uncomplicated candidal PVE is similar whether treatment is combined medical-surgical (33%) or medical alone (40%). In addition, 5 patients who were successfully treated with oral fluconazole alone were described.[32] Likewise, fluconazole has been successfully used to suppress candida PVE in patients who are not surgical candidates.[3] The numbers of patients in all of these reports are small, and more experience will be needed before such therapy can be regarded as standard of care.

Monitoring Therapy

In native valve endocarditis, blood cultures should be obtained shortly after antimicrobial therapy is initiated and repeated if positive. In PVE, cultures should be obtained daily for the first few days and then weekly until the end of therapy. Cultures should become negative within 3 to 5 days of initiating effective treatment.[40]

Blood levels of vancomycin, gentamicin and streptomycin should be checked at least once during the course of therapy when these agents are used, and they may require intermittent monitoring in the event of renal function or fluid balance problems. In elderly patients, vancomycin may accumulate in spite of safe levels obtained earlier on therapy. Monitoring should be ongoing in geriatric patients. Likewise, in patients with large body mass, vancomycin levels may fall to less than adequate levels after several days of therapy. Ongoing monitoring of peak levels as well as trough levels may be helpful in confirming the adequacy of therapy in such cases.

Controversy continues about the use of serum bactericidal assays as a means to confirm the effectiveness of therapy. Conflicting data from numerous studies have prevented any consensus regarding the value and interpretation of these tests.[41] A large, multicenter prospective trial showed that when serum bactericidal titers of 1:64 and 1:32 were achieved at peak and trough antibiotic levels, respectively, bacteriologic cure was virtually assured.[42] Unfortunately, this study did not confirm the value of the assay in predicting bacteriologic failure. This author tends to rely on these tests in cases involving usual pathogens or nonconventional drug combinations, and corrects dosing to achieve a titer of at least 1:8 or greater during the dosing interval (although there is admittedly little experiential support for this practice).

Prevention of Endocarditis

General Principles

Antimicrobial prophylaxis for all infectious diseases works best when it is: 1) given to a definable subset of patients at risk; 2) required for only a limited period of time; and 3) directed at a specific microbial agent or agents. When these criteria are met, prophylaxis is most likely to be effective in preventing infection with the target microorganisms and least likely to be associated with breakthrough of resistant microorganisms. In concept, antimicrobial prophylaxis to prevent subacute bacterial endocarditis meets these criteria. It is therefore presumed to be efficacious and has become recommended practice, even though direct proof of its efficacy is lacking and would be very difficult to obtain.

The subset of patients requiring prophylaxis are those with underlying cardiac conditions that increase their risk of endocarditis. For example, patients with prosthetic heart valves have an estimated incidence of endocarditis of 630 cases per 100,000 person-years (or 0.63% per year). Rheumatic heart disease and mitral valve prolapse with and without valvular regurgitation are associated with descending risks of endocarditis, i.e., from 440 to 55 and 4.9 cases per 100,000 person-years.[43] Antimicrobial prophylaxis is most likely to be effective for those patients with the greatest risk. Accordingly, the patients with prosthetic valves and complex congenital cyanotic cardiac disorders are always given prophylaxis for events associated with bacteremia, whereas patients who have mitral valve prolapse without valvular redundancy, thickening, or murmur are not given prophylaxis, because their risk is only marginally greater than that of the general population. The current American Heart Association guidelines propose giving prophylaxis for the high- and moderate-risk conditions listed in Table 3.[44]

In the pathogenesis of endocarditis, valvular vegetations develop after seeding of microorganisms from the bloodstream. Accordingly, prophylaxis is indicated for periods of time when bacteremia is anticipated. Most spontaneous bacteremias cannot be anticipated; however, certain medical procedures are known to cause transient bacteremia and are potentially associated with postprocedural endocarditis. For example, bacteremia can be documented after 18% to 85% of dental extractions. The peak bacteremia occurs within 30 seconds of the extraction and typically resolves after 10 minutes.[45] Transient bacteremias have been documented during

---

Table 3
Assessment of Cardiac Conditions for Endocarditis Prophylaxis

High Risk
- Prosthetic cardiac valves
- Previous bacterial endocarditis
- Complex cyanotic congenital heart disease
- Surgically constructed systemic-pulmonary shunts or conduits

Moderate Risk
- Most other congenital cardiac malformations
- Acquired valvular dysfunction (e.g., rheumatic heart disease)
- Hypertrophic cardiomyopathy
- Mitral valve prolapse with valvular regurgitation and/or thickened or redundant leaflets

*Low-risk conditions **not** requiring prophylaxis*
- Isolated secundum ASD
- Surgically repaired ASD, VSD, or PDA (after 6 months)
- Previous coronary bypass surgery
- Mitral valve prolapse, no valvular regurgitation, thickened or redundant leaflets
- Innocent heart murmurs
- Previous rheumatic fever or Kawasaki disease with no valvular dysfunction
- Cardiac pacemakers and implanted defibrillators

various other dental, respiratory, gastrointestinal, and genitourinary procedures. In general, dental procedures that involve manipulations below the gum line and that are likely to cause bleeding are associated with high rates of bacteremia with oral flora. Nondental procedures are most likely to produce bacteremia when they involve manipulation of potentially infected, heavily colonized, or obstructed viscera. For example, fiber-optic endoscopy rarely causes significant bacteremia, but the risk increases significantly with additional invasive procedures. Thus, the risk of bacteremia associated with esophagoscopy increases from 4% to 31% when combined with variceal sclerotherapy. Likewise, endoscopic retrograde choledoctropancreatography has a relatively low rate of bacteremia (5.6%) unless the biliary tract is obstructed (11%).[46] The American Heart Association recommends antimicrobial prophylaxis in patients with high- or moderate-risk cardiac conditions who will undergo dental or medical procedures associated with a high risk of bacteremia with microorganisms likely to cause endocarditis (Tables 4 and 5).

The mechanism of antimicrobial prophylaxis has been studied in animal models of endocarditis. Initially, it was assumed that only bactericidal levels of antimicrobials would prevent vegetations from forming. Subsequent experiments have shown that bacteriostatic antibiotics and suble-

---

Table 4
Dental Procedures and Endocarditis Prophylaxis

Prophylaxis recommended
- Dental extractions
- Periodontal surgery, scaling, planing, or recall maintenance
- Implants and reimplantation
- Root canal
- Insertion of subgingival antibiotic strips
- Placement of orthodontic bands, but not brackets
- Intraligamentary injections of local anesthetic
- Cleaning of teeth or implants where bleeding is anticipated

*Prophylaxis **not** recommended*
- Restorative dentistry
- Injection of local anesthetic
- Intracanal endodontic therapy
- Placement of rubber dams
- Suture removal
- Placement of removable prosthodontic/orthodontic appliances
- Electrosurgery
- Taking of oral impressions
- Fluoride treatment
- Taking of oral radiographs
- Orthodontic appliance adjustment
- Shedding of primary teeth

Table 5
Medical Procedures and Endocarditis Prophylaxis

	Prophylaxis recommended	Prophylaxis **not** recommended
Respiratory tract	• Tonsillectomy/adenoidectomy • Surgery of respiratory mucosa • Rigid bronchoscopy	• Endotracheal intubation • Tympanostomy tube insertion • Flexible bronchoscopy
Gastrointestinal tract	• Esophageal sclerotherapy • Esophageal dilation • ERCP with biliary obstruction • Biliary tract surgery • Surgery on intestinal mucosa	• Transesophageal echocardiography • Endoscopy with or without biopsy
Genitourinary tract	• Prostatic surgery • Cystoscopy • Urethral dilation	• Vaginal hysterectomy • Vaginal delivery or C-section • Surgery on uninfected tissues
Other		• Cardiac catheterization • Implantation of cardiac devices • Incision or biopsy of skin

thal levels of bactericidal antibiotics are also effective in preventing endocarditis, but only when the bacterial inoculum is low (i.e., less than the number of bacteria that would induce endocarditis in 90% of animals).[45] It is known that subinhibitory levels of bactericidal antibiotics or bacteriostatic antibiotics may impair bacterial adherence mechanisms in vitro. It therefore follows that sublethal doses of endocarditis prophylaxis may work by interfering with adherence to the endothelium or to fibrin. These findings suggest that bactericidal levels of an antibiotic need not be uniformly present to prevent endocarditis in most postprocedural settings, where the intensity of bacteremia and the probability of seeding the valve is statistically low. Thus, the antibacterial levels achieved with oral doses of recommended antimicrobials are assumed to be adequate.

Animal model studies also showed that antibiotic prophylaxis may be effective even when given up to 2 hours after the induction of bacteremia.[47] Since these experimental bacteremias (like the bacteremia following tooth extraction) last only a few minutes, it is assumed that prophylactic antibiotics do not kill the organisms before they make contact with a valve. Presumably, they exert their principal action upon organisms that are already adherent to the endocardium. This has significance for the practicing proceduralist. An operating dentist, medical proceduralist, or surgeon who intends to perform a noninvasive procedure is occasionally confronted with the necessity to extend the scope of the surgery. When the bacteremic risk in a high- or moderate- risk patient changes in midprocedure, it is not too late to give effective prophylaxis. It is recommended that prophylaxis still be administered as soon as possible, up to 2 hours after the presumed bacteremia.

Subacute Bacterial Endocarditis

Most procedure-related subacute bacterial endocarditis is associated with dental procedures and is thus caused by oral streptococci. Other bacteria, such as gram-negative enterics or staphylococci, are very rarely implicated. Consequently, prophylaxis for dental, otolaryngology, and respiratory procedures is designed primarily for activity against the oral streptococci.

For most situations, a single dose of oral amoxicillin is recommended; alternatives for allergic patients and those who cannot take oral medications are shown in Table 6.[44] Parenteral prophylaxis should be reserved for patients with cardiac conditions presenting a substantial risk of infection, rather than conditions such as mitral valve prolapse, where the risk of postprocedural endocarditis is extremely low. A recent meta-analysis of patients with mitral valve prolapse suggests that parenteral prophylaxis in this group may actually cause more deaths (due to fatal anaphylaxis) than it prevents (due to endocarditis).[48] Obviously, the clinician must judge the relative risks in individual cases of moderate- or low-risk cardiac conditions before prescribing intravenous antibiotics.

The oral streptococci are normally sensitive to amoxicillin and the other antimicrobials listed in Table 6. However, after patients have been taking these antimicrobials for a few days, the mouth may become populated with resistant organisms, and the ongoing antibiotic therapy cannot be assumed to represent adequate endocarditis prophylaxis. Therefore,

---

Table 6

Antimicrobial Regimens for Dental, Otolaryngology, and Respiratory Procedures*

	Adults	Children
Standard prophylaxis	Amoxicillin 2.0 g p.o.	Amoxicillin 50 mg/kg p.o.
Unable to take oral medications†	Ampicillin 2.0 g IM or IV	Ampicillin 50 mg/kg IM or IV
Penicillin-allergic	Clindamycin 600 mg p.o. or 1st generation cephalosporin 2.0 g p.o. OR Azithromycin or Clarithromycin 500 mg p.o.	Clindamycin 20 mg/kg p.o. or 1st generation cephalosporin 50 mg/kg p.o. OR Azithromycin or Clarithromycin 15 mg/kg p.o.
Penicillin-allergic AND unable to take oral medications	Clindamycin 600 mg IV OR Cefazolin 1.0 g IM or IV	Clindamycin 20 mg/kg IV OR Cefazolin 25 mg/kg IM or IV

* Oral medications are given 1 hour before procedures; parenteral medications are given 30 minutes before procedure.
† Other special circumstances may justify the use of parenterally administered prophylaxis at the judgment of the physician.

for patients at risk who are already taking antibiotics for another reason, it is recommended that bacteremia-inducing procedures be postponed whenever possible. Two weeks off an antibiotic should be sufficient to repopulate the oral flora with antibiotic-sensitive bacteria.

During gastrointestinal and genitourinary procedures, bacteremias may occur with enterococci or gram-negative enterics. In spite of documented bacteremias, postprocedural endocarditis with gram-negative enterics is an extremely rare event. Enterococci, however, present a real danger for the high-risk cardiac patient. Prophylaxis for gastrointestinal and genitourinary procedures is primarily focused on the prevention of enterococcal endocarditis. For these procedures, the intensity of the antimicrobial prophylaxis depends on the amount of risk presented by the underlying cardiac condition (Table 7). Patients with high-risk conditions, such as prosthetic valves, are given parenteral ampicillin and gentamicin in combination. This combination ensures that antibiotic levels bactericidal for enterococci will be circulating during the procedure. In moderate risk conditions, beta-lactam therapy alone is judged to be sufficient. The practitioner may individualize therapy to either parenteral ampicillin or oral amoxicillin as dictated by the individual case. Since enterococci are poorly susceptible to macrolides and cephalosporins, vancomycin is the appropriate substitute for ampicillin or amoxicillin when there is serious penicillin allergy.

Tables 3 to 7 summarize the 1997 recommendations of the American Heart Association committee on prevention of bacterial endocarditis.[44] These recommendations were not offered as a standard of care or as a substitute for clinical judgment, since definitive evidence that these regi-

---

Table 7
Antimicrobial Regimens for Gastrointestinal and Genitourinary Procedures*

	Adults	Children
High risk patients	Ampicillin 2.0 g IV PLUS gentamicin 1.5 mg/kg (up to 120 mg) IV *6 hours later:* ampicillin 1.0 g IV OR amoxicillin 1.0 g p.o.	Ampicillin 50 mg/kg IV PLUS gentamicin 1.5 mg/kg IV *6 hours later:* ampicillin 25 mg/kg IV OR amoxicillin 25 mg/kg p.o.
Moderate risk patients	Amoxicillin 2.0 g p.o. OR Ampicillin 2.0 g IM or IV (no gentamicin indicated)	Amoxicillin 2.0 g p.o. OR Ampicillin 2.0 g IM or IV (no gentamicin indicated)
Penicillin-allergic	Substitute vancomycin 1.0 g IV over 1–2 hours in the appropriate regimen above	Substitute vancomycin 20 mg/kg IV over 1–2 hours in the appropriate regimen above

* Oral medications are given 1 hour before procedures; parenteral medications are given 30 minutes before procedure.

mens actually protect against endocarditis is lacking. In fact, definitively proving the efficacy of prophylaxis in humans would be a daunting experimental task. A retrospective cohort analysis of over 500 patients with prosthetic valves showed that 6 of 223 patients (2.7%) who did not receive prophylaxis developed endocarditis, whereas 304 patients who were given prophylaxis remained infection-free (p = .04).[49] It has been estimated that a proper, prospective trial to assess efficacy in all patients at risk would require the random assignment and follow-up of over 6000 patients.[45]

Given the prevalence of underlying heart conditions and the frequency of dental and medical procedures in this country, the number of patients requiring antibiotic prophylaxis will be quite large. Owing to the relative rarity of procedure-related endocarditis, the number of endocarditis cases will be quite small. Most of these cases will be related to dental procedures; endocarditis related to the other medical procedures is quite rare. National surveillance of all endocarditis cases in the Netherlands showed that only 31 of 427 total cases (7.3%) were associated with dental procedures within 30 days of the onset of symptoms.[50] If the same proportion of the estimated 4000 to 8000 cases in the United States are associated with dental procedures, then only between 300 and 600 endocarditis cases a year are potentially preventable.

Acute Bacterial Endocarditis

Cases of acute bacterial endocarditis are very rarely associated with medical procedures and are therefore difficult to predict. Accordingly, there are no specific circumstances that require preventive therapy for these infections and no specific recommendations for prophylaxis. The regimens outlined in the American Heart Association guidelines for subacute bacterial endocarditis are mostly inactive against the principal agent of acute bacterial endocarditis, *Staphylococcus aureus*.

For patients with cardiac conditions placing them at risk for endocarditis, any potential source of *S. aureus* bacteremia should be treated promptly with antistaphylococcal antibiotics. These include pyodermas, abscesses, and suspected line-related bacteremias, each of which can serve as a source for valvular seeding. Standard treatment for these infectious problems should minimize the risk of subsequent endocarditis.

Summary

Treatment of bacterial endocarditis requires bactericidal levels of antibiotics over a sustained period of time to sterilize vegetations. Effective, standard regimens have been established for the more common etiologies of endocarditis. Much of the course of therapy is now routinely administered at home in stable patients. Abbreviated courses of therapy may be used in specific circumstances, and oral therapies are now being evaluated.

New guidelines for the prevention of bacterial endocarditis have recently been released by the American Heart Association. Continuous bactericidal antibiotic levels are not thought to be essential for preventing the formation of cardiac vegetations. Consequently, oral prophylaxis is now recommended in most instances. The indications for prophylaxis and appropriate regimens are summarized above.

References

1. Durack DT, Beeson PB. Experimental bacterial endocarditis. II. Survival of bacteria in endocardial vegetations. *Br J Exp Path* 1972;53:50–53.
2. Heldman AW, Hartert TV, Ray SC, et al. Oral antibiotic treatment of right-sided staphylococcal endocarditis in injection drug users: Prospective randomized comparison with parenteral therapy. *Am J Med* 1996;101:68–76.
3. Parker RH, Fossieck BE Jr. Intravenous followed by oral antimicrobial therapy for staphylococcal endocarditis. *Ann Intern Med* 1980;93:832–834.
4. Fuller RE, Hayward SL. Oral antibiotic therapy in infective endocarditis. *Ann Pharmacother* 1996;30:676–678.
5. Carbon C, Cremieux AC, Fantin B. Pharmacokinetic and pharmacodynamic aspects of therapy of experimental endocarditis. *Infect Dis Clin North Am* 1993; 7:37–51.
6. Karchmer AW, Moellering RC Jr, Maki DG, et al. Single-antibiotic therapy for streptococcal endocarditis. *JAMA* 1979;241:1801–1806.
7. Francioli P, Etienne J, Hoigne R, et al. Treatment of streptococcal endocarditis with a single daily dose of ceftriaxone sodium for 4 weeks. Efficacy and outpatient treatment feasibility. *JAMA* 1992;267:264–267.
8. Wilson WR, Karchmer AW, Dajani AS, et al. Antibiotic treatment of adults with infective endocarditis due to streptococci, enterococci, staphylococci, and HACEK microorganisms: American Heart Association. *JAMA* 1995;274: 1706–1713.
9. Wilson WR, Thompson RL, Wilkowske CJ, et al. Short-term therapy for streptococcal infective endocarditis: Combined intramuscular administration of penicillin and streptomycin. *JAMA* 1981;245:360–363.
10. Francioli P, Ruch W, Stamboulian D. Treatment of streptococcal endocarditis with a single daily dose of ceftriaxone and netilmicin for 14 days: A prospective multicenter study. *Clin Infect Dis* 1995;21:1406–1410.
11. Roberts RB. Streptococcal endocarditis: The viridans and beta-hemolytic streptococci. In Kaye D (ed.) *Infective Endocarditis*. New York, NY. Raven Press, 1992. pp 191–208.
12. Geraci JE, Martin WJ. Antibiotic therapy of bacterial endocarditis. VI. Subacute enterococcal endocarditis: Clinical, pathological, and therapeutic considerations of 33 cases. *Circulation* 1954;10:173–183.

13. Goldstein JA, Cohen H, Bia FJ. The ineffectiveness of tobramycin combination therapy in *Streptococcus faecium* endocarditis. *Yale J Biol Med* 1983;56:243–249.
14. Eliopoulos GM. Aminoglycoside resistant enterococcal endocarditis. *Infect Dis Clin North Am* 1993;7:117–133.
15. Kaye D. Treatment of infective endocarditis. *Ann Intern Med* 1996;124:606–608.
16. Nicolau DP, Marangos MN, Nightingale CH, et al. Efficacy of vancomycin and teicoplanin alone and in combination with streptomycin in experimental, low-level vancomycin-resistant, VanB-type *Enterococcus faecalis* endocarditis. *Antimicrob Agents Chemother* 1996;40:55–60.
17. Furlong WB, Rakowski TA. Therapy with RP 59500 (quinupristin/dalfopristin) for prosthetic valve endocarditis due to enterococci with VanA/VanB resistance patterns. *Clin Infect Dis* 1997;25:163–164.
18. Chow JW, Davidson A, Sanford E, et al. Superinfection with *Enterococcus faecalis* during quinupristin/dalfopristin therapy. *Clin Infect Dis* 1997;24:91–92.
19. Korzeniowski O, Sande MA. Combination antimicrobial therapy for *Staphylococcus aureus* endocarditis in patients addicted to parenteral drugs and in nonaddicts: A prospective study. *Ann Intern Med* 1982;97:496–503.
20. Abrams B, Sklaver A, Hoffman T, et al. Single or combination therapy of staphylococcal endocarditis in intravenous drug abusers. *Ann Intern Med* 1979; 90:789–791.
21. Small PM, Chambers HF. Vancomycin for *Staphylococcus aureus* endocarditis in intravenous drug users. *Antimicrob Agents Chemother* 1990;34:1227–1231.
22. Chambers HF, Miller RT, Newman MD. Right-sided *Staphylococcus aureus* endocarditis in intravenous drug abusers: Two-week combination therapy. *Ann Intern Med* 1988;109:619–624.
23. Ribera E, Gomez-Jimenez J, Cortes E, et al. Effectiveness of cloxacillin with and without gentamicin in short term therapy for right-sided *Staphylococcus aureus* endocarditis: A randomized, controlled trial. *Ann Intern Med* 1996;125: 969–974.
24. DiNubile MJ. Short-course antibiotic therapy for right-sided endocarditis caused by *Staphylococcus aureus* in injection drug users. *Ann Intern Med* 1994; 121:873–876.
25. Torres-Tortosa M, de Cueto M, Vergara A, et al. Prospective evaluation of a two-week course of intravenous antibiotics in intravenous drug addicts with infective endocarditis: Grupo de Estudio de Enfermedades Infecciosas de la Provincia de Cadiz. *Eur J Clin Microbiol Infect Dis* 1994;13:559–564.
26. Dworkin RJ, Lee BL, Sande MA, et al. Treatment of right-sided *Staphylococcus aureus* endocarditis in intravenous drug users with ciprofloxacin and rifampicin. *Lancet* 1989;2:1071–1073.
27. Entenza JM, Vouillamoz J, Glauser MP, et al. Levofloxacin versus ciprofloxacin, flucloxacillin, or vancomycin for treatment of experimental endocarditis due to methicillin- susceptible or -resistant*Staphylococcus aureus*. *Antimicrob Agents Chemother* 1997;41:1662–1667.
28. Levine DP, Fromm BS, Reddy BR. Slow response to vancomycin or vancomycin plus rifampin in methicillin-resistant*Staphylococcus aureus* endocarditis. *Ann Intern Med* 1991;115:674–680.
29. Xiong YQ, Caillon J, Kergueris MF, et al. Adaptive resistance of *Pseudomonas aeruginosa* induced by aminoglycosides and killing kinetics in a rabbit endocarditis model. *Antimicrob Agents Chemother* 1997;41:823–826.
30. Sanati H, Ramos CF, Bayer AS, et al. Combination therapy with amphotericin

B and fluconazole against invasive candidiasis in neutropenic-mouse and in-fective-endocarditis rabbit models. *Antimicrob Agents Chemother* 1997;41: 1345–1348.

31. Venditti M, De Bernardis F, Micozzi A, et al. Fluconazole treatment of catheter-related right- sided endocarditis caused by *Candida albicans* and associated with endophthalmitis and folliculitis. *Clin Infect Dis* 1992;14:422–426.

32. Nguyen MH, Nguyen ML, Yu VL, et al. Candida prosthetic valve endocarditis: Prospective study of six cases and review of the literature. *Clin Infect Dis* 1996; 22:262–267.

33. Van Scoy RE. Culture-negative endocarditis. *Mayo Clin Proc* 1982;57:149–154.

34. Magilligan DJ. Bioprosthetic valve endocarditis. In Magilligan DJ, Quinn EL (eds.) *Endocarditis: Medical and Surgical Management*. New York, NY. Marcel Dekker, Inc., 1986. pp 253–263.

35. Hammond GW, Stiver HG. Combination antibiotic therapy in an outbreak of prosthetic endocarditis caused by *Staphylococcus epidermidis*. *Can Med Assoc J* 1978;118:524–530.

36. Karchmer AW, Archer GL, Dismukes WE. *Staphylococcus epidermidis* causing prosthetic valve endocarditis: Microbiologic and clinical observations as guides to therapy. *Ann Intern Med* 1983;98:447–455.

37. Daikos GL, Kathpalia SB, Lolans VT, et al. Long-term oral ciprofloxacin: Expe-rience in the treatment of incurable infective endocarditis. *Am J Med* 1988;84: 786–790.

38. Uzun O, Akalin HE, Unal S, et al. Long-term oral ciprofloxacin in the treatment of prosthetic valve endocarditis due to *Pseudomonas aeruginosa*. *Scand J Infect Dis* 1992;24:797–800.

39. Muehrcke DD, Lytle BW, Cosgrove DM. Surgical and long-term antifungal therapy for fungal prosthetic valve endocarditis. *Ann Thorac Surg* 1995;60: 538–543.

40. Threlkeld MG, Cobbs CG. Infectious disorders of prosthetic valves and intra-vascular devices. In Mandell GL, Bennett JE, Dolin R (eds.) *Principles and Practice of Infectious Diseases*. New York, NY. Churchill Livingston, 1995. pp 783–793.

41. Coleman DL, Horwitz RI, Andriole VT. Association between serum inhibitory and bactericidal concentrations and therapeutic outcome in bacterial endocar-ditis. *Am J Med* 1982;73:260–267.

42. Weinstein MP, Stratton CW, Ackley A, et al. Multicenter collaborative evalua-tion of a standardized serum bactericidal test as a prognostic indicator in infective endocarditis. *Am J Med* 1985;78:262–269.

43. Steckelberg JM, Wilson WR. Risk factors for infective endocarditis. *Infect Dis Clin North Am* 1993;7:9–20.

44. Dajani AS, Taubert KA, Wilson W, et al. Prevention of bacterial endocarditis: Recommendations by the American Heart Association. *JAMA* 1997;277: 1794–1801.

45. Durack DT. Prevention of infective endocarditis. *N Engl J Med* 1995;332:38–44.

46. Botoman V, Surawicz C. Bacteremia with gastrointestinal procedures. *Gas-trointest Endosc* 1986;32:342–346.

47. Berney P, Francioli P. Successful prophylaxis of experimental streptococcal endocarditis with single-dose amoxicillin administered after bacterial chal-lenge. *J Infect Dis* 1990;161:281–285.

48. Devereux RB, Frary CJ, Kramer-Fox R, et al. Cost-effectiveness of infective

endocarditis prophylaxis for mitral valve prolapse with or without a mitral regurgitant murmur. *Am J Cardiol* 1994;74:1024–1029.

49. Horskotte D, Rosin H, Friedrichs W, et al. Contribution for choosing the optimal prophylaxis of bacterial endocarditis. *Eur Heart J* 1987;8 (Suppl J):379–381.

50. Van der Meer JTM, Thompson J, Valkenburg HA, et al. Epidemiology of bacterial endocarditis in the Netherlands. II. Antecedent procedures and use of prophylaxis. *Arch Intern Med* 1992;152:1869–1873.

Chapter 9
Aortic Valve Endocarditis

Lishan Aklog, M.D.
Reuben Gobezie, M.D.
David H. Adams, M.D.

Introduction

Definition

Aortic valve endocarditis is characterized by microbial infection of the endothelial surface of the aortic valve, often with extension into surrounding structures. Despite major advances in the diagnosis and treatment of this condition it remains a challenging disease with a high mortality rate. It tends to be more virulent than endocarditis originating from the mitral valve or from right heart structures. The successful management of this condition requires close collaboration among cardiologists, infectious disease specialists and cardiac surgeons. A systematic approach to this disease that emphasizes accurate microbiological and echocardiographic diagnosis, aggressive antimicrobial therapy and optimal timing of surgical intervention remains the mainstay of clinical care.

History

The earliest description of aortic valve endocarditis, by Lazare Reviere at the University of Montpelier, dates back to the 17th century. Over the next several hundred years, others including Corvisart, Laennac, Bouillaud, Virchow and Kirkes slowly unraveled the complex clinical and pathologi-

From: Vlessis AA, Bolling S (eds): *Endocarditis: A Multidisciplinary Approach to Modern Treatment.* © Futura Publishing Co., Armonk, NY, 1999.

cal characteristics of the disease.[1,2] Finally, William Osler, in his Gulstonian lectures delivered to the Royal College of Physicians in London in 1895, synthesized the findings of his predecessors to present the first comprehensive account of the clinical syndrome.[3] He also acknowledged the lack of effective treatment and lamented the fact that, whether it presented in its acute or subacute form, it was nearly universally fatal.

The introduction of penicillin in the early 1940s led to the first successful treatment of this disease.[4] Despite the dramatic impact of the introduction of antimicrobial therapy, a significant number of patients continued to succumb to ongoing sepsis or to congestive heart failure (CHF) resulting from structural damage to the valve. In the early 1960s the overall mortality remained up to 50% in patients who developed aortic insufficiency.[5,6]

The first reports of successful surgical intervention in aortic valve endocarditis did not occur until the mid-1960s. Many of the fundamental principles in the surgical management of this disease were well appreciated at that time. In 1964, Yeh and colleagues at the Medical College of Georgia reported on 6 patients who developed severe aortic insufficiency resulting in progressive, intractable congestive heart failure 4 to 30 months after successful antibiotic treatment of an episode of bacterial aortic valve endocarditis.[7] Five patients underwent suture valve repair, 4 with a Bahnson leaflet replacement. One patient underwent valve replacement with the recently introduced Starr-Edwards valve. Four patients survived, one died of cardiac tamponade and one died of sepsis. One patient who had undergone valve repair required reoperation and valve replacement for recurrent aortic insufficiency. The authors concluded that "in the course of bacterial endocarditis, if dynamic aortic regurgitation develops, the patient should be seriously considered for valve surgery soon after the blood stream has been sterilized [and] before the left ventricular myocardium sustains irreversible damage...."

In 1965, Wallace and colleagues at Duke University presented a patient who developed aortic valve endocarditis 5 weeks after urologic surgery and progressed to severe aortic insufficiency and persistent gram-negative sepsis despite 6 weeks of aggressive antibiotic therapy.[8] (Figure 1.) At exploration they found soft vegetations confined to the leaflets and performed a successful aortic valve replacement with a Starr-Edwards valve.

These landmark reports showed for the first time that surgery could salvage patients who had failed medical therapy or had developed anatomic complications despite successful control of the infectious process. They emphasized the importance of early surgery after the onset of congestive heart failure, removal of all infected tissue and aggressive pre- and postoperative antimicrobial therapy. These remain the cornerstones of the modern surgical treatment of the disease. Nearly 30 years later,

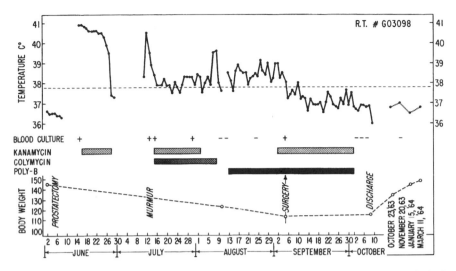

Figure 1. Graph of the clinical course (June 1963 through March 1964.) Included are the temperature curve, blood cultures, antibiotic data, body weight, and note of major events.

Wallace noted that his group's most important contribution was "demonstrating as invalid the then widely held assumption that prosthetic material could not be inserted into a site of active infection without inevitably becoming a source of continuing infection."[9] Other centers soon followed their lead and presented series of patients with aortic valve endocarditis treated surgically with good results.[10] Innovations such as the use of homograft and autograft replacement and the development of complex re constructive procedures for aortic root abscesses and annular destruction were introduced over the next 2 decades.[11] Improvements in antimicrobial therapy and in surgical and anesthetic techniques have reduced the operative mortality in recent reports to less than 10%.[12]

Epidemiology

Incidence

The incidence of aortic valve endocarditis is difficult to accurately measure as it is greatly influenced by the demographics of the patient population and the diagnostic criteria. Although reliable data are difficult to find, the overall incidence of infective endocarditis appears to have remained relatively stable and has been estimated to range from 1 to 6 per 100,000 per year.[13] The disease has evolved significantly over the past 50 years.[14,15]

This evolution has been attributed to several factors including 1) the decreasing incidence of rheumatic heart disease; 2) technological advances such as prosthetic devices, surgical repair of congenital defects and the increasing use of indwelling intravenous catheters; 3) increasing life expectancy resulting in more degenerative valve lesions; and 4) intravenous drug use.

Part of this evolution has been an increasing proportion of cases involving the aortic valve, from less than 10% in the earlier part of the century to over 50% in more recent reports.[16] The microbiology of the disease has also shifted from typical streptococci species to a variety of other organisms, including staphylococci, enterococci and fungi, many of which are more invasive and virulent than streptococci. This microbiological shift has resulted in a greater incidence of the more acute and aggressive form of the disease which has a greater likelihood of requiring surgical intervention.

The majority of cases of aortic valve endocarditis can be traced to a specific predisposing condition. However, in up to 30% of patients, no underlying cause can be identified. Each of these predisposing conditions carries its own epidemiological profile.

Specific Predisposing Conditions

Valvular Heart Disease

Aortic valve disease continues to remain the most common predisposing cause of aortic valve endocarditis. The proportion of rheumatic lesions has decreased from about 40% to 10% and has primarily been replaced by an increase in degenerative lesions. Congenital lesions of the aortic valve also contribute to the overall incidence. Up to 20% of cases of aortic valve endocarditis occur in patients with a bicuspid aortic valve. Congenital aortic stenosis carries a particularly high risk of endocarditis if it is not repaired.[16]

Hemodynamically significant lesions, including both aortic stenosis and aortic insufficiency, are particularly likely to develop endocarditis; their relative risk has been estimated at 10 to 50 times baseline.[16] Some authors have suggested that aortic insufficiency carries a higher risk since it appears to be more prevalent in most published series, but in many of these patients aortic insufficiency may have been a result of the infectious process and not the initiating cause.

Prosthetic Valves

The first reports of prosthetic valve endocarditis (PVE) appeared early in the valve replacement experience. The overall incidence of PVE in the early experience was as high as 10%[17] but has now decreased to about 3%.[18] This decline has been attributed to improved antibiotic prophylaxis at the time of implantation, which has been clearly shown to decrease the incidence of PVE.[18] However, given the increasing volume of valve surgery, the relative proportion of PVE has increased dramatically to over 50% in some recent reports.[12]

The epidemiology of PVE has been well studied in multiple reports. There has been a suggestion that valves in the aortic position carry a higher risk of PVE but not all studies support this. The risk of PVE is much greater in the early postoperative period with up to 50% of cases classified as "early" PVE, defined as PVE occurring less than 60 days after implantation. The hazard function, which provides a measure of the instantaneous risk of PVE over time, consistently shows an early peak that settles down to a relatively constant low-level risk of less than 1% per year at about 6 to 9 months.[19] It has been suggested that the risk of early PVE, as demonstrated by this peak, has gradually decreased over the years, presumably as a result of improved operative techniques and preoperative antibiotic prophylaxis, while the risk of late PVE has remained relatively constant.[20] The risk of early PVE after reoperative valve surgery was significantly higher than in primary operations.[19]

Other

Other conditions such as idiopathic hypertrophic subaortic stenosis (IHSS), certain congenital heart lesions, intravenous drug use and indwelling intravenous catheters also increase the overall incidence of infectious endocarditis but do not specifically target the aortic valve. In fact, endocarditis arising from intravenous drug use or catheters generally involves right heart valves, with only 13.5% involving the aortic valve.

Antibiotic Prophylaxis

The risk of infectious endocarditis from certain invasive procedures is a function of the amount and type of bacteremia encountered with that procedure and any specific predisposing condition. Oral and upper airway procedures are generally considered more risky than genitourinary and gastrointestinal procedures. High risk predisposing conditions include a prior history of infectious endocarditis, prosthetic valves and hemodynamically significant aortic stenosis or insufficiency. Native aortic valve disease without hemodynamic compromise carries an intermediate risk.[14] Specific recommendations on prophylaxis have been developed by the American Heart Association.[21] Oral regimens include amoxicillin or erythromycin. The most common intravenous regimens include ampicillin or vancomycin combined with gentamicin. The actual impact of pre-procedural antibiotic prophylaxis on the incidence of infectious endocarditis is controversial.

Pathology

Pathogenesis

Experimental studies have indicated that endothelial damage and bacteremia are necessary for the development of infective endocarditis.[22] Hemodynamic factors such as high velocity jets and turbulence cause endothelial damage which leads to deposition of platelets and fibrin. The platelet-fibrin complexes are then susceptible to bacterial colonization during episodes of transient bacteremia. The bacteremia can be spontaneous or related to a dental, genitourinary or gastrointestinal procedure. The bacteria's ability to colonize this fibrin-platelet complex is a function of the specific organism involved. Only a small subset of organisms that cause bacteremia accounts for the vast majority of cases of infective endocarditis. Certain organisms such as enteric gram-negative rods frequently cause bacteremia but rarely cause endocarditis.

Once a critical mass of bacteria has been deposited, one or more vegetations begin to develop over an incubation period typically lasting 1 to 2 weeks. The precise mechanism involved in the progression from colonization of the platelet-fibrin complex to the formation of vegetations is poorly understood and results from a complex interaction between bacterial and host factors. On native valves, the vegetations typically occur at the line of valve closure, usually on the ventricular side.[19] (Figure 2.) This results from the Venturi effect as blood flows during diastole from high pressure (aorta) to low pressure (ventricle). This phenomenon also occurs on bioprosthetic and homograft valves. The sewing ring of both mechanical and bioprosthetic valves is also a common site of infection and infection here can lead to periprosthetic leaks (Figure 3). Continuous shedding of bacteria from these vegetations leads to a sustained, low-grade bacteremia. Immunologic factors account for many of the signs and symptoms of the more classic, subacute form of bacterial endocarditis.

The infectious process can then lead to structural damage, typically leaflet perforation or destruction resulting in aortic regurgitation. Congestive heart failure resulting from aortic insufficiency remains the leading cause of death and the most frequent indication for surgery in this disease. Large vegetations can also cause hemodynamically significant aortic stenosis. Local extension, especially by *Staphylococcus aureus*, can lead to ab-

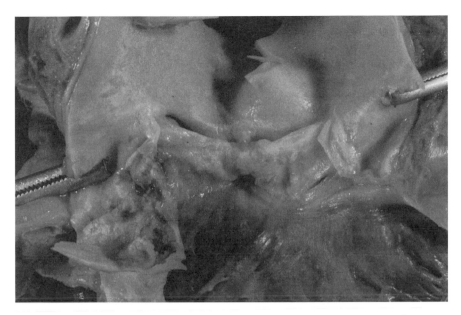

Figure 2. Native aortic valve demonstrating the vegetations that typically occur at the line of valve closure on the ventricular side. (See color appendix.)

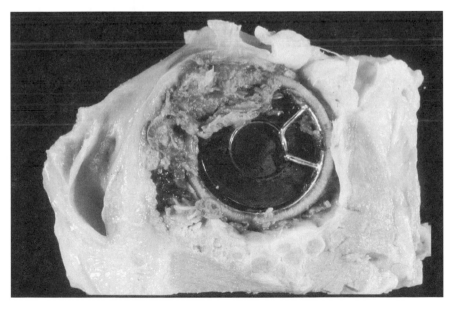

Figure 3. Vegetations on a prosthetic valve in the aortic position. The vegetations in PVE commonly occur along the sewing ring, which can lead to periprosthetic leaks. (See color appendix.)

scess formation, annular destruction, extension onto the mitral valve, pseudo-aneurysms or fistulization to other cardiac chambers. Pericarditis can be reactive or purulent from rupture of a paravalvular abscess into the pericardial space. Embolization can lead to catastrophic cerebral or visceral complications or metastatic sites of infection including myocotic aneurysms.

Microbiology

As previously mentioned, the microbiology of aortic valve endocarditis has changed significantly since its early description. The spectrum of organisms varies in native valve endocarditis (NVE), early PVE and late PVE. Three major genera of microorganisms—*Streptococcus*, *Staphylococcus* and *Enterococcus*—account for nearly all cases of NVE and the majority of early and late PVE.[23] (Table 1.) Polymicrobial infection is uncommon except in patients with a history of intravenous drug use.

Streptococcus

The viridans group of streptococci are oral flora that possess a specific predilection for diseased valves. *S. bovis* is another streptococcal species that often appears in patients with gastrointestinal malignancy. Com-

Table 1
Causes of Native and Prosthetic Valve Infective Endocarditis*

Microorganism	Frequency (%)		
	NVE	Early PVE	Late PVE
Streptococci	50	10†	30
Viridans streptococci	35	—	25
S. bovis	15	—	5
Enterococci	10	—	5
Staphylococci	25	50	40
S. aureus	23	15	10
Coagulase-negative	2	35	30
Diphtheroids	—	10	5
Gram-negative bacilli	6	15	10
Fungi	1	10	5
Other and culture-negative	8	5	5

* Data from multiple sources; frequencies are approximate.
† Includes enterococci.
NVE = native valve endocarditis; PVE = prosthetic valve endocarditis.

bined, these organisms formerly accounted for up to 80% of cases of infectious endocarditis which typically presented in its classic, subacute form. Although their relative incidence has decreased, the streptococci organisms are still the most common cause of NVE and remain a major organism in late PVE.

Staphylococcus

S. aureus and coagulase-negative staphylococci, including *S. epidermidis*, are skin flora which can infect diseased and normal valves. They are the most frequent cause of nosocomial endocarditis as well as endocarditis resulting from intravenous drug use. *S. aureus* is a major cause of NVE. It tends to produce an acute, more virulent form of the disease including local suppurative complications (e.g. abscesses, fistulas) and metastatic infection. Its presence has been shown in several studies to be a major risk factor for mortality and the need for surgery. *S. epidermis*, an uncommon cause of NVE, is the most common organism identified in both early and late PVE, probably from contamination of the valve at the time of implantation.

Enterococcus

Enterococci, primarily *E. fecalis,* are gastrointestinal and genitourinary flora that typically cause a subacute course in patients who often do not have an underlying lesion. They tend to occur in elderly patients (especially men) after genitourinary procedures.

Other

Gram-negative organisms are infrequent causes of endocarditis. Most cases result from members of the HACEK group of fastidious coccobacilli which are common oropharyngeal flora. Enteric gram-negative rods rarely cause endocarditis. Diptheroids and fungi (*Candida albicans* and *Aspergillus*) are important causes of PVE.

Diagnosis

Clinical Presentation

Signs and Symptoms

The classic signs and symptoms of aortic valve endocarditis result from low grade persistent bacteremia, the hemodynamic effects of valvular destruction, the host's immunologic response, and embolic phenomena. As the disease has evolved, fewer patients have presented with this classic picture, thereby making the diagnosis more difficult. The time course of the disease can vary from subacute to a rapidly progressive, acute, fulminant form depending on the infecting organism and host factors.

Fever is present in nearly all patients and is commonly associated with other constitutional symptoms such as rigors, chills, night sweats, malaise, arthralgia and myalgia. Most also present with *heart murmur* which can change or progress as the disease evolves. *Congestive heart failure* can appear when valvular destruction leads to acute aortic insufficiency. *Embolic events* can occur in nearly any organ system including the central nervous system (stroke, hemorrhage, abscess), kidney (hematuria, renal failure), eyes (Roth spots, monocular blindness), coronary arteries (myocardial infarction), and skin (petechia, Osler's nodes, splinter hemorrhages, Janeway's lesions).

Laboratory Tests

Abnormalities in routine laboratory tests are commonly encountered but are nonspecific. A normocytic, normochromic anemia is present in the majority of cases. Leukocytosis is also common. An elevated erythrocyte sedimentation rate is nearly always present.

Careful microbiological diagnosis with multiple blood cultures remains critically important in the diagnosis and management of patients. Multiple positive blood cultures within a 24-hour period can be useful in documenting the sustained bacteremia of infectious endocarditis and distinguishing it from other causes of transient bacteremia. About 5% of cases are culture- negative, usually as a result of prior treatment with antibiotics or fastidious organisms including the HACEK organisms, variant streptococci and fungi.

Echocardiography

Transesophageal echocardiography (TEE) has become a critical tool in the accurate diagnosis of aortic valve endocarditis. Newer technologies such as biplane and multiplane imaging and color Doppler have further expanded its role. The major goals of echocardiography are to 1) identify and characterize vegetations; 2) assess valvular dysfunction; and 3) document any perivalvular extension. TEE may also play a role in risk stratification and in predicting complications.

Vegetations

Vegetations typically appear as shaggy, oscillating echogenic structures attached to the valve leaflets. The development of TEE has dramatically improved the sensitivity of echocardiography in detecting vegetations. The improved image quality over transthoracic echocardiography (TTE) has lowered the size threshold for detection and improved the ability to determine the relationship of the vegetation to the valve. TEE has a particular advantage over TTE in detecting PVE, especially with mechanical valves where acoustic shadowing can significantly degrade image quality.

The overall sensitivity is over 90% for TEE compared to only about 60% for TTE. The negative predictive value of TEE is nearly 100% for native valve endocarditis and about 90% for prosthetic valve endocarditis. Both modalities have specificities of over 95%, with false positives usually resulting from thickened valve leaflets or difficulty in distinguishing vegetations from thrombi or other degenerative lesions. The advantages of TEE are most dramatic in PVE and in small (less than 5 mm) vegetations where the sensitivity of TTE is significantly less than 50%.[24] In patients with a negative TEE but with a high clinical suspicion of endocarditis, a follow-up study will often detect the vegetations.

Although TEE has become the gold standard, it is an invasive procedure that is more expensive and requires greater monitoring and sedation than TTE. Since TTE will detect up to 60% of cases and has a high specificity, it is reasonable to proceed to TEE only if the TTE is nondiagnostic, if a prosthetic valve is being evaluated or if paravalvular complications are suspected. If an operative indication has been identified by TTE, TEE can usually be performed in the operating room.

Valvular Dysfunction

Aortic insufficiency, with or without hemodynamic compromise, is present and easily demonstrated by echocardiography in nearly all cases of NVE and in most cases of PVE. TEE will usually visualize the actual area of valve perforation or destruction. Color Doppler can precisely document regurgitant jets and periprosthetic leaks. Aortic stenosis as a result of large vegetations can also be demonstrated when present.

Paravalvular Complications

Complications arising from local extension of the infectious process include myocardial or para-aortic abscesses, subaortic involvement including involvement of the anterior leaflet of the mitral valve, pseudoaneurysms and fistulae. These complications are more common in PVE and in cases caused by *S. aureus*. TTE is poor at detecting these complications; sensitivities of less than 30% have been reported. In the past these complications were generally discovered at surgery or at autopsy. However, with the advent of TEE, preoperative detection and characterization of these paravalvular complications have become possible in up to 90% of patients. This has allowed earlier operative intervention and better operative planning. Color Doppler is an important adjunct in distinguishing abscesses from pseudoaneurysms and in evaluating fistula tracts.

Risk Stratification

Several groups have tried to use echocardiography to identify patients with endocarditis who are at high risk of developed embolic and local complications. The results have been somewhat controversial. However, it does appear that patients with large (greater than 10 mm), mobile vegetations do have an increased risk of embolic complications. Monitoring the size of vegetations during the course of antimicrobial treatment may also be helpful. Patients whose vegetations do not decrease in size during treatment appear to have more complications. Whether early operative intervention in these high-risk patients results in improved outcome is not yet clear.

Other Radiological Tests

Cardiac catheterization is rarely indicated in the diagnosis of aortic valve endocarditis unless concomitant coronary artery disease is suspected. It can lead to embolization from manipulation of the catheter near the vegetation. A few recent reports have suggested a role for cross-sectional imaging including fast spiral CT scanning and cine-MR scanning in evaluating paravalvular structures; however, these modalities are not yet commonly performed for this indication. CT scanning may be an important aid in evaluating metastatic sites of infection, particularly the spleen and brain.

Diagnostic Criteria

Despite the advances in microbiological and echocardiographic techniques, aortic valve endocarditis remains a clinical diagnosis. Early studies of endocarditis were hampered by inconsistent and often inaccurate diagnostic criteria. The development of precise, prospectively tested criteria was a major breakthrough. The recently developed Duke criteria represent a significant improvement from prior systems because they incorporate echocardiographic data in the diagnosis.

Using the Duke criteria, the diagnosis of endocarditis is rejected if 1) another diagnosis is identified; 2) pathological evaluation clearly rules out endocarditis; or 3) symptoms resolve within 4 days of the initiation of treatment. A definitive diagnosis of endocarditis requires a positive pathological diagnosis, the presence of 2 major criteria or a combination of major and minor criteria. The major criteria are 2 positive blood cultures and echocardiographic evidence of endocarditis or a new murmur.

Treatment

Medical Therapy

The goal of antimicrobial therapy for aortic valve endocarditis is to sterilize or preferably to eliminate the vegetations. Since the vegetations are avascular, host defenses cannot penetrate them. Therefore, prolonged courses of intravenous antibiotics, often with multiple synergistic agents at high bactericidal doses are usually necessary to control or eradicate the disease. The minimal bactericidal concentration (MBC) can be significantly greater than the more commonly reported minimal inhibitory concentration (MIC) and is therefore useful in guiding therapy.

The most common regimen for streptococcal endocarditis is high-dose penicillin G for 4 weeks. Other 4-week regimens include ceftriaxone for its convenient once daily dosing, cefazolin and vancomycin for patients with beta-lactam allergies. In low-risk patients, a 2-week course of penicillin G and gentamicin appears to have equal efficacy. Enterococcal endocarditis is generally treated with ampicillin or vancomycin for 4 to 6 weeks with the addition of gentamycin during the first 2 weeks. *S. aureus* endocarditis can usually be treated with 4 to 6 weeks of naficillin, oxacillin or possibly cefazolin. Vancomycin is reserved for cases of methicillin-resistant *S. aureus* and coagulase-negative staphylococci and is often supplemented with rifampin or gentamicin. The HACEK group of gram-negative coccobacilli are usually treated with ampicillin and gentamicin. Fungal endocarditis usually requires a prolonged course of amphotericin B.

Medical therapy alone is successful at treating many cases of native valve endocarditis. In several recent reports, 75% of patients were cured with medical therapy alone.[25] However, the medical cure rate varies depending on the organism. In a significant number of the remaining patients, medical therapy can eradicate the active infectious process and allow surgical intervention for structural damage during the so-called "healed" phase of the disease. Prosthetic valve endocarditis (PVE) is rarely cured by medical therapy, almost always requiring surgical intervention.

Indications for Surgery

Approximately 35% of patients with aortic native valve endocarditis and essentially all patients with PVE will ultimately require surgery.[26,27] This rate of surgery is higher than the rate in cases involving other types of endocarditis. The following discussion will focus on the surgical treatment of native valve endocarditis. Surgical aspects of PVE will be discussed separately in a later section.

Despite thorough clinical evaluation including careful microbiological and echocardiographic diagnosis, determining if and when to operate on patients with NVE can be extremely difficult and requires sound clinical judgment. Undue attempts to avoid or delay surgery can lead to complications that significantly affect morbidity and mortality. However, premature surgical intervention can expose the patient to the increased operative mortality of emergency surgery and possibly to a higher risk of PVE.

Generally accepted indications for surgery include 1) congestive heart failure; 2) persistent sepsis; 3) recurrent systemic embolization including ischemia or infarction from coronary embolization; and 4) evidence of paravalvular extension including major conduction abnormalities. Multiple indications often exist and congestive heart failure is almost always a factor in the decision to operate. Other possible or relative indications for surgery include specific virulent organisms including *S. aureus*, gram-negative rods and fungi and high-risk echocardiographic findings including severe aortic insufficiency and large, mobile, enlarging or obstructing vegetations.

Congestive Heart Failure

Congestive heart failure is the most common indication for surgery and the most common cause of death in patients with aortic valve endocarditis. It is usually the result of valve perforation or destruction leading to aortic insufficiency. It can also result from arrythmias, ischemia or fistulas. It can be acute and fulminant, occurring early in the course of the disease and resulting in shock, acute pulmonary edema and end-organ failure. It can also be relatively well compensated, presenting months to years after the infectious process has cleared.

The mortality rate of these patients with antibiotic treatment alone is extremely high, in the 65% to 90% range, and surgical intervention is therefore indicated. Careful documentation of the anatomic defects using echocardiography is essential in operative planning. Patients with acute, uncompensated CHF that does not respond to medical therapy usually require emergency surgery despite the presence of active infection. Many patients will present with a single episode of CHF which resolves with appropriate treatment. These patients have a poor prognosis with medical treatment alone and will ultimately require surgery. However, surgery can often be delayed until after 2 to 3 weeks of antibiotic therapy as long as the patient remains stable. Patients with well compensated aortic insufficiency without CHF can usually complete a 4 to 6 week course of antibiotics before surgery is considered.

Persistent Sepsis

Careful microbiological diagnosis and sensitivity testing using MBC and aggressive treatment with adequate levels of appropriate antibiotics would result in clinical improvement in 3 to 5 days. Persistence of sepsis after 7 days of appropriate antibiotic therapy can result from 1) microorganism resistance, especially with fungal, staphylococcal and gram-negative infection; 2) extension of infection into sites that are inaccessible to antibiotics such as paravalvular abscesses; and 3) metastatic infection including distant abscesses (brain, spleen) and mycotic aneurysms.

TEE should be performed to identify paravalvular extension and CT scans should be obtained if distant abscesses are suspected. Surgery is indicated if the persistent sepsis is arising from a valvular or paravalvular focus. Uncontrolled sepsis, alone, in the absence of hemodynamic compromise from valvular destruction, is an uncommon indication for surgery.

Paravalvular Extension

Extension of the infectious process beyond the valve leaflets is relatively common in aortic valve endocarditis, occurring in up to 40% of cases, particularly in patients with *S. aureus* infection. Abscesses in aortic annulus, root or myocardium, pseudo-aneurysms, purulent pericarditis and fistula tracts represent absolute indications for urgent surgery. In the past, these lesions were rarely identified preoperatively, and these patients simply presented with congestive heart failure or persistent sepsis. With the advent of TEE, however, paravalvular extension can be documented preoperatively. The operative procedures required to treat these conditions are complex and carry a relatively high operative mortality. Every effort should therefore be made to intervene before these complications develop.

High grade *atrioventricular block* is included in this category since it results from extension of infection into the membranous interventricular septum. It carries a grave prognosis and is an absolute indication for urgent surgery.

Systemic Embolization

Systemic emboli are common in aortic valve endocarditis with clinically apparent emboli occurring in 4.2% of patients.[28] Autopsy studies have indicated that silent emboli are even more common. Certain organisms such as *S. aureus* have a higher incidence of embolization. Sites of embolization include central nervous system, spleen and other abdominal viscera, coronary arteries, ocular and peripheral. Embolization, especially cerebral embolization, can result in devastating morbidity and is a significant contributor to overall mortality.

Surgery has generally been recommended after a second clinically significant embolic event. Some authors, however, have recommended surgery after a single major embolic event. They argue that improvements in operative results and the potentially devastating impact of a second embolic event justify a more aggressive approach. This may be especially true if another risk factor for embolization, such as a large, mobile vegetation or *S. aureus* infection, is present.

Virulent Organisms

As mentioned previously, certain organisms—*S. aureus*, fungi and the gram-negative bacilli *Pseudomonas*, *Serratia* and *Hemophilus* species—are more virulent, produce a more rapidly progressive disease, lead to more complications and carry a higher mortality rate. Patients with these organisms frequently also have another major, absolute indication for surgery such as congestive heart failure, paravalvular extension or recurrent embolization. It is unclear whether or not the presence of one of these organisms alone, in the absence of one of the above complications, should be an indication for surgery.

Most authors agree that almost all patients with fungal endocarditis will require surgery, especially since most of these cases arise in prosthetic valves. The data on gram-negative infection are limited. The management of *S. aureus* aortic valve endocarditis, however, remains controversial. Proponents of early surgical intervention in all patients with *S. aureus* argue that a large number of these patients will progress to complications that will ultimately require surgery. Early intervention in these high-risk patients will, they argue, decrease operative morbidity and mortality and avoid potentially devastating embolic complications. Others state that there are no data documenting a long-term benefit to mandatory surgery in these patients and that many patients with staphylococcal endocarditis can be cured with antibiotics alone, avoiding the risks of surgery and possible subsequent prosthetic valve complications.

It is probably reasonable to continue medical treatment in a hemodynamically stable patient with *S. aureus* aortic valve endocarditis who quickly responds to aggressive antibiotic treatment, does not demonstrate paravalvular extension by TEE and does not show clinical evidence of embolization. Nonetheless, extreme vigilance is necessary to identify complications as early as possible, with a very low threshold to proceed to surgery in these high-risk patients.

High Risk Echocardiographic Findings

Severe aortic insufficiency, even in the absence of congestive heart failure, carries a poor prognosis and usually requires surgical intervention. However, if the patient remains well compensated without significant symptoms, completion of a 4 to 6 week course of antibiotic therapy may be possible. The decision on whether to intervene after completion of antibiotic therapy in patients with lesser degrees of aortic insufficiency is more difficult. Careful echocardiographic imaging of the valve leaflets is important. Patients with perforation or laceration of a leaflet will likely progress and should therefore be operated on, even in the absence of clinical signs or left ventricular dilatation.

Many studies have been conducted in an attempt to determine whether *high-risk vegetations* could be identified by echocardiography. Several studies have indicated that large vegetations (greater than 10 mm) that are mobile and are not decreasing in size despite antibiotic treatment carry a high risk of complications. They have suggested that these patients should be operated on early, even in the absence of other, more defined, indications for surgery. Others, however, have criticized the methods used in these studies, especially the unclear temporal relationship between echocardiographic identification of the vegetation, the initiation of antibiotic therapy and the actual embolic events. They also point to the lack of evidence that early surgery can actually change the long-term outcome in these patients.

It is not clear whether asymptomatic patients with these echocardiographic findings should undergo early surgery, but these factors should certainly be taken into consideration if other relative indications for surgery are present. For example, a patient with *S. aureus* endocarditis, in whom TEE shows moderately severe aortic insufficiency and an enlarging, mobile vegetation on the aortic valve, will very likely develop complications before completion of antibiotic therapy and will likely benefit from early surgical intervention.

Timing of Surgery

Although the major indications for surgical intervention in aortic valve endocarditis are relatively well established, the proper timing of surgery remains controversial. Ultimately the decision on when to operate requires sound clinical judgment and close collaboration among all of the specialties involved in the care of these complex patients. The decision requires sound clinical judgment with thorough assessment of all clinical data, especially the echocardiographic findings, and careful balancing of the relative risks and benefits of early and late surgery.

Certain facts that have an impact on the decision of when to operate are generally accepted and supported by the majority of the literature. The development of complications in these patients, including severe congestive heart failure, paravalvular extension and major systemic embolization significantly increases overall and operative mortality. However, operative mortality and subsequent complications, including prosthetic valve endocarditis, appear to be higher in patients operated on during the acute phase of their disease (before completion of antibiotic therapy) when compared to the healed phase. Predicting which patients will progress to complications and which patients will be able to achieve a healed state with antibiotic therapy is difficult, and this is the primary basis for the controversy surrounding the timing of surgery. Proponents of liberal indications for early surgery argue that the operative results are acceptable and that any increase in operative morbidity and mortality outweighs the benefits of avoiding the development of further complications. Proponents of trying to achieve a healed state claim that with aggressive medical therapy, this strategy is often successful and avoids exposing many patients to the added risks of operating in an acutely infected field.

Most clinicians agree on the management of patients on either end of the acuity spectrum. The patient with mild to moderate aortic insufficiency who responds quickly to antibiotic treatment and has not developed complications should complete antibiotic therapy before consideration is given to surgery. The patient with documented paravalvular extension, persistent sepsis or severe refractory congestive heart failure should be considered for urgent or emergent surgery. The controversy on the timing of surgery mainly concerns those patients in the "gray zone"—for example, the patient with an episode of congestive heart failure that has responded to medical therapy.

There are no randomized, prospective trials comparing early and late surgery in the treatment of aortic valve endocarditis. Many centers have retrospectively analyzed their experience with this disease and have made recommendations regarding the timing of surgery from their findings. Synthesizing this body of literature into a cogent set of criteria has been made difficult by many factors including 1) relatively small sample size; 2) the mixing of mitral and prosthetic valve cases with native, aortic valve endocarditis in many studies; 3) the long time period spanned during most of these studies—a period characterized by major changes in the diagnosis and management of these patients, particularly in the use of echocardiography and in operative techniques; 4) incomplete temporal data concerning the time between the onset of disease, initiation of antibiotic therapy and surgical intervention; 5) the inconsistent use of standard, multivariate statistical techniques. Nonetheless, several recently published, relatively large series do provide significant insight on the pros and cons of early surgery and are worth reviewing.

The largest study of aortic valve endocarditis was presented by Aranki et al.[12] The authors reviewed 200 patients who underwent aortic valve replacement for NVE and PVE over a 20-year period. Dr. Aranki's group examined predictors of early survival and late morbidity to formulate a strategy for determining the optimal timing of surgery in these patients. They found a significant difference in operative mortality between active and healed endocarditis: 15% and 7% respectively. The operative mortality for healed NVE was comparable to elective aortic valve replacement for other causes. NYHA Class IV and PVE were the only independent predictors of operative mortality. The other major finding was that the only independent predictor of recurrent endocarditis was the active endocarditis at the time of operation. It carried a relative risk of 3.0 when compared to those with healed endocarditis. They concluded that the significantly higher operative mortality and risk of recurrent endocarditis in patients undergoing valve replacement during active endocarditis justifies attempts to postpone surgery until a healed state can be achieved. They felt that this was particularly true given the high operative mortality of PVE to which patients who develop recurrent endocarditis are exposed. Although they accept that urgent surgery is justified in patients with septic emboli, large vegetations or deep tissue involvement, they felt that many patients with congestive heart failure alone could be maintained on aggressive medical therapy until the completion of antibiotic therapy, at which time aortic valve replacement would be safer.

Reinhartz et al[29] reviewed 89 patients with acute endocarditis who underwent valve replacement and compared them to 41 patients who were operated on after completing antibiotic treatment. Although this was an inhomogeneous group that included patients with mitral valve endocarditis and PVE, the majority of patients had NVE involving the aortic valve. Their results were similar to Aranki et al,[12] with a higher operative mortality for active endocarditis than for healed endocarditis although their results were not statistically significant. They also found that NYHA class and paravalvular extension were significant risk factors for operative mortality. They, however, did not feel that the difference in operative mortality was high enough to discourage early surgery.

Middlemost et al[30] presented 203 patients who underwent early valve replacement in the 1980s for NVE with the aortic valve involved in 153 patients. All of these patients were in NYHA class III or IV on admission and most underwent surgery within 7 days of admission. A significant number were found to have extensive infection and abscess formation at surgery. Despite these high-risk factors, operative mortality was only 6%. The rate of early PVE was 3% and no cases of late PVE were reported at a mean follow-up of about 3 years. They use these results to justify early surgery in all patients with NVE who develop heart failure, even if symptoms can be controlled with medical therapy. They attribute their unusually good operative results directly to their strategy of early surgery which, they argue, resulted in a very low incidence of preoperative embolization and multiorgan failure.

It should be apparent from these 3 studies that a major difficulty in reconciling the literature on the timing of surgery in aortic valve endocarditis is the widely divergent data on the operative mortality of aortic valve replacement during acute endocarditis. Most authors report operative mortalities in the range of 10% to15%, similar to Aranki et al.[12] However, in addition to Middlemost et al,[30] others have reported relatively low operative mortalities for aortic valve surgery during acute endocarditis. David et al[31] reported on 62 patients (42 aortic) with active endocarditis who underwent surgery, many involving extensive reconstructive procedures, with an operative mortality of 4.8%. Amrani et al[32] reported on 101 patients with active aortic valve endocarditis, the majority of whom had paravalvular extension, with an operative mortality of 8.5%. Mullany et al[33] on the other hand, reported an operative mortality of 26% in a 30-year review of 151 patients (72% aortic) who underwent early surgery for active endocarditis.

These divergent data certainly reflect differences in patient populations, improvements in operative techniques in the modern era and probably statistical effects of what are generally small sample sizes. Clear guidelines on the timing of surgery in patients with mild to moderate heart failure will have to await a randomized, prospective, and probably multicenter, trial comparing early surgery to aggressive medical therapy and delayed surgery. Until then, the decision will remain difficult, requiring careful clinical assessment and judgment. It seems reasonable to consider delaying surgery in a patient with native aortic valve endocarditis, mild to moderate aortic insufficiency and mild to moderate congestive heart failure that is well compensated with aggressive medical therapy. However, if the patient has risk factors suggesting a high risk for progressive heart failure or paravalvular extension, early surgery should be strongly considered. These factors might include *S. aureus* infection, severe aortic insufficiency, and large, mobile vegetations. If the congestive heart failure is severe and refractory, or if the patient has documented paravalvular extension of recurrent emboli, the patient should undergo surgery as soon as he or she is stabilized.

One final controversy concerns the timing of valve surgery specifically in patients with aortic valve endocarditis complicated by an acute neurological event. Neurological events are common in this disease, occurring in approximately 20% to 30% of patients. They include transient ischemic attacks, embolic ischemic stroke with or without hemorrhage, hemorrhage due to a ruptured mycotic aneurysm, brain abscesses and meningitis. Cardiopulmonary bypass soon after an acute neurological event can exacerbate the deficit by causing hemorrhage from intra- operative anticoagulation, infarct extension from intraoperative hypotension and cerebral edema from fluid shifts. Unlike early surgery for other cases of acute endocarditis, early surgery in the context of an acute neurological event appears to carry a very high operative risk. This risk must be balanced against the urgency of valve surgery.

Eishi et al[28] recently published a large, retrospective multicenter study addressing optimal timing of surgery in patients with endocarditis complicated by an acute neurological event. They reviewed 181 patients with cerebral complications of endocarditis (56% involving the aortic valve) and found a highly significant relationship between time interval to valve surgery, operative mortality and neurological exacerbation. They found that patients operated on within 7 days had a 44% operative mortality and a 46% rate of neurological deterioration, with over 50% of the deaths attributable to the neurological event. In contrast, patients who were operated on more than 28 days after the event had only a 7% operative mortality and a 2% rate of neurological exacerbation. None of these patients' neurological conditions worsened while waiting for surgery. Dr. Eishi and colleagues conclude that valve surgery is safe after 4 weeks and that surgery should be delayed at least 2 weeks if possible to minimize the rate of neurological exacerbation to about 10%.

Gillinov et al[34] reviewed their experience with 34 patients with acute endocarditis (18 aortic) complicated by an acute neurological event who required valve surgery for other indications. They performed valve surgery an average of 22 days after the neurological event. Based on their experience they presented an algorithm for the diagnosis and management of these patients. Briefly, if CT scan rules out intracranial hemorrhage, they recommend a 2 to 3 week delay, if possible, before proceeding with valve surgery. Patients with hemorrhage should undergo cerebral angiogram to rule out a ruptured mycotic aneurysm, which would require immediate surgical intervention followed by valve surgery 2 to 3 weeks later if possible. Patients with hemorrhage from an embolic stroke are at greatest risk and should wait up to 4 weeks if possible before undergoing surgery. Patients without intracranial pathology on CT scan, including those with transient ischemic attacks and those with lumbar puncture-proven meningitis, can safely undergo urgent surgery if indicated for other reasons.

Choice of Valve Replacement

Once all infected tissue from the aorta and surrounding structures has been debrided, the next major decision facing the surgeon is how to repair or replace the valve. A wide variety of options exist including valve repair, mechanical valves, xenograft valves (stented or stentless), homograft valves or the Ross procedure. All of these options have been successfully used in the context of aortic valve endocarditis, and each has its advantages and disadvantages. The best choice for a given patient depends on several factors: 1) the presence of active infection; 2) the degree of paravalvular extension; 3) other operative risk factors including age, hemodynamic stability, comorbid conditions; 4) contraindications to long-term anticoagulation; 5) homograft availability; and 6) surgeon preference and experience.

Risk of Recurrent Endocarditis

Perhaps the most important consideration in the choice of a replacement valve is the risk of recurrent endocarditis. Although Wallace et al[8] proved over 30 years ago that a prosthetic valve can be successfully placed in an infected field without inevitably reinfecting the valve, the risk of recurrent endocarditis is significantly greater than for valve replacement for noninfectious causes. Furthermore, the lethality of prosthetic valve endocarditis justifies all measures to minimize its risk.

Several groups have published extensively on the risk of PVE after valve replacement, including Kirklin's group at the University of Alabama,[19] O'Brien's group[35] at the Prince Charles Hospital in Brisbane, Australia, and Barratt-Boyes's group[36] at the Green Lane Hospital in Auckland, New Zealand. Using sophisticated actuarial, multivariate and hazard function statistical techniques they have consistently shown that native valve endocarditis is a major risk factor for recurrent endocarditis.

They have also documented the early peaking phase and late constant phase of the hazard function for recurrent endocarditis after valve replacement. Finally, they have both shown that homograft replacement is characterized by a constant low-level risk, eliminating the early peaking phase. Both of these groups have recently published reports reviewing their experience with the subset of patients with aortic valve endocarditis.

O'Brien's group reviewed 195 patients who underwent aortic valve replacement for aortic valve endocarditis over a 22-year period and studied the risk of recurrent endocarditis and death as a function of the type of valve replacement.[35] Two thirds of these patients underwent surgery during the active phase of the disease and the remainder during the healed phase, usually well after the episode of endocarditis. The estimated actuarial incidence of recurrent endocarditis at 10 years was 21%. This is significantly higher than the 5% incidence reported for patients undergoing valve replacement for noninfectious causes. However, they found that the shape of the hazard functions for recurrent endocarditis was similar to those previously reported for all valve replacements. Mechanical and xenograft valves continued to show an early peaking phase that was eliminated by the use of a homograft valve. The homograft valve was an independent predictor of early phase survival and freedom from recurrent endocarditis. Although the numbers were too small to achieve statistical significance, it also appeared the infection status (active versus healed) played a role in the risk of recurrent endocarditis in the early phase. Only one of the 6 patients with early PVE was operated on during the healed phase while the numbers were relatively even for late PVE. Based on these results they contend that the homograft aortic valve is the valve of choice for acute endocarditis.

Barratt-Boyes's group had published similar results earlier on 108 patients who all underwent valve replacement for *acute* aortic valve endocarditis.[36] Their actuarial incidence of PVE was nearly identical to O'Brien's group at 20%. The hazard functions for recurrent endocarditis with homograft and prosthetic valves also showed similar characteristics. They also strongly recommended homograft valves for acute aortic valve endocarditis.

Prosthetic Valves

The majority of patients in most major series of aortic valve endocarditis have undergone prosthetic valve replacement with one of a variety of mechanical and xenograft valves. They are widely available, compared to homograft valves, and they carry relatively low incidence of PVE for valves inserted during the healed phase of endocarditis. Therefore, they remain an excellent choice for valve replacement during this phase. The relative risk of PVE for mechanical and xenograft valves is controversial. Some studies show a higher early risk for mechanical valves. Others show no difference with perhaps a slight long-term advantage to mechanical valves. Given these mixed results, the choice of a mechanical or tissue valve should be based on standard criteria including age, life expectancy, annular size and risks of anticoagulation.

Homograft Valves

The above data clearly demonstrate some of the major advantages of homograft valves in patients who require aortic valve replacement during acute aortic valve endocarditis. By eliminating the early phase of the hazard function for PVE, homograft valves can significantly decrease overall morbidity and mortality in these patients. The excess homograft tissue, particularly the anterior leaflet of the mitral valve can be extremely useful in reconstructing the annulus and other structures in patients with extensive paravalvular destruction. Given these facts, the homograft valve, if available, should be strongly considered in all patients with acute endocarditis, especially those with paravalvular extension, *S. aureus* infection and PVE.

The homograft valves can be either maintained at a local homograft bank or obtained from homograft banks. They can be inserted in the subcoronary position using the freehand technique or as a complete or mini-root replacement with coronary reimplantation. The specific technique used is a function of the extent of paravalvular destruction and surgeon preference.

The Ross Procedure

There is increasing popularity for the use of the pulmonary Ross procedure in the treatment of noninfective aortic valve disease due to several reports demonstrating excellent short-term and long-term results.[37,38] However, use of the Ross procedure for the treatment of aortic valve endocarditis has only recently been reported.

One of the potential advantages of using the pulmonary autograft in the treatment of infective aortic endocarditis is that it is the only modality that uses autologous tissue. This fact should theoretically make pulmonary autografts superior to nonviable tissue or artificial material in resisting recurrent infection. A series by Joyce et al[37] investigated the Ross procedure in the treatment of prosthetic aortic valve endocarditis in 11 patients and reported a 0% mortality and 0% reinfection rate.

Other important arguments for the use of the pulmonary root in the aortic position include 1) its purported long-term durability;[11] 2) the optimal or near-optimal alignment and function of the valve leaflets, since the sinuses of Valsalva are also transplanted; 3) the absence of substantial transvalvular pressure gradients; 4) the reduced risk of thromboembolism without the need for anticoagulant therapy;[39] 5) the fact that the pulmonary valve is approximately the same size as the aortic valve; and 6) that it retains the potential for growth when used as an autograft.

The major long-term problem that may develop with the Ross procedure is the progressive valvular degeneration resulting in the need for repair. This is a consequence of prolonged exposure to systemic pressure and dilation of the pulmonary artery wall. However, in a series of 43 patients by Gerosa et al,[11] there was no definite instance of primary tissue failure among the pulmonary autograft recipients.

The potential for misalignment of the valve cusps and commissures and noncompliance of the aortic wall when using a free graft argues for the transplant of the entire pulmonary root rather than the pulmonary valve. Misalignment of the valve commissures or cusps puts greater stress on the valve components, often resulting in regurgitation. Likewise, a calcified aorta would prevent the inward movement of the aortic wall during diastole that is necessary to absorb energy and reduce dynamic loading during closure.[39]

Critics of the Ross procedure point to the potential increased operative morbidity and mortality from what is clearly an extensive, complex operation. Centers with wide experience, however, report reasonable complication rates. For example, Kouchoukos et al[39] reported on 33 patients with an operative mortality of 0%.

Aortic Valve Repair

Aortic valve repair may be appropriate in highly selective cases with healed aortic endocarditis. The techniques for repair of the aortic valve in IE have dealt primarily with cusp perforations or destruction leading to acute regurgitation[41]. In these repairs, autologous pericardial patching was used for the perforations and valve repair was always reinforced by an annular running 2-0 suture to avoid diastolic distention.

References

1. Frater RW. Surgical management of endocarditis in drug addicts and long-term results. *J Cardiac Surg* 1990;5:63–67.
2. Major RH. Notes on the history of endocarditis. *Bull Med Hist* 351–359.

3. Pruitt RD. William Osler and his Gulstonian Lectures on malignant endocarditis. *Mayo Clin Proc* 1982;57:4–9.

4. Scott SM. A successful century in dealing with bacterial endocarditis [editorial]. *Ann Thorac Surg* 1985;40:421.

5. Lerner PI, Weinstein L. Infective endocarditis in the antibiotic era. *N Engl J Med* 1966;274:388–393.

6. Cohn LH. Valve replacement for infective endocarditis: An overview. *J Cardiac Surg* 1989;4:321–323.

7. Yeh TJ, Hall DP, Ellison RG. Surgical treatment of aortic valve perforation due to bacterial endocarditis: A report of six cases. *Am Surg* 1964;30:767–769.

8. Wallace AG, Young WG, Osterhout S. Treatment of acute bacterial endocarditis by valve excision and replacement. *Circulation* 1965;31:450–453.

9. Prager RL, Maples MD, Hammon JW Jr, et al. Early operative intervention in aortic bacterial endocarditis. *Ann Thorac Surg* 1981;32:347–350.

10. Braniff BA, Shumway NE, Harrison DC. Valve replacement in active bacterial endocarditis. *N Engl J Med* 1967;276:1464–1467.

11. Gerosa G. Comparison of the aortic homograft and the pulmonary autograft for aortic valve or root replacement in children. *J Thorac Cardiovasc Surg* 1991; 102:51–60.

12. Aranki SF, Santini F, Adams DH, et al. Aortic valve endocarditis: Determinants of early survival and late morbidity. *Circulation* 1994;90:II175–182.

13. Hogevik H, Olaison L, Andersson R, et al. Epidemiologic aspects of infective endocarditis in an urban population: A 5-year prospective study. *Medicine* 1995;74:324–339.

14. Durack DT. Prevention of infective endocarditis. *N Engl J Med* 1995;332:38–44.

15. Kaye D. Changing pattern of infective endocarditis. *Am J Med* 1985;78:157–162.

16. Michel PL, Acar J. Native cardiac disease predisposing to infective endocarditis. *Eur Heart J* 1995;16:2–6.

17. Geraci JE, Dale AJ, McGoon DC. Bacterial endocarditis and endarteritis following cardiac operations. *Wisconsin Medical Journal* 1963;62:303–315.

18. Chastre J. Early infective endocarditis on prosthetic valves. *Eur Heart J* 1995; 16:32–38.

19. Blackstone EH, Kirklin JW. Death and other time-related events after valve replacement. *Circulation* 1985;72:753–767.

20. Horstkotte D, Piper C, Niehues R, et al. Late prosthetic valve endocarditis. *Eur Heart J* 1995;16:39–47.

21. Dajani AS, Bisno AL, Chung KJ, et al. Prevention of bacterial endocarditis. Recommendations by the American Heart Association [see comments]. *JAMA* 1990;264:2919–2922.

22. Weinstein L, Schlesinger JJ. Pathoanatomic, pathophysiologic and clinical correlations in endocarditis (first of two parts). *N Engl J Med* 1974;291:832–837.

23. Saccente M, Cobbs CG. Clinical approach to infective endocarditis. *Cardiol Clin* 1996;14:351–362.

24. Krivokapich J, Child JS. Role of transthoracic and transesophageal echocardiography in diagnosis and management of infective endocarditis. *Cardiol Clin* 1996;14:363–382.

25. Whitener C. Endocarditis due to coagulase-negative staphylococci: Microbiologic, epidemiologic, and clinical considerations. *Infect Dis Clin North Am* 1993; 7:81–96.

26. Blaustein AS, Lee JR. Indications for and timing of surgical intervention in infective endocarditis *Cardiol Clin* 1996;14:393–404.

27. Abe T, Tsukamoto M, Komatsu S. Surgical treatment of active infective endo-carditis—early and late results of active native and prosthetic valve endocardi-tis. *Jpn Circ J* 1993;57:1080–1088.

28. Eishi K, Kawazoe K, Kuriyama Y, et al. Surgical management of infective endocarditis associated with cerebral complications. Multi-center retrospec-tive study. *Jpn J Thorac Cardiovasc Surg* 1995;110:1745–55.

29. Reinhartz O, Herrmann M, Redling F, et al. Timing of surgery in patients with acute infective endocarditis. *J Cardiovasc Surg* 1996;37:397–400.

30. Middlemost S, Wisenbaugh T, Meyerowitz C, et al. A case for early surgery in native left- sided endocarditis complicated by heart failure: results in 203 patients [see comments]. *J Am Coll Cardiol* 1991;18:663–667.

31. David TE, Bos J, Christakis GT, Brofman PR, Wong D, Feindel CM. Heart valve operations in patients with active infective endocarditis. *Ann Thorac Surg* 1990;49:701–705; discussion 12–3.

32. Amrani M, Schoevaerdts JC, Eucher P, et al. Extension of native aortic valve endocarditis: Surgical considerations. *Eur Heart J* 1995;16:103–106.

33. Mullany CJ, Chua YL, Schaff HV, et al. Early and late survival after surgical treatment of culture-positive active endocarditis [see comments]. *Mayo Clin Proc* 1995;70:517–525.

34. Gillinov AM, Shah RV, Curtis WE, et al. Valve replacement in patients with endocarditis and acute neurologic deficit. *Ann Thorac Surg* 1996;61:1125–1129; discussion 30.

35. Agnihotri AK, McGiffin DC, Galbraith AJ, MF OB. The prevalence of infective endocarditis after aortic valve replacement. *J Thorac Cardiovasc Surg* 1995;110: 1708–1720; discussion 20–4

36. Haydock D, Barratt-Boyes B, Macedo T, et al. Aortic valve replacement for active infectious endocarditis in 108 patients: A comparison of freehand allo-graft valves with mechanical prostheses and bioprostheses. *J Thorac Cardiovasc Surg* 1992;103:130–139.

37. Joyce F, Tingleff J, Pettersson G. The Ross operation in the treatment of pros-thetic aortic valve endocarditis. *Semin Thorac Cardiovasc Surg* 1995;7:38–46.

38. Oswalt J. Management of aortic infective endocarditis by autograft valve re-placement. *J Heart Valve Dis* 1994;3:377–379.

41. Kouchoukos N. Replacement of the aortic root with a pulmonary autograft in children and young adults with aortic-valve disease. *N Engl J Med* 1994; 330:1–6.

42. Dreyfus G, Serraf A, Jebara VA, et al. Valve repair in acute endocarditis. *Ann Thorac Surg* 1990;49:706–711; discussion 12–3.

Chapter 10
Mitral Valve Endocarditis

Charles F. Schwartz, M.D.
Steven F. Bolling, M.D.

Introduction

Endocarditis began to be recognized as a specific disease during the middle of the last century. In 1885, William Osler brought together bacterial infection as the root cause, the relation of valvular disease as a predisposing factor, valvular incompetence as one lethal consequence and embolism as another.[1] The disease was finally treated with some success after World War II at the dawn of the antibiotic era. Before the availability of antibiotics, infection accounted for 64% of deaths in these patients, with congestive heart failure being the cause of death in only 12%. After antibiotics became available, infection could be identified as the cause of death in only 16% of patients, whereas 61% of endocarditis patients died from congestive heart failure.[2]

However, success was limited to cases treated before hemodynamically significant valvular damage or the lethal consequences of embolism had occurred. The first case of active endocarditis undergoing a deliberate valve replacement was one of aortic endocarditis confined to the cusps reported by Wallace et al in 1965. The essential contribution of this operation was to demonstrate that, with the aid of antibiotics, a synthetic foreign body could be successfully implanted in the presence of bloodstream infection.[3]

From: Vlessis AA, Bolling S (eds): *Endocarditis: A Multidisciplinary Approach to Modern Treatment.* © Futura Publishing Co., Armonk, NY, 1999.

Incidence

The true incidence of native valve endocarditis is difficult to establish. The locus of involvement of native cardiac valves by infective endocarditis parallels the valvular involvement with rheumatic heart disease; mitral, aortic, aortic and mitral combined, tricuspid, and pulmonary valves. The mitral valve is the most frequent site of native valve endocarditis in most series. A diseased native valve is at increased risk for the development of endocarditis, although infection of normal valves is occurring with increasing frequency. Mitral valve prolapse associated with a murmur and mitral annular calcification are also factors in the development of endocarditis. In one recent study, of all patients with endocarditis, 24% had rheumatic heart disease, 23% had congenital deformities, and 32% had normal valves.[4] Right-sided endocarditis, often associated with intravenous drug use, usually affects normal or congenitally deformed valves.

Endocarditis may develop in a normal valve when a focus of growth for a virulent organism is established, or it may be incurred in an immunocompromised patient. Predisposing or etiologic factors leading to bacterial endocarditis include intravenous drug addiction, infectious processes in other parts of the body, and recent dental extractions. Nondiseased valves may also be affected from infected long-term venous catheters or pacemaker pockets. Involvement of normal heart valves usually presents as an acute, often fulminant, process.

Prosthetic valve endocarditis is reported to occur in 0.2% to 2% of implants, constituting 15% to 30% of all cases. This may develop as an early form (less than 2 months postoperatively), usually related to extracardiac contamination from sources such as skin infections, or a late form, usually related to bacteremic seeding of the valve. Important differences exist in the microbiology of native versus prosthetic valve endocarditis. *Staphylococcus epidermidis, Staphylococcus aureus*, and gram-negative rods are most commonly seen in the early form of prosthetic endocarditis, and streptococcal, staphylococcal, or gram-negative rod infections in the late form.[5] Overall, *S. aureus* infections are more common in patients with native valve disease.

Pathology

Endocarditis of diseased valves may be precipitated by a transient bacteremia and characteristically runs an indolent, subacute course. *Streptococcus viridans*, followed by *Enterococcus*, other streptococcal species and *Staphylococcus*, in that order, are most often responsible for the subacute form of endocarditis.[4] Acute endocarditis is caused most commonly by

Staphylococcus aureus and involves normal valves in 40% to 60% of cases. *S. aureus* is also the most common cause of infection in intravenous drug users.

The initial stage of valvular infection is the surface vegetation, composed of platelets, fibrin, and microorganisms. The organisms are protected from the host defense mechanisms and the action of antibiotics by this location. The organisms multiply within the vegetations, migrate into the bloodstream, and may destroy adjacent valves. Clinical manifestations may also be due to deposition of immune complex components and allergic vasculitis involving small arteries.[6] The specific lesion of infective endocarditis begins on the external surface of the valve rather than being deposited through the valve's own blood supply.[7] These implants are usually found on the atrial surface of mitral valves. The vegetations may vary in form from a thin, granular lesion to large, fragile, polypoid masses.

Infection involving the native mitral valve is localized primarily to the leaflet. Valvular pathology may include annular calcification, chordal rupture, leaflet vegetations, annular abscess, annular dilation, flail leaflet, leaflet prolapse, chordal shortening and mitral stenosis. In prosthetic valve endocarditis, extension beyond the valve into the annulus and perivalvular tissue is common. As a result, dehiscence of the prosthesis with consequent regurgitation and myocardial abscess is often encountered. Large vegetations partially obstructing the prosthetic orifice are often associated with infection of a mitral valve prosthesis.[5]

Importantly, the larger the vegetation, the more likely the embolism, valve destruction, and failure of antibiotic cure. Penetration of antibiotics into the core of vegetations is inversely related to size. Vegetations of greater than 1 cm in diameter are significantly more often associated with failed treatment.[8] A series of 42 patients from the University of Michigan demonstrated that the presence of a vegetation was associated with a higher incidence of major complications (100% versus 67% in the absence of a large vegetation).[9] The presence of a large vegetation was associated with a higher likelihood of progression to congestive heart failure and death. Vegetations which are multiple, pedunculated, or extending onto the extravalvular structures may also better predict the risk of further complications.

Presentation

The patient with endocarditis presents with fever, chills, or sweats. Septic emboli occur in about 30% of patients and produce a variety of symptoms. In general, infected emboli produce ischemia, abscesses, and mycotic aneurysms. Clinical features suggestive of embolism include shoulder tip or flank pain for one or more days, anterior tibial compartment pain, and mental confusion without localizing neurological signs. Emboli commonly affect the spleen, causing abdominal pain. Renal emboli may produce hematuria, middle cerebral artery emboli may cause hemiplegia, and coronary emboli can lead to myocardial infarction. The early application of antimicrobial therapy has decreased the frequency of the classic physical stigmata of subacute endocarditis, such as Osler's nodes, Janeway's lesions, and Roth spots.

Two thirds of patients will have a murmur at the time of presentation and some of the remaining will develop a murmur at some point in the course of their disease. Some patients have pre-existing murmurs associated with native valve disease or the presence of prosthetic valves. Changing murmurs are usually found with acute endocarditis and strongly correspond with tissue destruction.

Diagnosis

Blood culture remains the mainstay of diagnosis of infective endocarditis. Most accurate blood cultures are obtained with 3 to 6 sets of cultures within 24 hours of presentation. Premature administration of antibiotics may interfere with efforts to recover the causative organism. Intramyocardial abscess or fungal infections may cause false negative results.

Echocardiography has proven to be extremely valuable in the assessment of patients with suspected infective endocarditis. This noninvasive technique not only allows evaluation of the hemodynamic status of patients in whom cardiac catheterization may be hazardous but can directly image the vegetations on the valve leaflets. Overall, echocardiography is accurate in 55% to 80% of cases.[10] The axial resolution of most echocardiographic instruments is 1 mm to 2 mm and therefore all vegetations may not be perceptible.

Patients with a clinical diagnosis of infectious endocarditis will have a 20% to 35% likelihood of having a large vegetation when this methodology is used. In the absence of other risk factors such as congestive heart failure, persistent bacteremia, intramyocardial abscess, recurrent large artery emboli, or fungal infection, the presence of a large vegetation alone is not an indication for surgery. However, any patient with a large lesion should be followed closely and with a low threshold for using noninvasive and invasive tests to determine valvular integrity, ventricular function, and overall hemodynamic status. Mitral valve vegetations appear thick and echo dense. The quality of the appearance of vegetations on an echocardiogram is frequently described as "shaggy" or "velvety."[11] Vegetations detected by echocardiogram have been associated with an increased incidence of complications.

Management

The mainstay of treatment for bacterial endocarditis of the mitral valve is appropriate antibiotic prophylaxis. Medical therapy for established endocarditis consists of intravenous administration of appropriate antibiotics at bactericidal levels for a period of 4 to 6 weeks. This is effective in 50% to 80% of cases, depending upon the organism involved. When choosing between effective antimicrobial regimens, considerations to minimize toxicity must prevail. Once the etiology of infective endocarditis is known, there is no reason to delay therapy.

If the course of infective endocarditis has been indolent, and clinical findings do not suggest hemodynamic impairment requiring urgent surgical intervention, blood cultures should be obtained and administration of antibiotic therapy delayed.[5] If the initial cultures are negative, as often occurs when patients have received antibiotics, this delay provides an opportunity to repeat cultures or to use special culture techniques. However, if the infective endocarditis is acute or if the presence of valve dysfunction and congestive heart failure indicates a need for early valve repair or replacement, 4 to 6 separate blood cultures should be obtained over an hour and empirical antibiotic therapy begun immediately thereafter.

The treatment regimens recommended for infective endocarditis caused by a specific organism are based on the in vitro bactericidal activity of antibiotics against the organism and clinical experience. The treatment of native valve endocarditis caused by penicillin-susceptible (MIC less than or equal to 0.2 μg/mL) nonenterococcal streptococci, including *S. bovis*, is penicillin G, with or without streptomycin, for 4 to 6 weeks. The combination of penicillin G and streptomycin for 2 weeks, followed by 2 additional weeks of parenteral penicillin, is recommended for prosthetic valve endocarditis caused by penicillin-susceptible streptococci.[5] Penicillin-resistant streptococcal and enterococcal endocarditis, regardless of valve type, is treated with a synergistic bactericidal combination of penicillin and gentamicin. The frequency of high-level resistance to streptomycin (40% of enterococci) precludes the use of this drug for enterococci.

Endocarditis due to *S. aureus* is treated with a penicillinase-resistant penicillin, cephalosporin, or vancomycin. If the strain is confirmed to be penicillin-susceptible, penicillin may be used. Vancomycin is the only agent recommended for treatment of endocarditis caused by methicillin-resistant *S. aureus*.

S. epidermidis endocarditis is treated with a combination of antimicrobials. Native valve endocarditis caused by *S. epidermidis* is usually methicillin-susceptible and may be treated with the regimens designated for endocarditis caused by *S. aureus* with comparable susceptibilty to methicillin. Prosthetic valve endocarditis caused by *S. epidermidis* is commonly resistant to all beta-lactam antibiotics. Vancomycin, in combination with rifampin and gentamicin, is the treatment of choice.

A patient is exposed to multiple devices during the perioperative period, including the bypass machine, cardiac assist pumps, endotracheal tubes, arterial and venous lines, and Foley catheters. In this way, indolent organisms that rarely cause native valve infection, such as *S. epidermidis*, diphtheroids, and various *Candida* species, may cause prosthetic valve infections. Due to the low pathogenicity of these organisms, infection may not become apparent until months later.

Optimal treatment regimens for treating endocarditis caused by gram-negative organisms have not been established. High cure rates with the combination of ampicillin and streptomycin have been achieved. Experience in drug addicts with endocarditis due to *Pseudomonas aeruginosa* has shown a need for the combination of tobramycin and ticarcillin in high doses. The treatment of other gram-negative bacilli should be designed on the basis of in vitro susceptibility studies and the role of combinations of antibiotics.

Patients with infective endocarditis must be monitored closely while receiving antibiotic therapy. Blood cultures should be obtained during the initial 3 to 5 days of treatment to document that the bacteremia has been eradicated. Thereafter, if cultures are negative, repeat cultures are obtained only to assess complications or unexplained fever. In monitoring therapy, the serum bactericidal titer is determined at the time of expected highest (peak) and lowest (trough) serum antibiotic concentrations.

Indications for Surgery

Hemodynamic deterioration as a consequence of mitral valve dysfunction is a major cause of death in patients with infective endocarditis and is the cardinal derangement prompting surgical therapy. Electrocardiographic conduction abnormalities, particularly those which are new or persistent, suggest a myocardial abscess involving the conduction system and warrant placement of a demand pacemaker as well as surgery.

Continued medical therapy of mitral valve endocarditis in the face of cardiac deterioration carries an 80% to 90% mortality rate.[11] Mortality with early prosthetic valve infections with *Staphylococcus* or gram-negative rods is as high as 85%. Therefore, surgical treatment is indicated in these clinical situations. Debriding infected paravalvular tissue, removing infected mitral valves, and replacing dysfunctioning valves with prosthetic ones have become increasingly important in the management of native valve endocarditis and prosthetic valve endocarditis alike. In some patients, antibiotic therapy alone cannot eradicate infection or remedy intracardiac complications. In this population of patients, the survival rate of those undergoing surgery is higher than that of those treated medically.

The most common indication for surgical treatment of mitral valve endocarditis is hemodynamic deterioration due to valve dysfunction, either regurgitation or stenosis. When congestive heart failure is moderate to severe, surgery is required if mortality rates of 75% to 90% are to be avoided.[5] Once heart failure has developed in the course of the illness, it will always be progressive even though it may respond temporarily to medical measures. The most common error is to underestimate the degree of congestive failure present and to realize it only after surgery with the dramatic change in clinical status.[12] Other surgical indications include perivalvular abscess and pericarditis. Perivalvular abscesses can heal and stabilize so that they present as nonexpanding smooth-walled cavities, but this outcome cannot be predicted in the active phase. Therefore, echocardiographic demonstration of a perivalvular abscess should be followed by urgent surgery.

Patients with prosthetic mitral valve endocarditis who have invasive disease or who have a relapse of endocarditis usually require surgery. Much of the published literature on infection of artificial valves describes extremely high mortality from both medical and surgical treatment. This literature describes artificial valves that have developed a dehiscence or have extensive perivalvular infection. In general, when infection occurs in the presence of foreign material, it is more difficult to cure with antibiotics.

When patients with native or prosthetic mitral valve endocarditis caused by *S. aureus* do not show a prompt and progressive response to medical therapy, early surgical intervention may improve survival rates. *S. aureus* is generally regarded as an organism that virtually always requires surgery for cure. A similar approach should be used for patients with mitral valve endocarditis due to antibiotic-resistant gram-negative bacilli. Moreover, the presence of unusual organisms demands early consideration for surgery unless the patient is responding extremely well to conventional therapy. Infection extending beyond the valve leaflet is increasingly being accepted as an indication for surgery.

Persistent infection, with low-grade fever and leukocytosis, after 6 weeks of antibiotic therapy, with or without positive blood cultures, is an indication for surgery. The significance of bacteremia in the presence of an artificial heart valve was studied in 171 patients. During an observation period of 1 year, 43% of the patients developed endocarditis, 56 at the time of original bacteremia and 18 later.[13]

The sewing ring location of infection in mechanical valves presents a potential danger of early spread to the perivalvular tissues. Many clinicians believe that bioprosthetic valves do not produce surgical mortality much different from that of endocarditis on normal valves. Endocarditis of homografts may be less common than infection of other devices.[14] Moreover, a smaller presence of inorganic material will produce a response closer to that of a natural valve.

Recurrent systemic emboli are an additional indication for surgical treatment of mitral valve endocarditis. Emboli appear to be more common in mitral bacterial endocarditis than in aortic.[15] It is significant that the development of neurological manifestations of bacterial endocarditis is associated with a 50% mortality rate and that major cerebral emboli are generally preceded by manifestations of minor emboli. If embolism occurs, the presence or absence of vegetations must be determined by transthoracic echocardiography (TTE). If TTE is inconclusive, transesophageal echocardiography should be performed. As noted above, the presence of vegetations on the mitral valve seen on echocardiography defines a group of patients who are likely to have complicated courses of disease, to require surgery, or to die.

Additionally, the type of organism is important. The frequency of embolic events is greater with infections caused by indolent, slow-growing gram-negative bacilli such as *Hemophilus parainfluenzae*, nutritionally variant *Streptococcus viridans*, and fungi that have a tendency to form large, mobile vegetations.[1] The size of the vegetation alone does not preclude cure by antibiotic treatment, but may strengthen the argument to proceed to surgery. Stewart et al concluded that the presence of congestive heart failure, rather than the finding of vegetations, remains the most important indication for surgical therapy for patients with infective endocarditis.[16]

Preoperative Investigation

The benefits of surgery for patients with mitral valve endocarditis depend upon the timing of the procedure. When surgery is unequivocally indicated, the results are strikingly better than the results of medical treatment. Operative mortality is directly proportional to the patient's preoperative hemodynamic status. Of particular importance are multiple system abnormalities, including myocardial dysfunction, renal failure, recent cerebral infarction and pulmonary abnormalities. The occurrence and rate of progression of such complications secondary to acute valvular disruption is often difficult to predict. These points serve to emphasize the concept that delay of operation in an attempt to achieve bacteriological cure in patients with unstable heart failure may impose greater jeopardy than "premature" surgical intervention.[17]

The development of perivalvular extension, during an attempt at avoiding surgery, should be regarded as a mark of bad decision-making: the surgery will be less beneficial to the patient and its risk will be increased.[1] Ideally, patients receive 7 to 10 days of antibiotic therapy prior to surgery. However, if absolute indications for surgical treatment exist, the procedure should not be delayed. Prolonged medical therapy prior to surgery has not been associated with a more favorable outcome in patients with native or prosthetic valve endocarditis. A strong correlation between surgical success and the duration of preoperative antibiotic treatment has not been demonstrated.

The preoperative investigation of patients with endocarditis is no different from that of other cardiac patients. It is necessary to quantitate any cardiac physiologic disorder and the valvular pathology should be precisely defined. If time permits, evidence of extracardial infection should be sought, and if possible, eradicated. For example, a renal or splenic abscess should be drained or removed prior to valve replacement. The risks of surgery, including operative mortality, recurrence of original endocarditis, new onset prosthetic valve endocarditis and its associated mortality, and thromboembolic complications must be evaluated in each clinical situation. Acute central nervous system damage may be a reason for postponing surgery.[18] Patients with endocarditis who are comatose at the time of cardiopulmonary bypass generally do not recover neurologically. The timing of surgery is dependent upon daily evaluation of both the patient's neurological and cardiac status.

Valve Replacement

Valve replacement in the hemodynamically stable patient results in an initially favorable outcome in 80% to 90% of cases.[10] Late mortality rates between 20% and 60% have previously been reported. The risk of recurrent endocarditis following mitral valve replacement is approximately 10% to 15% at 5 years. Hendren et al reported on the use of 12 prosthetic annuloplasty rings in 22 repairs with no instances of reinfection at 24 months of follow-up.[19] The choice between mechanical, bioprosthetic, and biological devices may be made according to the usual criteria. These include age, the presence of renal disease, risk of bleeding on anticoagulants, and patient preference. However, there is strong opinion that a homograft valve or a pulmonary autograft is less likely to be followed by recurrent infection than a xenograft or a mechanical valve.[20]

The exposure for a mitral valve replacement in this situation may require a more extensive cardiotomy since the critical hemodynamic disorder may have been acquired recently. The size of the chamber through which access is obtained may be small.[1] The left atrium may be normal size in cases of acute mitral endocarditis. A vertical trans- septal incision provides excellent exposure in this situation.

Extracardial extensions usually require repair before valve insertion. A tension- free closure of the margins of the defect may be achieved by using a patch of tanned pericardium. If this is not done, a common consequence is a defect with or without a perivalvular leak.

Valve Repair

Recently, mitral valve repair, rather than replacement, has yielded good functional results, and a low risk of recurrent disease in the surgical treatment of mitral valve endocarditis. The preservation of the native mitral valve functional apparatus and avoidance of long-term complications associated with valvular replacement would support the philosophy of operative treatment using techniques of mitral valve reconstruction. The life expectancy of bioprosthetic valves is limited, especially in the mitral position.[21] Lifelong anticoagulation will be required if a mechanical prosthesis is used and is associated with bleeding and thromboembolic complications. Women who wish to become pregnant cannot take oral anticoagulants because of their teratogenic effects.

Investigators have shown that left ventricular function is preserved when the subvalvular apparatus is not transected, which favors mitral valve repair. Cosgrove reported on successful mitral valve repair in 49% of patients with mitral regurgitation caused by endocarditis.[22] Muehrcke et al revealed that patients who could undergo mitral valve repair had a lower hospital mortality rate and better midterm durability than patients who did not have repair.[23]

Additionally, neurological complications including postoperative strokes may be reduced by valve repair rather than valve replacement. Ting et al reported that preoperative cerebral embolic events associated with hemorrhagic infarcts in the setting of left-sided valvular endocarditis were associated with an increased risk for postoperative strokes following valve replacement.[24] The decision to repair the valve is dependent upon the proportion of functional to destroyed tissue. Success is more likely if the disease occurs on a normal valve. In each case there is a necessity to substitute new material for that which has been destroyed. The development of new techniques has permitted many surgeons to enlarge the indications for mitral valve repair rather than replacement.

Valvular repair includes anterior and posterior leaflet resection, leaflet patching, and direct suture. Subvalvular repair may involve chordal shortening and transposition. Annular remodeling involves commissural refection and placement of prosthetic rings. Pagani et al demonstrated that reconstructive techniques including debridement of infected tissue, leafletoplasty and implantation of prosthetic annuloplasty rings can be performed in this setting with low operative mortality and morbidity.[25] Initially, all macroscopically involved tissue is resected without any concern for the possibility of repair. The valve may be widely resected, including a strip of normal valvular tissue (approximately 2 mm). Valve reconstruction may then be performed according to Carpentier's techniques and principles including ring annuloplasty, transposition of chordae and chordal elongation.[26]

Specific techniques are used for acute valve endocarditis. Perforations of the anterior leaflet of the mitral valve may be repaired with an autologous pericardial patch. A piece of pericardium is tanned intraoperatively with a glutaraldehyde solution and then washed in a saline bath. The smooth surface of the pericardium is turned toward the atrium for mitral valve repair.[27] Rupture of the marginal chordae of the anterior leaflet can be repaired with chordal transposition. Marginal chordae of the posterior leaflet are selected, detached with part of the posterior leaflet, and then transposed onto the anterior leaflet in an adequate position. Commissural refection is indicated when the commissural area of both the anterior and posterior leaflets are prolapsed from ruptured commissural chordae.

All of the techniques described are considered reproducible and stable. The essential requirement is the desire to conserve the mitral valve. The underlying pathology must be understood and a repair maneuver attempted. The limiting factor is the quality of tissue that must hold sutures to make the repair possible. Complete excision of all inflamed or weakened tissue must be performed. If a satisfactory result is not reached within an established time limit, valve replacement can be undertaken without undue risk to the patient. The most difficult question to decide is when a reconstruction, though not perfect, is nevertheless superior to a valve replacement.[28]

Postoperative Care

Postoperatively, a full course of antibiotics is indicated if persistent infection was the reason for surgery. At times, the decision to discontinue antibiotics is determined by the pathology at surgery. Antibiotics should be continued for 6 weeks if cultures of the valve or surrounding tissues are positive. Periannular involvement is also an indication for 6 weeks of treatment. If cultures and histology are negative and there was no perivalvular extension, then there is no need for more than completion of the original course of antibiotics.

Results of Treatment

Overall, the hospital mortality rate for patients with native valve endocarditis treated surgically ranges between 5% and 20%. The published mortality rate of antibiotic therapy remains 30% to 40%. Perivalvular infection, staphylococcal infection, renal and multiorgan failure are statistically significant risk factors for mortality.[29] Medical treatment for prosthetic valve endocarditis may cause a 70% mortality.[30] It is now evident that surgery should be performed early and should not be dependent upon an arbitrary period of antibiotic administration. Recent studies have reported 0% to 22% mortality with aggressive surgical treatment.

The prognosis for patients with native or prosthetic mitral valve endocarditis for whom surgery is indicated is clearly improved by appropriately timed surgical intervention. Patients with surgical treatment may experience late endocarditis-related complications, including relapse of disease and prosthetic valve dysfunction due to periprosthetic leakage. These complications are more commonly seen in patients with invasive perivalvular infection or with positive blood cultures or Gram's stain of excised material.

While the prognosis for patients with mitral valve endocarditis has improved with the increased availability of potent antibiotics and the increased frequency of early surgical intervention, morbidity and mortality remain high. Consequently, when treating this disease, the portal of entry for the causative organism should always be sought and corrected. Dental health should be assessed routinely. Moreover, patients remain at risk for recurrent mitral valve disease and must be instructed to use antibiotic regimens as prophylaxis against infective endocarditis.

References

1. Frater RW. Surgery for bacterial endocarditis. In Baue AE, Geha AS, Laks H, et al (eds.) *Glenn's Thoracic and Cardiovascular Surgery*, 6th ed. Stamford, CT. Appleton & Lange, 1996. pp 1915–1929.
2. Robinson MJ, Ruedy J. Sequelae of bacterial endocarditis. *Am J Med* 1962;32: 922–928.
3. Wallace AG, Young WG, Osterhout S. Treatment of acute bacterial endocarditis by valve excision and replacement. *Circulation* 1965;31:450–453.
4. Bayliss R, Clark C, Oakley CM, et al. Incidence, mortality, and the prevention of infective endocarditis. *J R Coll Physicians Lond* 1986;20:15.
5. Karchmer AW. Prosthetic and native valve endocarditis. In Grillo HC, Austen WG, Wilkins EW, et al (eds.) *Current Therapy in Cardiothoracic Surgery*. Philadelphia, PA. Mosby, 1989. pp 386–391.
6. Gutman RA, Striker GE, Gilliland BC. The immune complex glomerulonephritis of bacterial endocarditis. *Medicine* 1972;51:1–25.
7. Wilcox BR. The role of surgery in the management of infective endocarditis. In Roberts AJ (ed.) *Difficult Problems in Adult Cardiac Surgery*. Chicago, IL. Year Book Medical, 1985. pp 199–216.
8. Strom J, Becker RM, Davis R, et al. Echocardiographic and surgical correlations in bacterial endocarditis. *Circulation* 1980;62:164–167.

9. Buda AJ, Zotz RJ, Lemire MS, et al. Prognostic significance of vegetations detected by two-dimensional echocardiography in infective endocarditis. *Am Heart J* 1986;112:1291.

10. Isom OW, Rosengart TK. Valvular heart disease. In Greenfield LJ, Mulholland MW, Oldham KT, et al (eds.) *Surgery: Scientific Principles and Practice*. Philadelphia, PA. Lippincott, 1993. pp 1388–1390.

11. Bloomfield P, O'Boyle JE, Parisi AF. Non-invasive investigations for the diagnosis of mitral valve disease. In Ionescu MI, Cohn LH (eds.) *Mitral Valve Disease: Diagnosis and Treatment*. Boston, MA. Butterworth, 1985. p 72.

12. Becker RM, Frishman W, Frater RWM. Surgery for mitral valve endocarditis. *Chest* 1979;75:314–319.

13. Fang G, Keys TF, Gentry LO, et al. Prosthetic valve endocarditis resulting from nosocomial bacteremia: A prospective multicenter study. *Ann Intern Med* 1993;119:560–567.

14. Kirklin JK, Pacifico AD, Kirklin JW. Surgical treatment of prosthetic valve endocarditis with homograft aortic valve replacement. *J Cardiac Surg* 1989;4: 340–347.

15. Windsor HM, Golding LA, Shanahan MX. Cardiac surgery in bacterial endocarditis. *J Thorac Cardiovasc Surg* 1972;64:282.

16. Stewart JA, Silimpen D, Harris P, et al. Echocardiographic documentation of vegetative lesions in infective endocarditis: Clinical implications. *Circulation* 1980;61:374.

17. Stinson EB, Griepp RB, Vosti K, et al. Operative treatment for infective endocarditis. *J Thorac Cardiovasc Surg* 1976;71:659–665.

18. Ting W, Silverman NA, Levitsky S. Right and left side endocarditis: Cerebral emboli. In Gabbay S., Bonchek LI, Bortolotti U (eds.) *Infective Endocarditis of Heart Valves*. Austin, TX. Silent Partners, 1991. pp 3–15.

19. Hendren WG, Morris AS, Rosenkranz ER, et al. Mitral valve repair for bacterial endocarditis. *J Thorac Cardiovasc Surg* 1992;103:124–128; discussion 128–129.

20. Donaldson RM, Ross DN. Homograft aortic root replacement for complicated prosthetic valve endocarditis. *Circulation* 1984;70 (suppl I):178–181.

21. Grover FL, Cohen DJ, Oprian C, et al. Determinants of the occurrence of and survival from prosthetic valve endocarditis: Experience of the Veterans Affairs Cooperative Study on Valvular Heart Disease. *J Thorac Cardiovasc Surg* 1982; 108:207–214.

22. Cosgrove DM. Surgery for degenerative mitral valve disease. *Semin Thorac Cardiovasc Surg* 1989;1:183–193.

23. Muehrcke DD, Cosgrove DM III, Lytle BW, et al. Is there an advantage to repairing infected mitral valves? *Ann Thorac Surg* 1997;63(6):1718–1724.

24. Ting W, Silverman N, Levitsky S. Valve replacement in patients with endocarditis and cerebral septic emboli. *Ann Thorac Surg* 1991;51:18–21.

25. Pagani FD, Monoghan HL, Deeb GM, Bolling SF. Mitral valve replacement for active and healed endocarditis. *Circulation* 1996;94 (9 suppl):II133–138.

26. Carpentier A. Cardiac valve surgery—the "French correction." *J Thorac Cardiovasc Surg* 1983;86:323–337.

27. Dreyfus G, Serraf A, Jebara VA, et al. Valve repair in acute endocarditis. *Ann Thorac Surg* 1990;49:706–713.

28. Duran CM. Techniques in mitral valve reconstruction. In Starek PJ (ed.) *Heart*

Valve Replacement and Reconstruction. Chicago, IL. Year Book Medical, 1987. pp 119–123.

29. Miller DC. Determinants of outcome in surgically treated patients with native valve endocarditis. *J Card Surg* 1989;4:331–339.

30. Petheram IS, Boyce JMH. Prosthetic valve endocarditis: A review of 24 cases. *Thorax* 1977;32:478–485.

Chapter 11

Right Heart Endocarditis

Agustin Arbulu, M.D.
Steven Gellman, M.D.
Donald Levine, M.D.
Larry W. Stephenson, M.D.

Right-sided Infective Endocarditis

Introduction

In his classic Gulstonian Lectures on malignant endocarditis, Osler described only 9 cases of endocarditis isolated to the right side of the heart, or 3.8% of the cases.[1] The incidence increased only slightly over decades. In 1977 Pelletier and Petersdorf recognized isolated right heart infection in 14% of 125 patients at the University of Washington.[2] By 1983 the prevalence of right-sided infection among intravenous drug users in our medical center climbed to 51 of 74 cases (69%).[3] This increasing incidence reflects not only improved recognition but also an increase in associated risk factors, details of which will be discussed below. This chapter will also describe the unique features of right-sided endocarditis and the current approach to management.

Epidemiology

For reasons that are not entirely clear, injection drug use is the most important risk factor for right-sided endocarditis. With the exception of reports

From: Vlessis AA, Bolling S (eds): *Endocarditis: A Multidisciplinary Approach to Modern Treatment.* © Futura Publishing Co., Armonk, NY, 1999.

excluding addicts from consideration, injection of illicit drugs is the primary risk factor cited in virtually every study.[4] Even among addicts, recognition of right-sided infection was delayed. In 1944, Hussey et al stated that localization to the tricuspid valve alone in 3 cases was "noteworthy because of its rarity."[5] Cherubin and others in 1968 studied medical examiners' files and reported a prevalence in addicts of left-sided infection, finding tricuspid involvement alone in only 9%.[6] It is now clearly established that addiction-related endocarditis affects the right side of the heart quite frequently and that despite the absence of underlying heart disease, the tricuspid valve, including most leaflets, is almost exclusively involved.[7] In populations where drug use is not prevalent, cases of right-sided infection are seen, albeit infrequently, and are associated with congenital heart disease. It is noteworthy that in a population in which rheumatic fever is prevalent and responsible for most cases of left-sided infective endocarditis (IE), congenital disease—not post-rheumatic disease—is associated with right-sided infection.[8] In an earlier study, Kaplan et al found that endocarditis in pediatric patients was most often associated with nonvalvular congenital heart disease.[9] They found an increased risk among cyanotic patients with systemic-to-pulmonary artery shunts. In older subjects, either congenital or acquired valvular disease was the most common risk factor.

Endocarditis is now also recognized as an important complication of modern medical advances. Several reports document an association between long-term indwelling catheters and right-sided infection, involving both the cardiac valves and the mural endocardium.[10–16] Most patients with long-term indwelling catheters have a serious underlying medical problem, but there may be an increased incidence among patients who 1) suffer from severe liver disease and receive total parenteral nutrition;[11] 2) have had bone marrow transplant; or 3) suffer from leukemia.[12] Pulmonary artery flow directed catheters are additional risk factors for right-sided endocarditis in hospitalized patients with an incidence ranging from 3.4% to 33%.[15–18] Patients with such catheters commonly develop noninfected intracardiac lesions; the longer the duration of catheterization, the greater the likelihood of damage occurring.[19,20] Perhaps the most striking feature of these catheter-related infections is the fact that the majority involve the pulmonic valve, a location seldom seen in other circumstances. The various components of cardiac pacemakers are also recognized as risk factors for right-sided endocarditis.[21,22] The majority of these lesions are on the tricuspid valve, although disease may be confined to the ventricular septal wall. Infections probably originate at the pacemaker insertion site and extend along the pacing lead, although on occasion they originate at a distant site and spread to the heart via the bloodstream.

Pathophysiology

The pathophysiology of infective endocarditis has been discussed in a previous chapter. In some cases right heart endocarditis infection is preceded by the classic pathway of valvular damage leading to a sterile thrombotic vegetation. Undoubtedly infections associated with central venous catheters, pacemakers, and pulmonary artery catheters arise in this fashion in a situation analogous to the animal model of endocarditis.[10-23] Indeed, the formation of bland thrombi in relation to intracardiac catheters has been described.[10] Abnormalities of the right heart valves are also known to be a focal point for infective endocarditis, undoubtedly due to the classic mechanism noted earlier.[8]

In drug users, endocarditis is more difficult to understand. A full discussion is beyond the scope of this chapter, but the subject has recently been discussed in detail.[24] At issue is the initiation of infection in the absence of valvular damage. In one study, 13 of 26 intravenous drug users were found to have echocardiographically abnormal right-side valves despite the absence of any known history of endocarditis.[25] Careful analysis of patients with *Pseudomonas* endocarditis failed to reveal any evidence of underlying valve pathology.[26] One intriguing study reported an increased frequency of endocarditis in drug users addicted to cocaine.[25] The association between cocaine use and valve disease is unclear, but the authors speculated that the intensity of cocaine use (i.e., frequency of injections per day) and/or the fact that the drug, unlike heroin, is not cooked, may predispose the user to infection.

The finding of normal valves in drug users with endocarditis has led to the "particle" theory, which suggests that particulate impurities injected by addicts induce microscopic damage to the endocardial surface which may then initiate the classic pathway of thrombosis, vegetation formation and subsequent infection if the patient becomes bacteremic.[23-28]

Regardless of etiology, addicts with right-sided endocarditis have disease almost exclusively restricted to the tricuspid valve. In addition, despite the absence of underlying valve disease, all 3 leaflets on the valve may become infected.[7] Myocardial and valve ring abscesses and valvular perforations are uncommon. Although right-sided heart failure occurs, it is usually not clinically apparent. Thus, recognition of right-sided endocarditis, particularly in the drug user, is dependent upon clinical suspicion in the presence of extracardial findings such as pulmonary signs and symptoms.

Microbiology

The microbial etiology of right-sided endocarditis is varied and differs somewhat from left- sided infection. The difference is primarily due to the associated factors which are often absent in aortic or mitral infection. Overall, various species of staphylococci are responsible for the majority of cases, regardless of the underlying process. Patients with congenital or acquired valvular disease (like their counterparts suffering from mitral or aortic disease) are frequently infected with *Streptococcus viridans*,[29] although *Staphylococcus aureus* was the predominant pathogen in at least one study.[8] Fungal endocarditis affects either side of the heart, but is seen most frequently as a complication of intravenous drug use, valve replacement surgery, indwelling catheters, and, more recently, liver transplantation.[20,30] Endocarditis associated with indwelling catheters is most often due to gram-positive cocci. Of these, coagulase-negative staphylococci are most frequently reported,[12,13,15,16] but *S. aureus*, and enterococci[11] are also encountered. Gram-negative bacilli[16] and *Candida* are occasional isolates. Pacemaker-induced infections are likewise most often due to staphylococci;[22] however, an unusual gram-positive bacillus, *Corynebacterium striatum*, was recently described.[31] A comprehensive list of organisms causing endocarditis in illicit drug users is far beyond the scope of this chapter and would include representation from the entire spectrum of microbiology. Nevertheless, virtually all studies verify that *S. aureus* is the predominant pathogen.[3-6,32-34] Streptococci, predominantly groups A, C and G, are commonly seen and enterococci are frequent isolates, but rarely involve the right heart. Gram-negative bacilli, notably *Pseudomonas aeruginosa* in Detroit, Chicago and New York and *Serratia marcescens*, once common in the Oakland, California, area, are seen sporadically. Among the fungi, *Candida* (often non-*albicans*) is the commonest cause of endocarditis.

Clinical Features

The clinical features of right-sided endocarditis are quite different from the findings in left- sided infection. Disease of the tricuspid or pulmonic valves is usually not manifest by cardiac signs and symptoms. As indicated earlier, although right-sided heart failure occurs, symptoms are usually mild and are rarely the predominant feature. Pulmonary signs and symptoms dominate the clinical picture, and are usually the result of septic pulmonary emboli.[4,7,28,33] Some patients have evidence of severe sepsis at presentation.[8] In most cases, nonspecific findings consistent with any infectious process are present, such as chills, fever and myalgia, but are unlikely to suggest the diagnosis.

The physical findings in right-sided infection are minimal and few of the signs classically associated with endocarditis are present. Characteristic skin lesions are rare, as are ophthalmologic signs, mucous membrane changes, and splenomegaly.[3,28] Murmurs of tricuspid endocarditis are present in the majority and may be augmented by the Rivero-Carvallo maneuver (accentuation of the murmur by deep inspiration). When combined with hepato-jugular reflux, the sensitivity for diagnosing tricuspid insufficiency is 93% and the specificity 100%.[26]

The laboratory is not particularly helpful in making the diagnosis, other than the finding of blood cultures positive for the offending pathogen. Since bacteremia in endocarditis is constant, virtually every organ is affected and almost any screening test is likely to be abnormal during the acute phase. Renal failure may be severe and often progresses during treatment due to immune complex nephritis.[33] Coagulopathy occasionally occurs and may take the form of thrombocytopenia, vasculitis or hemolytic anemia. Additional common, but nonspecific findings are elevated erythrocyte sedimentation rate, leukocytosis, anemia and hematuria.[22]

Perhaps the most characteristic evidence of right-sided endocarditis is the finding of multiple nodular or segmental pulmonary infiltrates, indicative of septic pulmonary emboli. These lesions are predominantly in the lower lobes, usually bilateral, and often cavitate.[4] A more serious lesion, mycotic aneurysm of the pulmonary artery, presents as a perihilar coin lesion with definite vascular connection. Alternatively, rapid change in the contour of the pulmonary artery may be observed. On right anterior oblique views, there may be an encroachment of the aneurysm shadow on the retrosternal space between the aortic arch and the left atrial shadow. Left anterior oblique views may show impingement of the interior aspect of the aortic window. Pulmonary angiography is diagnostic.[35] Indeed, the broad array of hematologic and serological abnormalities, coupled with bacteremia and the absence of localized findings outside of the lungs are so striking that they should make endocarditis a consideration.

Ultimately, the diagnosis depends on a strong clinical suspicion and a sufficient number of compatible signs and symptoms. Recently, Durack et al published a set of diagnostic criteria (commonly called the Duke criteria) that have gained wide acceptance.[36] These have been discussed in an earlier chapter and will not be repeated here, save to say that careful application can help to clarify an otherwise confusing case. Prominent in the Duke criteria is the contribution of echocardiography.

Echocardiography in Right-sided Infective Endocarditis

Many clinical series on right-sided IE that include echocardiographic findings report good sensitivity of the transthoracic two-dimensional technique for the diagnosis of vegetations. In a series of 16 patients with clinical tricuspid valve endocarditis, Ginzton et al[37] report 100% sensitivity for tricuspid valve vegetations. In a series of 12 narcotic addicts with right-sided IE, Berger et al[38] reported sensitivity of 83% for vegetations (9 tricuspid and one pulmonic). In a literature review compilation of 28 cases of isolated pulmonic valve IE, Cassling et al[39] reported that of the 15 patients on whom echocardiography was performed, the sensitivity for vegetations was 100%. In all of the above series, two-dimensional exam was superior to M-mode exam.

Whereas several investigations have concluded that transesophageal echocardiography (TEE) is superior to transthoracic echocardiography (TTE) for the detection of vegetations in left-sided IE and prosthetic valve IE, no such conclusion can yet be firmly drawn for right-sided IE as it usually presents. In a prospective series of 48 intravenous drug users with clinically suspected right-sided IE, San Roman et al[40] compared TEE to TTE for the detection of vegetations. In almost all patients, the TEE exam immediately followed the TTE exam. Sensitivities of the 2 examinations were identical, although the authors note that their young patients had good acoustic windows during TTE exam, and that their TEE probes were monoplane. In TEE the probe is closer to the mitral valve, and in TTE, the probe is closer to the tricuspid valve. Another plausible explanation for the comparability of TTE and TEE exams in right-sided IE is the fact that tricuspid vegetations are larger than left-sided vegetations. San Roman[40] reported a mean tricuspid valve vegetation diameter of 17 mm. Mügge et al[41] reported a mean tricuspid valve vegetation diameter of 18 mm, significantly larger than mean vegetation diameters of 10 mm for the aortic valve, 11 mm for the mitral valve, and 7 mm for prosthetic valves.

While TEE has been shown to be superior to TTE in diagnosing many of the complications of left-sided IE, such complications are either extremely rare or are less relevant clinically in right- sided IE. In a series of 118 consecutive patients with IE studied by both TTE and TEE for detection of abscess, Daniel et al[42] reported clear superiority of TEE over TTE for abscess detection. However, of 44 patients with abscess confirmed at surgery or autopsy, only one was associated with right-sided IE. For the diagnosis of leaflet perforation, Cziner et al[43] reported superiority of TEE over TTE in a series of 10 patients with mitral valve IE. However, leaflet perforation in right-sided IE is ordinarily well-tolerated hemodynamically, and does not of itself constitute an indication for surgery. While TEE is likely to be useful when applied to patients in whom right-sided IE is clinically suspected but in whom TTE images are inadequate or raise questions answerable by improved magnification, other indications for the more invasive technique remain best defined on a case-by-case basis.

Medical Management

The therapy of right-sided endocarditis is based on the offending pathogen, just as it is with left-sided infection. Recommendations for treatment of the usual organisms have been established by a committee of the American Heart Association.[44] The overriding principle to apply is the need for bactericidal drugs which must be given in high concentrations, and usually for prolonged periods. No specific recommendations exist for some of the gram-negative organisms encountered in drug users; however, the same rules apply. In addition, a combination of antibiotics is often used in an attempt to achieve synergy. Data exist that support the use of nafcillin plus an aminoglycoside for only 2 weeks in patients with uncomplicated right-sided *S. aureus* endocarditis, and this is a routine practice in our medical center.[45]

The most challenging question regarding right-sided endocarditis pertains to the use of anticoagulants in patients with septic pulmonary emboli. Generally these emboli pose much less of a problem than the systemic emboli associated with left-sided disease. Nevertheless, they can lead to respiratory compromise and, at the very least, may result in substantial pleuritic pain. There are in vitro and animal model data suggesting a potential benefit to the use of anticoagulants.[46,47] Currently, a multicenter trial is in progress and so no recommendations can be made at this time. It is important to note that for years, anticoagulants have been considered as contraindications for fear that they may result in fatal cerebral hemorrhage in patients with mycotic aneurysms, a well-known complication of endocarditis. Hence, until the results of the above mentioned study are known, most clinicians would refrain from their use.

Surgery for Right Heart Endocarditis in Non-intravenous Drug Users

Indications for Valve Surgery

The indications for surgery with right heart endocarditis include persistent sepsis, which may include fever, elevated white blood count, persistent septicemia despite appropriate antibiotic coverage, infectious involvement of the valve leaflets, and usually seeding of the lungs with bacteria-causing abscess formation. Documentation of valvular vegetations or valve destruction must be demonstrated with echocardiography. The greater the destruction of the valve by the septic process, and/or the larger the vegetation, the earlier surgical intervention may be considered.

Congestive heart failure may also be a further indication for surgical intervention.

One of the dilemmas in the management of patients with tricuspid valve endocarditis is whether surgical intervention is necessary, and if so, when. With appropriate antibiotic therapy alone, most patients can be treated successfully. When an indwelling venous catheter is present, removal of the catheter along with the appropriate antibiotic treatment will frequently result in a rapid cure. Some have recommended surgery if sepsis persists beyond 1 to 2 weeks in cases with documented valvular involvement,[48,49] whereas others feel 6 to 8 weeks of antibiotic treatment are necessary before surgical intervention.[50] Obviously, this must be tempered by the degree of valvular involvement and the degree of sepsis. For example, if a heart valve is largely destroyed as demonstrated by echocardiogram and large vegetations are present, or major bacterial seeding of the lungs continues to occur, one would intervene surgically sooner than in a person with minimal vegetations on the valve and low-grade sepsis.

Some have recommended surgical intervention when vegetations are larger than 1 cm on a native heart valve and there is continued evidence of sepsis,[37,51–55] while others have shown that the size of vegetation does not correlate with the need for surgery.[56] With fungal endocarditis, bulky, friable vegetations can measure many centimeters in diameter and are the source of large emboli.[30,57,58] Emboli are frequently multiple and commonly cause significant pathology. In a review of this subject by Rubinstein and Lang, they recommend surgery as soon as bulky vegetations are diagnosed in order to avoid embolization.[30]

When one is operating for valvular involvement, the options include valve-sparing debridement and possibly repair, valvulectomy without prosthetic replacement and valvulectomy with prosthetic valve replacement.

Valve-sparing operations with debridement are limited to cases in which the involvement of the valve and destruction is limited. Both Carpentier et al and Pearlman et al recommend valve repair when feasible.[59,60] In Carpentier's series of 40 patients undergoing valve repair for acute native valve endocarditis, the tricuspid valve alone was involved only twice. The lesions were similar to those found with the mitral valve, namely chordal ruptures and leaflet perforation. The tricuspid valve was involved with the mitral valve in 3 other patients. The lesions were chordal rupture. When leaflet perforation occurred, autogenous pericardial patching was used after the pericardium had been treated with a glutaraldehyde solution.

The surgical principles used by Carpentier included removing all macroscopically involved tissue without concern for possibilities of repair.[59] The involved valve tissue was widely resected including a strip of at least 2 mm of normal-appearing valvular tissue. Valve reconstruction was then performed according to Carpentier's techniques and principles. The use of a Carpentier ring was indicated when the annulus was dilated by previous underlying pathology, particularly degenerative lesions or for reinforcement of the annular remodeling after extensive resection. According to Carpentier, immediate hemodynamic improvements were shown in all survivors. Continuous antibiotic therapy was used for up to 2 months. With late follow-up in Carpentier's series, there was one hospital death in a patient with mitral valve repair who died of persistent sepsis leading to cardiogenic shock. In a follow-up from 6 to 94 months, there was no return of endocarditis, there was one late death 2½ years after repair. The cause of the death was unclear. Carpentier stated that the infectious organism involved should not influence the surgical policy.

Pearlman and associates reported on 4 patients with tricuspid valve endocarditis, all having grade 3 to 4 tricuspid regurgitation.[60] Evidence of right ventricular enlargement and mobile vegetations was also present. In each case up to three quarters of the anterior leaflet was excised en bloc with infected chordae and papillary muscle head. The surgical procedures included standard quadrangle resection, conversion to bicuspid valve and pericardial patch replacement of the anterior leaflet with mobilization of basal chordae to replace resected marginal chordae. All repaired valves were successfully sterilized without recurrent infections. Two of the 4 patients continued to have postoperative 3+ tricuspid regurgitation. Two of the patients were intravenous drug users. All patients completed full courses of antibiotics for 2 to 6 months postoperatively. The specific time of follow-up is not mentioned, but they do state that there was no evidence of recurrent endocarditis.

Yee and Ullyot have also reported on tricuspid valve repair for endocarditis in 12 patients with encouraging results[61]. Although persistent tricuspid valve regurgitation was present in many, their feeling was that there was still a lesser degree of regurgitation than when tricuspid valvulectomy by itself was used.

David and associates reported on 62 consecutive patients who underwent heart valve operation for active infective endocarditis[62]. Annular abscess was encountered in 33 patients. Complex valve procedures involving reconstruction of the left ventricular outflow tract were performed in 31 patients. In 2 of the 62 patients, the tricuspid valve was involved. Twenty-four patients had prosthetic valve endocarditis; 8 with mechanical valves and 16 with tissue valves. In their series, 37 patients had aortic valve endocarditis. Operations mainly included aortic valve replacement, frequently with reconstruction of the left ventricular outflow tract, and some replacement of the ascending aorta. Some also underwent mitral valve replacement. Two also underwent mitral valve repair and one also underwent tricuspid valve replacement. Of 18 patients presenting with primary mitral valve endocarditis, 13 underwent mitral valve replacement, some with additional cardiac procedures. In the 2 presenting with only tricuspid endocarditis, both underwent tricuspid valve repair. The overall mortality for the 62 patients was 4.8%. Both patients undergoing tricuspid valve repair survived. There were no operative deaths among the patients with native valve endocarditis (as opposed to prosthetic valve endocarditis). They recommended that with mechanical valve endocarditis, these patients should undergo operation as soon as the diagnosis is established. An exception to this would be patients who develop septicemia early after prosthetic valve replacement. These patients can frequently be managed with antibiotics alone.

Heimberger and Duma reviewed 4 major studies of 10,660 patients receiving cardiac valves.[63] The overall incidence of prosthetic valve endocarditis ranged from 0.98% to 4.4%. They arbitrarily defined early prosthetic valve endocarditis as occurring less than 60 days after cardiac valve replacement and late as 60 or more days following valve replacement. They found that 18% to 36% of the infections occurred early, and 64% to 82% of the infections occurred late. The risk of acquiring prosthetic valve endocarditis was highest within 5 to 6 months after valve replacement and the risk was lowest at one year after valve replacement. After that, the risk remained constant. They point out that one of the dilemmas in patients with a prosthetic heart valve is determining whether the bacteremia represents endocarditis. The Heimberger and Duma review did not specifically mention prosthetic tricuspid valve endocarditis; nonetheless, the principles would apply to the tricuspid valve.[63] An important component of management is early surgical intervention when prosthetic valve endocarditis is documented.

Sande et al studied 22 patients with prosthetic valves.[64] They had 24 episodes of sustained bacteremia. All were suspected of having prosthetic valve endocarditis. The patients were divided into 2 groups; those with definite prosthetic valve endocarditis based on autopsy or surgical findings, which included 11 patients; and those with no clinical (9 patients) or pathological evidence of prosthetic valve endocarditis. They found that a short duration (less than 25 days) between surgery and the documentation of bacteremia, absence of new murmurs and evidence of extracardial source of bacteremia suggested that bacteremia, rather than prosthetic valve endocarditis was present. They also found that all of the patients in Group I died of causes related to prosthetic valve endocarditis. In contrast, 7 of 13 in Group II survived with the antibiotic treatment alone and had no evidence of heart failure over a median follow-up of 2 years.

Rubinstein and Lang found that mechanical and bioprosthetic valves were associated with the same rate of relapse for candida endocarditis, and therefore had no recommendation as to whether to use a mechanical or biological prosthesis.[30]

Our recommendation for patients with tricuspid endocarditis who are not intravenous drug users is to attempt to repair the valve when the damage is not extensive, and to replace the valve when it is. We make no recommendation in favor of a mechanical or a biological prosthesis. This decision should be individualized to the patient. Valvulectomy alone should be considered in patients with fairly good ventricular function where there is extensive annular involvement. When prosthetic valve endocarditis is documented, we recommend early surgical intervention.

Surgery for Endocarditis in Patients with Congenital Heart Disease

Patients with congenital cardiac lesions are prone to develop endocarditis, frequently involving the right heart, as are patients who have undergone palliative and reparative procedures of their congenital heart lesions. Kaplan et al surveyed 26 major cardiovascular centers where congenital cardiac procedures were performed.[9] They found 278 patients who developed infective endocarditis in the year of their survey. An in-depth review of this subject is presented. Indications for surgical intervention must be individualized for each patient. Clearly, if the patient can be treated medically and gotten over the acute episode of endocarditis, this is preferable, particularly when a prosthetic valve or other prosthetic material will be required for the repair. Nonetheless, in some cases, the surgeon must proceed during an acute episode of bacterial endocarditis.[65]

Pacemaker Lead Infections

A review by Heimberger and Duma found that greater than 6% of patients undergoing permanent pacemaker insertion developed infectious complications.[63] They found that the risks were increased in patients with diabetes mellitus, corticosteroid therapy, anticoagulants, postoperative hematoma, malignancy, generator replacement and dermatologic diseases. Infections may involve the pacemaker pocket and lead portion in the pocket, or the lead within the vascular system and surrounding tissue. *Staphylococcus* organisms were responsible for 75% of all pacemaker infections. Although some have reported successful eradication of pacemaker pocket infections using various closed or open irrigation techniques, most studies indicate that pacemaker pocket infections will require removal of the pacemaker and eventually removal of the pacemaker leads to eradicate the infection.

A dilemma for the clinician is the patient with a permanent endocardial pacemaker or defibrillator device who has developed bacteremia. It is often difficult to prove that the pacemaker lead itself is infected, particularly in a case where there is no evidence of pacemaker pocket infection. Removal of the leads, particularly after they have been in for a long period of time, cannot be taken lightly. In some cases, lead extraction requires open-heart surgery. Intravascular pacer lead infections are more prone to occur late after pacemaker replacement as opposed to pacemaker pocket infections which tend to occur early.[66–68] In fact, pacemaker pocket infections are usually diagnosed within a few weeks after the pacemaker system has been implanted or the pulse generator battery changed. In patients with recurrent bacteremia with no other source for infection, pacemaker lead infections should strongly be considered, particularly if there are vegetations on the lead or if there is evidence of right-sided endocarditis in conjunction with the pacemaker leads. Courses of appropriate antibiotics can be tried in patients with an endocardial pacemaker system and bacteremia and may be successful.

Camus et al studied data on 26 patients with permanent endocardial pacemakers who had 28 episodes of bacteremia to determine whether removal of the pacer lead was necessary.[21] They concluded that the high rate of uncontrolled infection or relapse among patients with staphylococcal bacteremia confirmed the need for immediate removal of the entire pacemaker system when obvious infections of the pulse generator pocket or the subcutaneous part of the wire is observed, or when vegetations exist on the pacing lead. They also found that even after prompt removal of the wire, the occurrence of endocarditis or persistently positive blood cultures suggest that intravenous antibiotic therapy should be given for a minimum period of one month.

Arber et al reviewed records of 10 major hospitals over a 10-year period where 8303 permanent pacemaker procedures were performed.[22] There were 468 diagnosed cases of infection. Of these, 44 were associated with pacemaker endocarditis. They stated that although their analysis was not sufficient to conclude that pacemaker endocarditis is an absolute indication for electrode removal, their data strongly suggested the need for electrode removal. The mortality rate was 13% in the group that underwent electrode removal and 32% in the medically managed group.

Surgical Treatment of Intractable Right-sided Endocarditis in Drug Addicts

It is important to stress that drug addiction is the primary illness that affects this group of patients; endocarditis is the secondary illness. With this in mind, it is possible to evolve a rational plan for surgical management of intractable endocarditis among drug addicts.

The great majority of patients affected with these infections have normal hearts. A normal heart is defined as a heart that has no previous congenital or acquired disease. The function of the heart in most of these patients is normal: the right-sided pressures as well as the hemodynamics are normal. The infection of the heart is the result of the self-administration of intravenous drugs. Our procedure of choice during the past 30 years in the management of intractable right-sided endocarditis in drug addicts is the removal of the tricuspid valve without replacement. This represents the preferred surgical treatment among this population of patients.

Brief Historical Review

Our experience with this group of patients started in 1967. Initially following the classic approach, we excised the infected tricuspid valve and inserted a prosthesis. This resulted in 100% failure for the following reasons: 1) inability to control the endocarditis in 80% of patients; 2) reinfection of the prosthetic valve due to patient's return to drug abuse; and 3) fatal complications due to patient noncompliance with the anticoagulant therapy.

Our experimental work in 1968 was aimed at answering the following questions. 1) Is it possible to resect the tricuspid valve without replacement? 2) If this is possible, what are the conditions that allow this operation to succeed? We operated on 7 dogs and removed the tricuspid valve using cardiopulmonary bypass. Five of the animals survived the operation with minimal or no hemodynamic difficulties. The dogs were able to have a normal existence with a trivalvular heart. The liver, renal, pulmonary and endocrine functions remained within normal range.

On September 3, 1970, we operated upon our first surviving patient with intractable tricuspid endocarditis due to *Pseudomonas aeruginosa*. A totally destroyed valve had been replaced by florid vegetations. These vegetations were removed including part of the annulus of the tricuspid valve. The operation was basically a debridement type of procedure. No prosthetic valve was inserted in the tricuspid position. At the time of the operation, the patient was moribund, with a temperature of 104°F. The patient was comatose because of severe sepsis; his hemoglobin was 7 gm%. He required prolonged postoperative care including intravenous administration of the appropriate antibiotics. This patient survived for 24 years. About 12 years following the removal of the tricuspid valve without replacement, he suffered a stab wound, resulting in severe injury of the liver. He was treated at another institution and the patient survived this problem and continued in satisfactory health. Most important during his 24 years of survival, he had numerous relapses into drug abuse, including alcohol, tobacco, and cocaine intermittently. In fact, his demise was most likely related to an overdose of cocaine.

This initial patient exemplifies the problem of the drug-addicted patient. In addition, during the past 30 years we have received numerous telephone calls and letters from cardiac surgeons asking us what to do with an infected prosthesis in a patient who, after being cured by our approach, underwent a second cardiac operation with insertion of a prosthesis in the tricuspid position.

Patient Material and Methods

Our 55 patients had been heroin addicts for periods ranging from 1 year to 20 years before their heart surgery, with an average of 9 years. Forty were men and 15 were women. Their ages ranged from 20 to 55 years with a median age of 30 years. Extended intravenous antibiotic treatment failed to control the infection in each. They received antibiotics for periods ranging from 1 to 11 months, averaging 3 months. Surgery was indicated in all as a life-saving measure (Table 1).

Of the 55 patients, 30 had *P. aeruginosa* infection, and 4 of those also had *Staphylococcus aureus* infection (3 methicillin resistant). Another patient had *Candida albicans* infection in addition to the infection caused by *P. aeruginosa*. In 28 patients, *S. aureus* was the infecting organism. In 15 patients, this microorganism was the only pathogen isolated from the blood cultures. Of the staphylococcal infections, 20, or 80%, were due to bacteria resistant to methicillin. Ten (36%) of the gram-positive infections had 1 or 2 additional microorganisms, and in 4 the organism was fungus

Table 1
55 Patients: All Had Intractable Right-Sided Endocarditis

Sex	Age (yrs)	Bacteriology*	Operation	Deaths
40 M	Median 30	PSA = 30	TVE = 53	Total = 17 Early = 6
15 F	(20–55)	SA = 28	TVE + PVE = 2	Late = 11

* Predominant microorganism. See text for description of various mixed infections.
M = Male
F = Female
PSA = *Pseudomonas aeruginosa*
SA = *Staphylococcus aureus*
TVE = Tricuspid valvulectomy without replacement
PVE = Pulmonic valvulectomy without replacement

(2 *C. albicans* and 2 *C. tropicalis*). A total of 8 patients had fungal infections. In 7 of these (88%), the endocarditis was due to mixed microorganisms. Only 1, or 12%, had *C. albicans* as the only infecting organism. Of the total of 55 patients, 14 (25%) were infected by multiple organisms.

In all 55 patients, the diagnosis of right-sided endocarditis was made by: 1) history of intravenous drug addiction for periods that ranged from 1 to 20 years; 2) fever and prostration; 3) chest pain and chest radiographic manifestation of septic embolic lesions of the lungs such as parenchymal infiltrates, pleural effusion or both; and 4) positive blood cultures.[69,70] When echocardiography became available, it was used routinely and is very helpful in the diagnosis of right-sided tricuspid endocarditis.

Fifty-three patients underwent total excision of the tricuspid valve without replacement and 2 had both the tricuspid and pulmonary valves removed without replacement. All patients received postoperative intravenous antibiotics for 2 to 6 weeks. Twenty-four of the 49 patients (49%) who survived the valvulectomy are known to have returned to the use of intravenous drugs after their operation.

Six patients (11%) required prosthetic valve insertion in the tricuspid position from 3 days to 13 years after the excision of the valve. Five had the tricuspid valve only excised, and 1 had both the tricuspid and pulmonary valves excised. These patients are summarized in Table 2. (Patient numbers reflect their chronological location in our registry.) Patient 4 had insertion of a Starr-Edwards prosthetic valve 6 months after his tricuspid valvulectomy without replacement. This operation was performed at another institution and the indication for valve replacement was "absence of the tricuspid valve." Unfortunately, the patient returned to his intravenous drug habit and developed a second endocarditis that involved the mitral and aortic valves which caused his death.

In patients 11, 16, 23 and 31, the indication for insertion of a prosthetic valve in the tricuspid position was intractable right heart failure 2 to 13 years after tricuspid valve excision without replacement. Patient 11 died 5 weeks after tricuspid valve replacement, which was completed 13 years after tricuspid and pulmonary valve removal without replacement. He died suddenly, and no postmortem examination was carried out. Arrhythmia or pulmonary embolism were considered as possible causes of death. The patient had been using cocaine. His sudden death occurred as he was carrying a television set. The next patient, number 16, was 33 years old at the time of his tricuspid valvulectomy without replacement on July 16, 1973. He had used heroin for 10 years. He recovered well from this operation and 5 years later was able to free himself from drugs. In 1981, he developed symptoms and signs of right heart failure. Initially, he responded to medical treatment. However, his condition continued to deteriorate. In an attempt to control his refractory right heart failure, on July

Table 2

Intractable Right-sided Endocarditis: Patients Who Had a Prosthesis Inserted After Valvulectomy

Patient Number*	Age/Sex	Cured by Valvulectomy Insertion	Time Interval	Indication for Valve Inserted	2nd Operation Prosthesis	Results
4	24/M	Yes	6 months	Absence of tricuspid valve	Starr-Edwards	Died 7 months after valve insertion.
11	22/M	Yes	13 years	Enlarged heart intractable right-sided heart failure	35 mm Carpentier-Edwards	Died suddenly 5 weeks after valve insertion.
16	33/M	Yes	10 years	Intractable right heart failure	35 mm Carpentier-Edwards	Died 2 months after valve insertion.
23	27/F	Yes	4 years	Intractable right heart failure	35 mm Carpentier-Edwards DDD epicardial pacemaker	Alive, using drugs, now HIV positive.
31	29/M	Yes	2 years	Intractable right heart failure	Repair of iatrogenic inter-ventricular septal defect 31 mm Carpentier-Edwards pacemaker	Alive, has required change of pacemaker.
39	33/F	No	3rd P.O. day	Low cardiac output	Repair of iatrogenic interventricular septal defect 31 mm Ionescou-Shiley valve	Died 2 days after second operation.

* Numbers correspond to registry
PO = postoperative.

16, 1983, 10 years after his tricuspid valvulectomy without replacement, he had a Carpentier-Edwards bioprosthetic valve inserted in the tricuspid position. Initially, he improved after his second cardiac operation, but then developed symptoms and signs of uncontrollable right heart failure and died 2 months after the tricuspid bioprosthetic valve insertion. Autopsy was not granted by the family.

Patient 23 had her second cardiac operation 4 years after the initial operation. She is still alive, but uses drugs and has been tested positive for the human immune deficiency virus (HIV). Patient 31 was operated upon 2 years after his tricuspid valvulectomy. He had a ventricular septal defect as a result of debridement of the tricuspid annulus during the initial operation and he has required insertion of a permanent single chamber (VVI) pacemaker. He is alive with failure of his tricuspid bioprosthesis and has twice undergone pulse generator replacement. The sixth patient, number 39, had methicillin-resistant S. aureus infection and received 3 months of unsuccessful intravenous antibiotic therapy. She was in a moribund state when she underwent tricuspid valvulectomy. As a result of the tricuspid annular debridement, a ventricular septal defect was created. She developed a low cardiac output and underwent a second cardiac operation on her third postoperative day. The iatrogenic ventricular septal defect was closed and a bioprosthetic valve was inserted in the tricuspid position. The patient died 2 days later; that is, 5 days after the initial operation. The autopsy showed acute endocarditis, acute myocarditis and a large acute posterior myocardial infarction.

Of the 55 patients, a total of 17 died, giving an overall mortality rate of 31%. Six of the deaths, or 11%, occurred within 45 days following the operation. All had endocarditis that could not be controlled by tricuspid valvulectomy. One case, that of patient 39, is mentioned above. Two cases had gram-negative infections due to P. aeruginosa. Both had long preoperative courses of antibiotic treatment lasting 5 and 6 months respectively. They were referred to surgery in a moribund condition. Another 2 had endocarditis due to methicillin-resistant S. aureus. They had intravenous therapy lasting 1 and 2 months respectively. Both developed diffuse intravascular coagulopathy secondary to uncontrollable infection. In one case the blood cultures grew P. aeruginosa, S. aureus (methicillin resistant) and C. albicans. This patient died on the third postoperative day as a consequence of the uncontrollable infection.

Eleven patients, or 20%, died 9 to 24 years after tricuspid valve excision without replacement (10 tricuspid and 1 tricuspid and pulmonary valve excision). In 10 of these 11 patients, the late deaths were related to the recurrent use of intravenous drugs in 8 and cocaine via the nasal route in 2.

In only 1 patient was the death related to uncontrollable right heart failure, 2 months after the insertion of a prosthetic valve in the tricuspid position (see case number 16 above).

Literature Review

During the past 30 years, several articles have been published on right-sided infective endocarditis in intravenous drug addicts.[28,50,69,71-76] None of these reports have supplied long-term follow-up of the operations proposed in the management of intractable right-sided endocarditis in intravenous drug addicts.

Several operations have been recommended.[60,61,74,77-81] The classic concept of infected valve excision followed by prosthetic replacement, in the same operation or in staged operations, is championed by some experienced surgeons. Preservation of the different components of the tricuspid valve has recently been re-advocated by others. These conservative operations consist of excision of the vegetations with involved portions of the tricuspid valve, and reconstruction either by valve repair or by insertion of autologous tissues (fascia lata or pericardium), reestablishing the integrity of the tricuspid valve.

We think it is necessary to compare these other operations to our surgical approach: Single (tricuspid) or double (tricuspid and pulmonary) valve excision without inserting a replacement valve. It is our aim to compare these other operations and answer the following questions:

1. Were all the patients intravenous drug addicts? For how long?
2. What microorganisms were involved in the infections?
3. How many of the reported cases of endocarditis were intractable?
4. How many patients returned to their intravenous drug addiction after the initial operation and what were the consequences?
5. How long have the reported patients been followed?
6. Was there a need to use anticoagulants? If so, what was the degree of patient compliance?

We believe that this approach will allow realistic conclusions and recommendations in the surgical treatment of intractable right-sided infective endocarditis in the intravenous drug- addicted patient.[69,75,81-86]

There are 6 publications in the literature that suggest a surgical approach different from ours. In the early report of Alexander and associates,[78] a 24-year-old woman developed right-sided endocarditis 6 weeks prior to admission. The patient had been "injecting stimulants into arm and leg veins." The drug most often used in those days (the late 1960s) was methylphenidate (ritalin hydrochloride). The description of the patient's addiction suggests that she had also been using amphetamines for 2 years. During her hospitalization, she was treated with a combination of antibiotics. Blood cultures grew S. *marcescens*. Finally, on her 69th hospital day, she underwent cardiac surgery. Loose, friable vegetations were found at the junction of the posterior and anterior leaflet of the tricuspid valve, and the chordae tendinae were disrupted for approximately 2 cm along the valve junction. This area of the valve was debrided and a tricuspid annuloplasty accomplished, leaving a 2.5 cm orifice. Eighteen months after the onset of the infection, the patient was well and without evidence of recurrent infection.

This report[78] documents that the patient was an intravenous drug user for at least 2 years. The microorganism, S. *marcescens*, could not be eradicated. The gross anatomy of the tricuspid valvular lesion lent itself to the conservative operation that the authors successfully performed. The patient follow-up extended to only 18 months. We agree with the authors' plan of therapy. However, none of the patients upon whom we operated had such a limited pathological anatomy of the tricuspid valve as that which was described by Alexander.

In 1974, Simberkoff[77] published the case of a 28-year-old heroin addict with an intractable tricuspid endocarditis secondary to coagulase positive S. *aureus* and Enterobacter organisms. On his 75th day of hospitalization, the patient underwent a tricuspid valvulectomy without prosthetic replacement. At surgery, one of the tricuspid valve leaflets was found to be replaced by a pink, rounded vegetation measuring 1 cm in diameter. Stain showed gram-positive cocci and gram- negative rods. S. *aureus* and Enterobacter were cultured from the vegetation. The patient was given intravenous antibiotics and was cured of his endocarditis. His exercise tolerance was severely limited and cardiac catheterization showed a cardiac index of 1.9 L/min/m2. Twenty- seven days after his tricuspid valvulectomy, he underwent a second cardiac operation. A Starr- Edwards prosthetic valve was inserted in the tricuspid position. Cultures taken at surgery and blood cultures obtained subsequently in the absence of antibiotic therapy were sterile. The patient was discharged 3 months after his second cardiac operation on warfarin sodium (coumadin) and methadone hydrochloride. He was asymptomatic and without evidence of recurrent infection 8 months and 10 days after insertion of the Starr-Edwards prosthetic valve. No further follow-up is given.

In 1986 Stern and associates published a paper recommending immediate tricuspid valve replacement for endocarditis.[74] They reviewed their experience with 10 intravenous drug users who were operated upon between March 1981 and October 1984. The length of drug addiction of these patients is not stated. Apparently, all had intractable tricuspid endocarditis due to S. *aureus*. All received a bioprosthetic valve after excision of the infected native tricuspid valve (5 Carpentier-Edwards and 5 Hancock). The mean duration of observation was 12.5 months (range from 4 to 36 months). One patient was lost to follow-up after 5 months; 3 returned to intravenous drug use and all died. In this paper, the authors wrote an addendum stating that "a fourth patient has returned to drug addiction 2 years after valve replacement. He is currently receiving antibiotic therapy for infection of the aortic valve and probably the tricuspid prosthesis."

We do not believe that the report of Stern and associates supports their recommendations of immediate tricuspid valve replacement for endocarditis among intravenous drug addicts. If 50% of their patients were either dead, dying or lost to follow-up at a mean duration of observation of 12.5 months, one wonders what may be the fate of any surviving patients at the present time.

In 1987[61] and later in 1989,[79] Yee reiterated Alexander's recommendations[78] of a reparative approach to the tricuspid valve for right sided endocarditis. Of Yee's 15 patients, 7 were intravenous drug addicts. In this subset of patients, the length of addiction is not clearly stated, nor is the length of intravenous antibiotic administration evident. The microorganisms involved were *Streptococcus fecalis*, *S. aureus* (methicillin-resistant in 4 cases) and *Torulopsis globatra*. Among these drug addicted patients it appeared that the endocarditis had become intractable. The reparative operation was applicable in 3 or 4 of the 7 who had "grade I and II infections." According to the authors, grade I or II might be lesions "involving only one major leaflet and/or the minor leaflet." The authors also stated that "extensive annular invasions and multileaflet infections were technical limitations in the remaining patients." This statement probably indicates that almost half of their 7 drug addicted patients with intractable tricuspid endocarditis were not candidates for tricuspid valve repair. The follow-up of their patients extended to a mean period of 24 months.

In 1991, Allen[60] reported on 4 patients in whom the principles of mitral valve repair were applied in the surgical management of tricuspid valve endocarditis. The drug to which they were addicted is not mentioned, nor is the length of addiction. The endocarditis was due to *S. aureus*, *Streptococcus viridans* and *Hemophilus parainfluenza* in one, and only *S. aureus* in the other. These authors do not state if the endocarditis was intractable. It is interesting to note that in the resected specimens, i.e., central portions of the tricuspid leaflet, *Staphylococcus epidermidis* was cultured from one of the patients, and from the other the cultures were negative. These findings suggest that the endocarditis of these 2 patients was most likely cured at the time of the tricuspid reconstruction. Although the 2 addicted patients received 6 weeks of postoperative antibiotic therapy, no length of follow-up beyond this period is stated.

In our patients the duration of their preoperative intravenous drug addiction averaged 9 years (range 1 to 20 years). All of these patients had prolonged preoperative intravenous antibiotic administration averaging 3 months (range 1 to 11 months). All were intractable and some were moribund. In the first 10 years of our experience, *P. aeruginosa* was the predominant microorganism causing the endocarditis. During the second 10 years, *S. aureus* predominated and we observed the emergence of methicillin-resistant strains, mixed infections and fungal infections. This microbiological evolution aggravated the severity and complexity of the infections.

At the time of the operation, the pathology of the infected tricuspid valve precluded any reparative approach. Perhaps the severity of infection was related to efforts to control the infection with intravenous antibiotic administration for longer periods than necessary. We have no argument with reports by others, but want to stress that statements related to the type of surgical treatment should take into account the specific conditions of patients under treatment. We also consider it important that the length of "good" or "satisfactory" results should be counted in years, extending to at least 10 to 20 years, and not in months.

Only 6 of our 55 patients subsequently required a prosthetic valve insertion in the tricuspid position after their valvulectomy. The clinical courses, including indications for valve replacement at the second operation and final outcomes, are outlined in Table 2. Endocarditis and drug addiction have been the most important determinants in the final outcome of these unfortunate patients. Only in patient 16 is there clinical evidence that the prolonged absence of the tricuspid valve was the most important factor contributing to his death.

In relation to right-sided valve(s) excision without replacement as a surgical treatment for intractable endocarditis in the intravenous drug user, we want to emphasize the following:

1) The patient must have an otherwise normal heart with normal cardiac function. Our patients fulfilled this criterion.
2) The operation is simple to perform. It requires cannulation of the superior and inferior vena cava. It can be performed with a beating heart or using anterograde cardioplegia. Normothermia or mild hypothermia can be used. It is a "debridement operation." It does not require unusual skills. All grossly infected endocardial structures (leaflets, cordi, papillary muscle, etc.) must be removed. Usually this operation takes 15 to 20 minutes of cardiopulmonary bypass.
3) The excellent tolerance by the patients and their rapid recovery is remarkable. Currently, hospitalization is short, 4 to 7 days if the patient's medical condition permits. Additional antibiotic therapy can be given

on an outpatient basis and combined with rehabilitation for the drug addiction.

4) Finally, compared to other cardiac operations, tricuspid valvulectomy is less expensive: there is no need for the use of artificial valves or other devices; and the postoperative care of the majority of the patients is relatively low cost—no special tests, anticoagulants, etc. The economic constrictions that currently affect the health care systems of many countries demand that physicians propose therapeutic measures that restore the good health of the patients and are cost effective.

Our experience is the best-documented large series involving intractable right-sided endocarditis among drug addicts. We have not observed this type of infection in nonaddicted patients. Our experience exceeds 27 years. The actuarial survival is 61%. (see Table 1). We think that tricuspid or tricuspid and pulmonary valve excision without replacement remains the operation of choice in the surgical treatment of intravenous drug addicts with intractable right-sided endocarditis. We recommend removing the entire tricuspid valve when at least 1 of the 2 major leaflets is destroyed, since leaving the other major leaflet does little to reduce the degree of tricuspid regurgitation and residual valve tissue could potentially become infected with subsequent drug use. Other authors share our recommendations.[87] Time has given us the strongest evidence to support our conclusion.

References

1. Osler W. Gulstonian lecture on malignant endocarditis. *Lancet* 1885;1: 415,159,505.
2. Pelletier LL, Petersdorf RG. Infective endocarditis: A review of 125 cases from the University of Washington hospitals. *Medicine* 1977;56:287–313.
3. Levine DP, Crane LR, and Zervos MJ. Bacteremia in narcotic addicts at the Detroit Medical Center. II. Infectious endocarditis: A prospective study: *Rev Infect Dis* 1986;8:374–395.
4. Reisberg BE. Infective endocarditis in the narcotic addict. *Prog Cardiovasc Dis* 1979;22:193–204.
5. Hussey HH, Keliher TF, Schefer BF, et al. Septicemia and bacterial endocarditis resulting from heroin addiction. *JAMA* 1944;126:535–538.
6. Cherubin CE, Baden M, Kavaler F, et al. Infective endocarditis in narcotic addicts. *Ann Intern Med* 1968;69:1091–1098.
7. Roberts WC, Buchbinder NA. Right-sided valvular infective endocarditis: A clinicopathologic study of twelve necropsy patients. *Am J Med* 1972;53:7–19.
8. Grover A, Anand IS, Varma J, et al. Profile of right-sided endocarditis: An Indian experience. *Int J Cardiol* 1991;33:83–88.
9. Kaplan EL, Rich MA, Welton G, et al. A collaborative study of infective endo-

carditis in the 1970s: Emphasis on infections in patients who have undergone cardiovascular surgery. *Circulation* 1979;59:327–335.

10. Becker AE, Becker MJ, Martin FH, et al. Bland thrombosis and infection in relation to intracardiac catheter. *Circulation* 1972;46:200–203.

11. Gatti JE, Reichele N, Mullan JL. Endocarditis complicating home hyperalimentation. *Arch Surg* 1981;116:933–935.

12. Liepman MK, Jones PG, Kauffman CA. Endocarditis as a complication of indwelling right atrial catheters in leukemic patients. *Cancer* 1984;54:804–807.

13. Power J, Wing EJ, Talamo TS, et al. Fatal bacterial endocarditis as a complication of permanent indwelling catheters: Report of two cases. *Am J Med* 1986; 81:166–168.

14. Putchell RA, White CL III, Clark AW, et al. Non-bacterial thrombotic endocarditis in bone marrow transplant recipients. *Cancer* 1988;55:631–635.

15. Quinn JP, Counts GW, Myers JD. Intracardiac infections due to coagulase-negative staphylococcus associated with Hickman catheters. *Cancer* 1986,57: 1079–1082.

16. Martino P, Micozzi A, Venditti M, et al. Catheter-related right-sided endocarditis in bone marrow transplant recipients. *Rev Infect Dis* 1990;12:250–257.

17. Ford, SE, Manley PN. Indwelling cardiac catheters: An autopsy study of associated endocardial lesions. *Arch Pathol Lab Med* 1982;106:314–317.

18. Lang HW, Galliani CA, Edwards JE. Local complications associated with indwelling Swan-Ganz catheters: Autopsy study of 36 cases. *Am J Cardiol* 1983; 52:1108–1111.

19. Rowley KM, Clubb KS, Smithe GJW, et al. Right-sided infective endocarditis as a consequence of flow-directed pulmonary-artery catheterization. A clinico-pathological study of 55 autopsied patients. *N Engl J Med* 1984;311:1152–1156.

20. Welty FK, McLeod GX, Ezratty C, et al. *Pseudoallescheria boydii* endocarditis of the pulmonic valve in a liver transplant recipient. *Clin Infect Dis* 1992;15: 858–860.

21. Camus C, Leport C, Raffi F, et al. Sustained bacteremia in 26 patients with a permanent endocardial pacemaker: Assessment of wire removal. *Clin Infect Dis* 1993;17:46–55.

22. Arber N, Pras E, Copperman Y, et al. Pacemaker endocarditis. Report of 44 cases and review of the literature. *Medicine* 1994;73:299–305.

23. Garrison PK, Freeman LR. Experimental endocarditis. I. Staphylococcal endocarditis in rabbits resulting from placement of a polyethylene catheter in the right side of the heart. *Yale J Biol Med* 1971;42:394–410.

24. Levine DP. Infectious endocarditis in intravenous drug abusers. In Levine DP, Sobel JD (eds.) *Infections in Intravenous Drug Abusers.* New York, NY. Oxford University Press, 1991. pp 255–257.

25. Robbins MJ, Soeiro R, Frishman WH, et al. Right-sided valvular endocarditis: Etiology, diagnosis, and an approach to therapy. *Am Heart J* 1986;111:128–135.

26. Reyes MP, Palutke WA, Wylin RF, et al. Pseudomonas endocarditis in the Detroit Medical Center, 1969–1972. *Medicine* 1973;52:173–194.

27. Chambers HF, Morris DL, Tauber MG, et al. Cocaine use and the risk for endocarditis in intravenous drug users. *Ann Intern Med* 1987;106:833–836.

28. Chan P, Ogilby JD, Segal B. Tricuspid valve endocarditis. *Am Heart J* 1989; 117:1140–1146.

29. Nakamura K, Satomi G, Sakai T, et al. Clinical and echocardiographic features of pulmonary valve endocarditis. *Circulation* 1983;67:198–204.

30. Rubinstein E, Lang R. Fungal endocarditis. *Eur Heart J* 1995;16(58):84–89.
31. Melero-Bascones M, Munoz P, Rodriguez-Creixems M, et al. *Corynebacterium striatum*: An undescribed agent of pacemaker-related endocarditis. *Clin Infect Dis* 1996;22:576–577.
32. Levine DP. Infectious endocarditis in intravenous drug abusers. In Levine DP, Sobel JD. *Infections in Drug Abusers. Infections in Drug Abusers*. New York, NY. Oxford University Press, 1991. pp 251–254.
33. Hecht, SR, Berger M. Right-sided endocarditis in intravenous drug users: Prognostic features in 102 episodes. *Ann Intern Med* 1992;117:560–566.
34. Matthew J, Addai T, Anand A, et al. Clinical features, site of involvement, bacteriologic findings, and outcome of infective endocarditis in intravenous drug users. *Arch Intern Med* 1995;155:1641–1648.
35. Navarro C, Dickinson PCT, Kondlapodi P, et al. Mycotic aneurysms of the pulmonary arteries in intravenous drug addicts. Report of three cases and review of the literature. *Am J Med* 1984;76:1124–1131.
36. Durack DT, Lukes AS, Bright DK. The Duke endocarditis service: New criteria for diagnosis of infective endocarditis: Utilization of specific echocardiographic findings. *Am J Med* 1994;96:200–209.
37. Ginzton LE, Siegel RJ, Criley JM. Natural history of tricuspid valve endocarditis: A two-dimensional echocardiographic study. *Am J Cardiol* 1982;49:1853–1859.
38. Berger M, Delfin LA, Jelveh M, et al. Two-dimensional echocardiographic findings in right- sided infective endocarditis. *Circulation* 1980;61:855–861.
39. Cassling RS, Rogler WC, McManus BM. Isolated pulmonic valve infective endocarditis: A diagnostically elusive entity. *Am Heart J* 1985;109:558–567.
40. San Roman JA, Vilacosta I, Zamorano JL, et al. Transesophageal echocardiography in right- sided endocarditis. *J Am Coll Cardiol* 1993;21:1226–1230.
41. Mügge A, Daniel WG, Frank G, et al. Echocardiography in infective endocarditis: Reassessment of prognostic implications of vegetation size determined by the transthoracic and the transesophageal approach. *J Am Coll Cardiol* 1989;14:631–638.
42. Daniel WG, Mügge A, Martin RP, et al. Improvement in the diagnosis of abscesses associated with endocarditis by transesophageal echocardiography. *N Engl J Med* 1991;324:795–800.
43. Cziner DG, Rosenzweig BD, Katz ES, et al. Transesophageal versus transthoracic echocardiography for diagnosing mitral valve perforation. *Am J Cardiol* 1992;69:1495–1497.
44. Wilson WR, Karchmer AW, Dajani AS, et al. Antibiotic treatment of adults with infective endocarditis due to streptococci, enterococci, staphylococci, and HACEK microorganisms. *JAMA* 1995;274(21):1706–1713.
45. Chambers HF, Miller RT, Newman MD. Right-sided *Staphylococcus aureus* endocarditis in intravenous drug abusers: Two-week combination therapy. *Ann Intern Med* 1988;109(8):619–624.
46. Nicolau DP, Freeman CD, Nightingale CH, et al. Reduction of bacterial titers by low-dose aspirin in experimental aortic valve endocarditis. *Infect Immun* 1993;61(4):1593–1595.
47. Nicolau DP, Marangos MN, Nightingale CH, et al. Influence of aspirin on development and treatment of experimental *Staphylococcus aureus* endocarditis. *Antimicrob Agents Chemother* 1995;39(8):1748–1751.

48. Newfeld GK, Branson CG, Marshall LW, et al. Infective endocarditis as a complication of heroin use. *South Med J* 1976;69:1148.
49. Silverman NA, Levitsky S. Right-sided endocarditis. In Magilligan DJ, Quinn EJ (eds.) *Endocarditis: Medical and Surgical Management.* New York, NY. Marcel Dekker, 1986. p 223.
50. DiNuble M. Surgery for addiction-related tricuspid valve endocarditis: Caveat emptor. *Am J Med* 1987;82:811.
51. Robbins MJ, Frater RWM, Soeiro R, et al. Influence of vegetation size on clinical outcome of right-sided infective endocarditis. *Am J Med* 1986;80:165.
52. Wong D, Chandraratna PAN, Wishnow RM, et al. Clinical implications of large vegetations in infectious endocarditis. *Arch Intern Med* 1983;143:1874.
53. Buda AJ, Zotz RJ, LeMire MS, et al. Prognostic significance of vegetations detected by two- dimensional echocardiography in infective endocarditis. *Am Heart J* 1986;112:1291.
54. Gilbert BW, Haney RS, Crawford F. Two-dimensional echocardiographic assessment of vegetative endocarditis. *Circulation* 1977;55:346.
55. Durack DT, Beeson PB. Experimental bacterial endocarditis II. Bacteria in endocardial vegetations. *Br J Exp Pathol* 1972;53:50.
56. Lutas EM, Roberts RB, Devereux RB, et al. Relation between the presence of echocardiographic vegetations and the complication rate in infective endocarditis. *Am Heart J* 1986;112:107.
57. Vo NM, Russel JC, Becker DR. Mycotic emboli of the peripheral vessels: Analysis of 44 cases. *Surgery* 1981;90:541–545.
58. Andriole VT, Kravetz HM, Roberts WC, et al. *Candida* endocarditis: Clinical and pathological studies. *Am J Med* 1962;32:251–285.
59. Dreyfus G, Serraf A, Jebara VA, et al. Valve repair in acute endocarditis. *Ann Thorac Surg* 1990;49:706–713.
60. Allen MD, Slachman F, Eddy C, et al. Tricuspid valve repair for tricuspid valve endocarditis: Tricuspid valve "recycling." *Ann Thorac Surg* 1991;51:593–598.
61. Yee ES, Ullyot DJ. Reparative approach for right-sided endocarditis. Operative considerations and results of valvuloplasty. *J Thorac Cardiovasc Surg* 1988;96: 133–140.
62. David TE, Bos J, Christakis G, et al. Heart valve operations in patients with active infective endocarditis. *Ann Thorac Surg* 1990;49:701–705.
63. Heimberger TS, Duma RJ. Infections of prosthetic heart valves and cardiac pacemakers. *Infect Dis Clin North Am* 1989;3:221–245.
64. Sande MA, Johnson WD, Hook EW, et al. Sustained bacteremia in patients with prosthetic cardiac valves. *N Engl J Med* 1972;286:1067–1070.
65. Oakley GDG, Carson PHM, Sanderson JM. Right-sided endocarditis involving both tricuspid and pulmonary valves in a patient with ventricular septal defect. *Br Heart J* 1977;39:323–325.
66. Beeler BA. Infections of permanent transvenous and epicardial pacemakers in adults. *Heart Lung* 1982;11:152–156.
67. Bluhm G. Pacemaker infections: A clinical study with special reference to prophylactic use of some isoxazolyl penicillins. Acta Med Scand 1985;699 (Suppl):1.
68. Kennelly BM, Piller LW. Management of infected transvenous permanent pacemakers. *Br Heart J* 1974;36:1133.
69. Arbulu A, Holmes RJ, Asfaw I. Tricuspid valvulectomy without replacement: Twenty years experience. *J Thorac Cardiovasc Surg* 1991;102:917–922.

70. Arbulu A, Thoms NW, Chiscano A, et al. Total tricuspid valvulectomy without replacement in the treatment of pseudomonas endocarditis. *Surg Forum* 1971; 22:62–64.
71. Arbulu A, Kafi A, Thoms NW, et al. Right-sided bacterial endocarditis: New concepts in the treatment of the uncontrollable infection. *Ann Thorac Surg* 1973; 16:136–140.
72. Reyes MP, Lerner AM. Current problems in the treatment of infective endocarditis due to *Pseudomonas aeruginosa*. *Rev Infect Dis* 1983;5:314–321.
73. Dressler FA, Roberts WC. Infective endocarditis in opiate addicts: Analysis of 80 cases studied at necropsy. *Am J Cardiol* 1989;63:1240–1257.
74. Stern HJ, Sisto DA, Strom JA, et al. Immediate tricuspid valve replacement for endocarditis: Indications and results. *J Thorac Cardiovasc Surg* 1986;91:163–167.
75. Ibarra RG, Villa JA, Goya IL, et al. Valvulectomia tricuspidea en un caso de endocarditis bacteriana por *Staphylococcus aureus* en un drogadicto. *Rev Esp Cardiol* 1983;36:179–183.
76. Dickens P, Chan AC, Lam KY. Isolated right-sided endocarditis in Hong Kong Chinese. *Am J Cardiovasc Pathol* 1993;4(4):367–370.
77. Simberkoff MS, Isom W, Smithivas T, et al. Two stage tricuspid valve replacement for mixed bacterial endocarditis. *Arch Intern Med* 1974;133:212–216.
78. Alexander R, Holloway A, Honsinger RW. Surgical debridement for resistant bacterial endocarditis: A case of antibiotic-refractory *serratia marcescens* infection on the tricuspid valve cured by operative excision. *JAMA* 1969;210: 1757–1759.
79. Yee ES, Khonsari S. Right-sided infective endocarditis: Valvuloplasty, valvectomy or replacement. *J Cardiovasc Surg* 1989;30:744–748.
80. Turley K. Surgery of right-sided endocarditis: Valve preservation vs. replacement. *J Cardiac Surg* 1989;4:317–320.
81. Arbulu A, Thomas NW, Wilson RF: Valvulectomy without prosthetic replacement: A lifesaving operation for tricuspid pseudomonas endocarditis. *J Thorac Cardiovasc Surg* 1972;64:103–107.
82. Robin E, Belamaric J, Thomas NW, et al. Consequences of total tricuspid valvulectomy without prosthetic replacement in treatment of pseudomonas endocarditis. *J Thorac Cardiovasc Surg* 1974;68:461–465.
83. Arbulu A, Asfaw I. Tricuspid valvulectomy without prosthetic replacement: Ten years of clinical experience. *J Thorac Cardiovasc Surg* 1981;82:684–690.
84. Varthakavi PK, Advani R, Parthasarathi R, et al. Tricuspid valvulectomy as therapy for spontaneous right-sided endocarditis. *J Assoc Physicians India* 1986; 873–876.
85. Barbour DJ, Roberts WC. Valve excision only versus valve excision plus replacement for active infective endocarditis involving the tricuspid valve. *Am J Cardiol* 1986;57:475–478.
86. Mesa JM, Oliver J, Dominguez F, et al. Endocarditis infecciosa derecha. *Rev Esp Cardiol* 1990;43:25–29.
87. Arbulu A, Holmes RJ, Asfaw I. Surgical treatment of intractable right-sided infective endocarditis in drug addicts: 25 years experience. *J Heart Valve Dis* 1993;2:129–137.

Chapter 12

Management of Annular Destruction, Fistulae and Abscesses

Angelo A. Vlessis, M.D., Ph.D.
G. Michael Deeb, M.D.
Suhas Bendre, M.D.
David Stuesse, M.D.

Introduction

Progression of native or prosthetic valve endocarditis from the valve leaflets or prosthetic valve apparatus into the surrounding cardiac tissue denotes an advanced stage of myocardial infection. The progressing infection destroys the muscular and fibrous portions of the heart leading to fistula and abscess formation, heart block, annular destruction with perivalvular leak or valve dehiscence, and even cardiac perforation with tamponade. Clinical, angiographic or echocardiographic signs of advanced infection are indications for operative intervention. At operation, the extent of tissue destruction is often worse than that predicted by preoperative studies. The debridement and ultimate repair can represent some of the most challenging problems encountered by cardiac surgeons today. This chapter reviews some guiding principles in the operative management of these often complex cases.

From: Vlessis AA, Bolling S (eds): *Endocarditis: A Multidisciplinary Approach to Modern Treatment.* © Futura Publishing Co., Armonk, NY, 1999.

Diagnosis

After the diagnosis of native or prosthetic valve endocarditis has been secured, the extent of the infection is best assessed by transthoracic or transesophageal echocardiogram. With color Doppler techniques, fistulae involving the cardiac chambers or aortic root are readily appreciated. Abscesses in the periannular tissues of the involved valve should be carefully sought out. Any degree of perivalvular prosthetic leaks should arouse suspicion of advancing infection, especially if associated with other clinical signs of infection such as fever, positive blood cultures, progressive renal dysfunction or shock. New onset of left bundle branch or complete heart block signifies involvement of the conduction system within the septal wall. Evidence of abscess formation, fistula formation, new or developing heart block and perivalvular leak are indications for operation.

Microbiology

Most microorganisms associated with native and prosthetic valve endocarditis can invade the cardiac tissues, leading to abscess and fistula formation as well as annular destruction. As in native and prosthetic valve endocarditis, staphylococcal and streptococcal species predominate and other less common pathogens represent only a minority of cases.

Generalized Approach to Operation

Broad spectrum or culture directed antibiotics should be given before, during and after the operative procedure. Familiarity with the various reconstructive techniques is essential, as the patient may require extensive debridement of the aortic root, annular, ventricular and atrial tissues. Effective myocardial protection is paramount to a successful outcome, as these procedures are often long and technically demanding. We prefer a combination of intermittent cold antegrade and retrograde cardioplegia to keep the myocardial temperature below 15° C. Antifibrinolytics before, during and after operation help control the diffuse coagulopathy incited by the infectious process, the long cardiopulmonary bypass run, and the extensive myocardial dissection and reconstruction.

Complete debridement of all infected tissues is a primary goal of the operation. We begin by placing clean drapes around the operative field, covering the retractor and cardiopulmonary bypass tubing prior to opening the heart or aorta and exposing the infected valve. All infected material is completely excised. A thorough search of the surrounding tissues is conducted for additional abscesses or fistulae. Anticipate encroachment towards major coronary artery branches during the debridement to avoid unnecessary or accidental injury. The area is then irrigated with copious amounts of cold saline. A pulse lavage irrigation system is ideal and provides additional debridement of loose and nonviable tissue. All instruments and superficial drapes used for the debridement and irrigation process are then removed from the field and the surgical gloves of all members of the operative team are changed prior to beginning the reconstructive phase of the operation.

The magnitude of the reconstruction is dictated by the extent of the debridement. Autologous or homograft tissues are preferred for the reconstruction. If these are not available or suitable, glutaraldehyde-treated bovine pericardium is preferred over Dacron or other synthetic materials. Abscesses and fistulae are obliterated or covered with the reconstructive material. Sutures are placed widely into the normal tissue surrounding the defect. Only nonabsorbable monofilament sutures are used.

Some case examples are presented below to illustrate these surgical guidelines.

Mitral Annular Destruction: Case 1

A 47-year-old forest ranger with known mitral regurgitation secondary to myxomatous degeneration presented with fever, florid septicemia and declining mental status. Transthoracic echocardiography revealed chordal rupture and mitral valve vegetations. A CT scan of the head showed several cerebral abscesses measuring 0.5 cm to 1 cm. The patient required intubation and inotropic support. He was taken immediately to the operating room, where it was found that the posterior and anterior leaflets of this myomatous valve were heavily involved with infection as noted by active vegetations and partially destroyed leaflet and chordal tissue. Cultures grew *Staphylococcus epidermidis*. The annulus was not involved. The mitral leaflets and subvalvular apparatus were excised and a 31 mm mechanical prosthesis was placed. The patient recovered from the acute process and was discharged to home in good condition. Two weeks after completing his 6-week course of intravenous antibiotics, he presented with fever and congestive heart failure requiring intra-aortic balloon pump placement, intubation with mechanical ventilation, and inotropic support. Transesophageal echocardiography showed a large perivalvular leak with valve dehiscence from the posterior annulus.

At operation, the valve was removed (Figure 1) and revealed an invasive infection of the posterior annulus involving the left ventricular and left atrial tissues. Debridement of all infected tissues required partial exci-

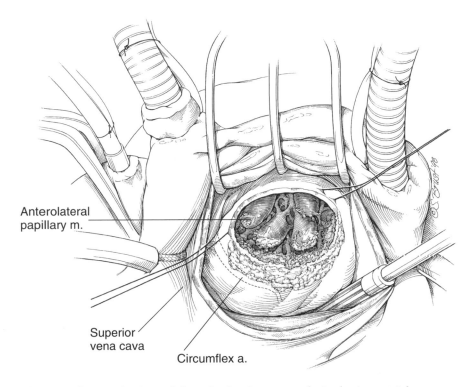

Figure 1. Surgeon's view of the mitral valve exposed via the interatrial groove. The mitral prosthesis has been removed exposing an extensive infection of the posterior annulus, left ventricular myocardium and the posterior left atrial wall. The dotted lines denote the location of the circumflex coronary artery beneath the area of infection.

sion of the posterior left ventricular and left atrial walls and exposed the circumflex artery in the atrioventricular groove. The entire area was reconstructed with a large elliptical bovine pericardial patch taking deep sutures into the posterior left ventricle and left atrium (Figure 2). Another 31 mm mechanical prosthesis was seated to the native anterior annulus and to the mid-portion of the pericardial patch (Figure 3). Postoperatively, the patient recovered quickly. Cultures grew the same *S. epidermidis* organism. The patient was discharged on vancomycin and oxacillin which he received for 8 weeks postoperatively. At 10-month follow-up, the patient continues to do well, is off antibiotics and is without signs of recurrent infection.

Aortic-Right Ventricular Fistula: Case 2

A 49-year-old male presented with fever and murmurs of aortic insufficiency and stenosis. Transthoracic echocardiography showed a bicuspid

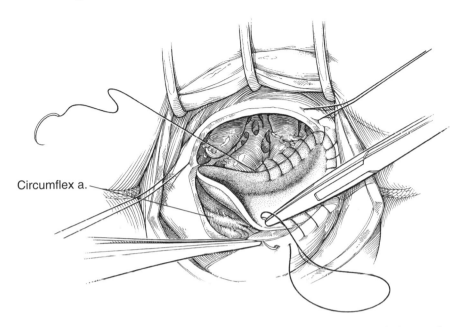

Circumflex a.

Figure 2. All infected tissues have been excised and the area irrigated vigorously with cold saline. Significant portions of the left ventricular and left atrial wall as well as the entire posterior annulus were debrided. A large pericardial patch is being sewn to the normal tissues around the perimeter of the defect. A portion of the circumflex coronary artery was exposed during the dissection and is about to be covered by the pericardial patch.

aortic valve and a 1 cm aortic valve vegetation. Blood cultures grew *S. epidermidis.* The patient was treated with intravenous antibiotics. After 1 week, fevers persisted and he was taken to the operating room where the aortic valve was excised and a small root abscess closed with glutaraldehyde-treated autologous pericardium. A mechanical prosthesis was seated to a normal appearing annulus. Antibiotics were continued postoperatively and the patient was discharged to home 1 week later. At 3-week follow-up, a continuous murmur was noted at the left upper sternal border and an echocardiogram showed a 2 cm abscess of the aortic root that bulged into the right ventricular outflow tract (Figure 4). There was a fistula that communicated with the abscess cavity and the right ventricular outflow tract producing a continuous jet on Doppler echocardiography. The protruding abscess was partially obstructive, producing a 30 mm peak gradient across the right ventricular outflow tract.

At operation, the pericardial patch repair had dehisced and a large defect in the right posterior aortic wall was visible above the aortic annulus. The aortic defect emptied into a large, complex, blood-filled abscess cavity. The mechanical valve sewing ring appeared infected; however, it

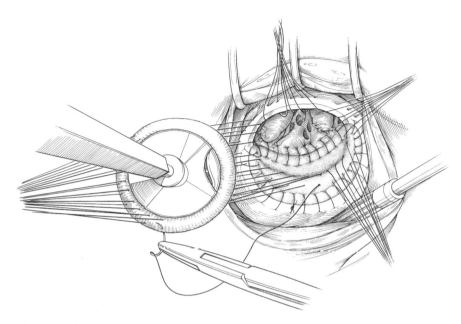

Figure 3. Once the pericardial patch is secured over the defect, valve sutures are placed through the normal annulus and the mid-portion of the pericardial patch. The new mechanical prosthesis is shown as the sutures are being passed through the sewing ring.

remained firmly seated to the aortic annulus. The valve was removed and the aortic annulus, aortic wall and abscess cavity were extensively debrided. The fistula opening to the right ventricular outflow tract was exposed through the tricuspid valve orifice and closed with a single non-absorbable monofilament suture. The aortic valve and ascending aorta were then replaced with a 25 mm homograft valve. The patient recovered uneventfully and was discharged to home on postoperative day 5. He remains without evidence of recurrent infection.

Valve Conduit (Bentall) Infection: Case 3

A 36-year-old female presented with fever, severe sinusitis and a right shoulder abscess. She had a previous history of aortic valve endocarditis 10 years prior following a dental infection. At that time, she underwent aortic valve replacement and did well for 2 years. She then developed prosthetic valve endocarditis and required replacement of the ascending aorta with a 25 mm mechanical valved conduit. She recovered uneventfully and was without signs of recurrent prosthetic valve infection for 8

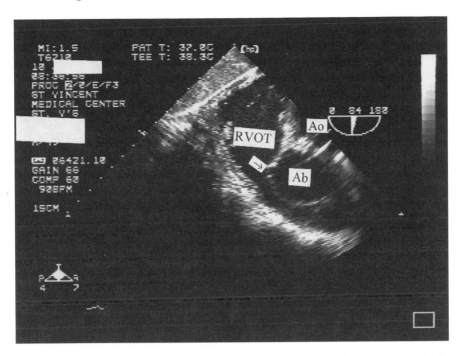

Figure 4. A transesophageal echocardiogram demonstrates a large aortic root abscess (Ab) bulging into the right ventricular outflow tract (RVOT). A portion of the aortic root (Ao) is seen in the upper right in transverse section. The arrow shows the location of the fistulous communication between the blood-filled abscess cavity and the right ventricular outflow tract.

years until presenting with the above mentioned fever, sinusitis, and right shoulder abscess. Blood cultures grew *Staphylococcus aureus* and she received intravenous oxacillin and gentamicin. Her shoulder abscess and sinuses were surgically drained. Transesophageal echocardiography showed a large abscess extending the entire length of the valved conduit posteriorly (Figure 5). The proximal posterior portion of the graft had dehisced from the posterior aortic annulus producing a large communication between the abscess cavity and the left ventricle (Figure 6). In addition, a prosthetic valve vegetation and a posterior perforation of the mitral leaflet with associated mitral regurgitation were noted.

The patient was taken to the operating room where the blood-filled abscess cavity was noted to be contained by scar tissue from her previous operations. The abscess extended across the dome of the left atrium compressing the right atrium and superior vena cava laterally. Right femoral cannulation was necessary and, with much difficulty, the infected prosthesis was removed with the perigraft felt and old suture material. The

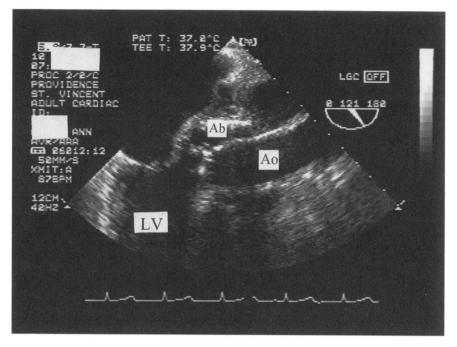

Figure 5. Transesophageal echocardiogram, long axis view, demonstrating a large abscess (Ab) located posterior to a prosthetic mechanical valved aortic conduit (Ao). The left ventricular (LV) cavity is seen in the lower left.

abscess cavity, aortic annulus, and coronary buttons were thoroughly debrided. After irrigation, a 25 mm homograft with a long ascending aortic segment was used for reconstruction. The attached anterior mitral leaflet was sewn to the native anterior mitral leaflet over the area of the perforation. The homograft annulus was then seated to the posterior ventricular septum and intact anterior aortic annulus with interrupted and running nonabsorbable monofilament suture. Inverting the homograft into the left ventricular cavity facilitated the proximal anastomosis. Coronary buttons were reattached and the distal graft anastomosis was accomplished to the native distal ascending aorta.

Postoperatively, the patient did well; she recovered without complications and was discharged home on postoperative day 7. She received 8 weeks of intravenous oxacillin and 2 weeks of intravenous gentamicin.

Results

Several retrospective studies have been published describing outcomes after various techniques of reconstruction for complex endocarditis.[1-21]

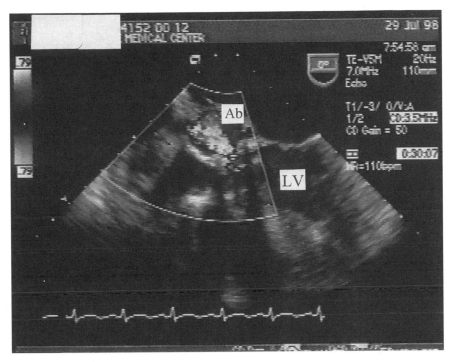

Figure 6. Color doppler demonstrates flow into the abscess cavity (Ab) from the left ventricle (LV) during systole. The left atrium is seen in the upper portion of the figure in close proximity to the abscess cavity. (See color appendix.)

The perioperative mortality rates in these studies range from 7% to 30%. These mortality rates reflect the combined effects of sepsis and hemodynamic compromise present in this patient population. The mean preoperative New York Heart Association heart failure class ranged from 2.8 to 4.0 in these studies. Interestingly, endocarditis recurrence after treatment is only 0% to 14% with a mean follow-up of 37 to 148 months. Actuarial 5-year survival ranged from 64% to 80%. These favorable outcome statistics justify the aggressive surgical approach advocated by the authors of these studies.

Dossche et al[15] compared the results of prosthetic reconstruction with homograft reconstruction using the data reported in several studies describing the surgical treatment of complicated aortic prosthetic valve endocarditis. Recurrent or persistent endocarditis ranged from 11% to 25% for prosthetic reconstruction compared to 3.4% to 6.5% for homograft reconstruction of the aortic root. Additionally, 5-year actuarial survival ranged from 54% to 75% in the prosthetic group versus 73% to 87% for the homograft group. Although these data were pooled from retrospective studies with differing patient populations and operative techniques, they provide support for the use of homograft material over prosthetic material for the surgical treatment of complicated aortic valve endocarditis.

Complications are common in patients with complex endocarditis. Conduction pathways may be injured by the infection or during surgical debridement. The incidence of postoperative heart block requiring permanent pacing ranges from 18% to 47%.[1,8,12,16] Reexploration for postoperative bleeding is higher than in the general cardiac surgery population, ranging from 5% to 37%.[1,6,16] Early valve dehiscence, paravalvular leak and pseudoaneurysm of suture lines are less common postoperative occurrences.

Several retrospective studies of complicated endocarditis have used univariate and multivariate analysis to identify factors associated with poor outcome.[1,5,9–14] Patients with complicated prosthetic valve endocarditis tend to have worse outcomes than patients with complicated native valve endocarditis.[11] The New York Heart Association functional class at presentation has a direct positive correlation with mortality.[6,9,12] In addition, the development of a new high-grade conduction defect has also has been correlated with a worse outcome.[5] Interestingly, one study did not find a statistically significant change in outcome when comparing cases of native valve endocarditis with and without abscess formation.[13] Other factors portending poor surgical outcome are the presence of staphylococcal infection,[1] early prosthetic valve infection,[5] advanced patient age[12] and multiple valve involvement.[1]

New York Heart Association functional class improves after surgery for complicated endocarditis. In a review of 49 patients who survived surgery for complicated endocarditis, 78% of the patients were class IV preoperatively while 92% were class I or II postoperatively and 8% were class III with a mean follow-up of 56 months.[1] In a similar study of patients undergoing homograft root reconstruction, 88% were class I or II and 12% were functional class III at 66 months postoperatively.[5]

In aortic valve endocarditis, homograft aortic valve replacement appears to be associated less frequently with early aortic valve insufficiency than mechanical valve replacement. In a study of mechanical device replacement of the aortic root for endocarditis, John et al[9] found clinically significant aortic insufficiency in 57% of the survivors 6 months postoperatively. In contrast, Dearani et al[10] reports that 81% of survivors of homograft aortic valve replacement for endocarditis had no immediate postoperative aortic regurgitation, while at follow-up (mean 2.6 years) 50% had no aortic regurgitation. In another study of homograft root reconstruction for endocarditis,[15] 80% of postoperative survivors had no aortic insufficiency, while18.5% had grade I and 3.5% had grade II insufficiency at a mean follow-up of 37 months.

Authors' Results

The electronic cardiac surgery database at St. Vincent Hospital and Medical Center was recently reviewed for surgical cases of endocarditis (1988–1998) requiring annular reconstruction and/or closure of abscesses and fistulae. Thirty-six cases were identified; of these, 28 were male patients and 8 were female. Destruction involved aortic (53%), mitral (19%), aortic-mitral (19%), aortic-tricuspid (6%) or aortic-mitral-tricuspid (3%) valves and their associated annuli. The microorganisms recovered with blood and tissue culture were streptococcal species (25%), staphylococcal species (39%), gram-negative bacilli (17%), fungus (6%) and no growth (14%). The majority of cases were prosthetic valve or prosthetic valved conduit endocarditis (53%). Intravenous drug use was involved in only 8%. Valve replacement devices included 17 mechanical aortic valves, 10 mechanical mitral valves, 8 homograft aortic valves, 4 bioprosthetic aortic valves and 1 bioprosthetic tricuspid valve. In addition, there were 5 mitral valve repairs and 3 tricuspid valve repairs. There were 2 reoperations for paravalvular leak. The overall mortality was 39% (14 of 36) with a mean follow-up of 3.82 years. The cause of death was unknown in 4 cases, recurrent endocarditis in 4, postoperative heart failure in 3 and unrelated (cancer, myocardial infarction, accidental) in 3. Therefore, the probable endocarditis-related mortality was 31%.

The superiority of autologous and homograft aortic root replacement for extensive aortic root infection has improved the outcome of complex aortic root endocarditis. Between 1994–1998, 29 patients with aortic annular destruction, abscesses and/or fistulae were treated with a Ross procedure (9 of 29) or homograft aortic valve/root replacement (20 of 29) at St. Vincent Hospital and Medical Center in Portland, Oregon, and the University of Michigan Medical Center in Ann Arbor. Abscesses were debrided and defects repaired with pericardial, autologous or homograft tissues. All patients received at least 6 weeks of postoperative antibiotics directed at the causative microorganism. There were 2 deaths with a mean follow-up of 18 months for a mortality rate of only 7%. The results with autologous, or homograft, valve replacement devices appear to be superior to other prosthetic valve replacement options. The technique of homograft valve replacement is illustrated in Figure 7 for a case of aortic endocarditis associated with annular destruction, abscess and fistula formation. In this illustrated case, the inclusion cylinder or "mini-root" technique was used. For more extensive destruction of the aortic root, the entire

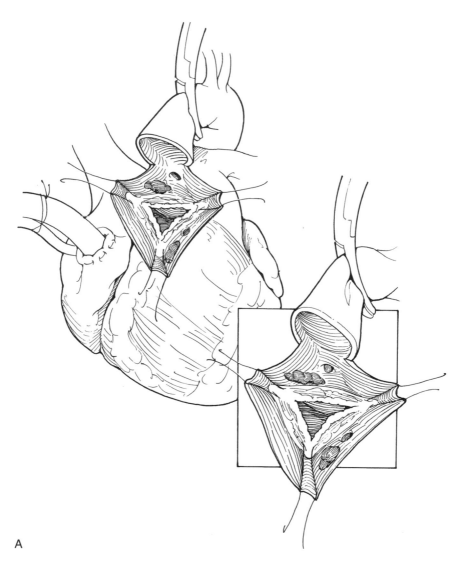

A

Figure 7. (**A**) Extensive native aortic valve endocarditis with near complete de-struction of all leaflet tissue and destruction of annular tissues is shown through a transverse aortotomy. An annular abscess is depicted next to the left coronary ostia. A defect near the right coronary ostia is also present which communicates with the right atrium through the base of the right and noncoronary commissure.

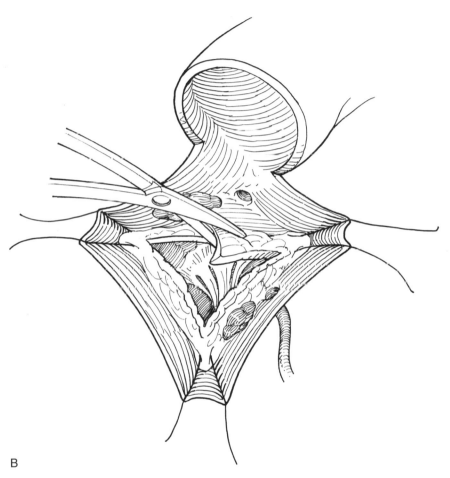

B

Figure 7. *(continued)* (**B**) The leaflet tissue and infected portions of the annulus are debrided sharply.

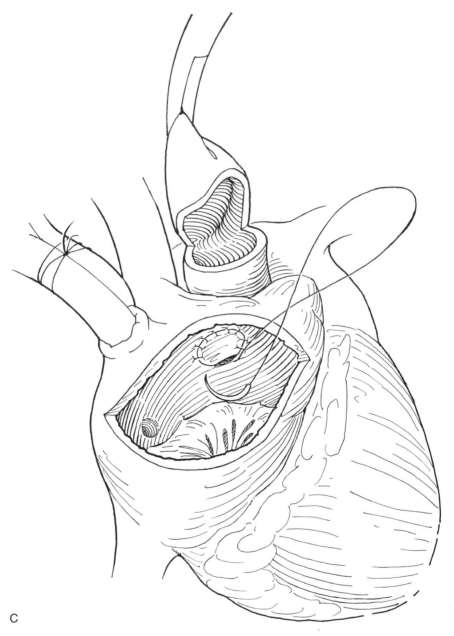

C

Figure 7. *(continued)* (**C**) The fistula opening in the right atrium is closed through a right atriotomy with a glutaraldehyde-fixed autologous pericardial patch.

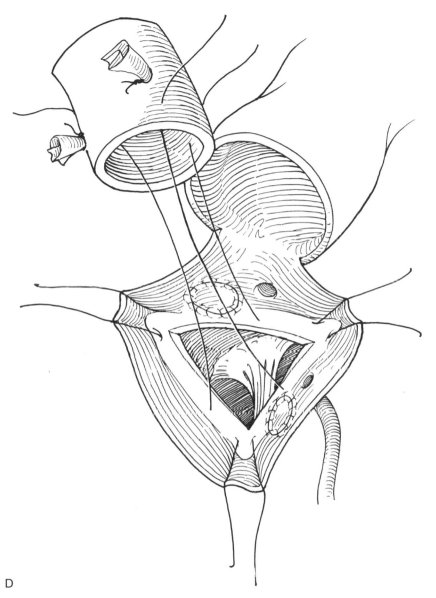

D

Figure 7. *(continued)* (**D**) The abscess cavities next to the right and left coronary ostia have been debrided sharply, irrigated thoroughly, and closed with glutaraldehyde-fixed autologous pericardial patches. Three nonabsorbable monofilament sutures are placed at the base of each of the homograft leaflets in order to line up the middle of coronary sinuses with the right and left coronary ostia. The homograft is then inverted into the left ventricular cavity and the base of the homograft is sewn to the subaortic annulus by running each of the 3 sutures to one another.

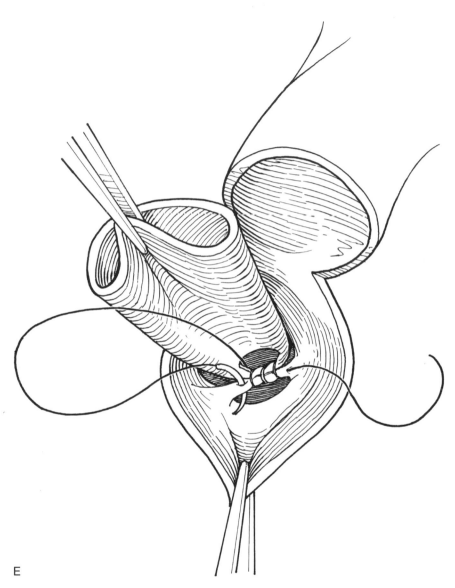

E

Figure 7. *(continued)* (**E**) The homograft is then reverted back into the natural position in the aortic root and each coronary ostia is sewn to a window created in the aortic homograft.

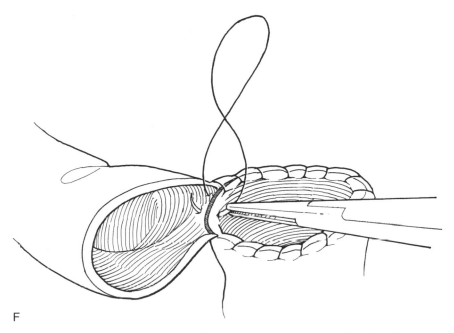

F

Figure 7. *(continued)* (**F**) The top of the homograft is trimmed back to the same height as the native aortic root. Using running nonabsorbable monofilament suture, the homograft and native aortic walls are sewn together. The aortotomy is then closed in 2 layers, completing the repair.

native aortic root should be completely excised and a complete homograft root replacement performed with reimplantation of coronary buttons onto the homograft root.

Concluding Remarks

Annular destruction with abscess and fistula formation secondary to endocarditis represents one of the most challenging aspects of cardiac surgical practice. When faced with these cases, one must be mentally prepared for a long, difficult operation. It is necessary to strive to completely remove all grossly infected tissues in order to decrease the risk of persistent infection postoperatively. We agree with the recommendations of David[2,16,20] which stress thorough debridement, irrigation, and changing of all surgical instruments and gloves prior to beginning the reconstructive phase of the operation. Reconstruction is undertaken with autologous or homograft tissue. Alternative choices include bovine pericardium followed by synthetic materials. Mortality remains high, but with widespread application of these principles by experienced surgeons, we expect overall survival will improve.

The utility of C-reactive protein (CRP) deserves further comment. A minimum of 6 weeks of post-repair intravenous antibiotics directed against the offending organism is recommended. Prior to stopping the antibiotics, a CRP level is drawn and antibiotics are continued if the CRP level is elevated above 10 mg/dL. If the CRP level is normal, we feel it is safe to stop the antibiotics after 6 weeks.

References

1. d'Udekem Y, David T, Feindel CM, et al. Long-term results of operation for paravalvular abscess. *Ann Thorac Surg* 1996;62:48–53.
2. David T. The surgical treatment of patients with prosthetic valve endocarditis. *Semin Thorac Cardiovasc Surg* 1995;7(1):47–53.
3. Vlessis AA, Khaki A, Grunkemeier GL, et al. Risk, diagnosis, and management of prosthetic valve endocarditis: A review. *J Heart Valve Dis* 1997;6:443–465.
4. Glazier JJ, Verwilghen J, Donaldson RM, et al. Treatment of complicated prosthetic aortic valve endocarditis with annular abscess formation by homograft aortic root replacement. *J Am Coll Cardiol* 1991;17:1177–1182.
5. Watanabe G, Haverich A, Speier R, et al. Surgical treatment of active infective endocarditis with paravalvular involvement. *J Thorac Cardiovasc Surg* 1994; 107:171–177.
6. Amrani M, Schoevaerdts JC, Eucher P, et al. Extension of native aortic valve endocarditis: Surgical considerations. *Eur Heart J* 1995;16 (suppl B):103–106.
7. Camacho MT, Cosgrove DM III. Homografts in the treatment of prosthetic valve endocarditis. *Semin Thorac Cardiovasc Surg* 1995;7:32–37.
8. Jault F, Gandjbakhch I, Chastre JC, et al. Prosthetic valve endocarditis with ring abscesses. *J Thorac Cardiovasc Surg* 1993;105:1106–1113.
9. John RM, Pugsley W, Treasure T, et al. Aortic root complications of infective endocarditis: Influence on surgical outcome. *Eur Heart J* 1991;12:241–248.
10. Dearani JA, Orszulak TA, Schaff HV, et al. Results of allograft aortic valve replacement for complex endocarditis. *J Thorac Cardiovasc Surg* 1997:113: 285–291.
11. Ergin MA, Raissi S, Follis F, et al. Annular destruction in acute bacterial endocarditis. *J Thorac Cardiovasc Surg* 1989;97:755–763.
12. Bauernschmitt R, Jakob HG, Vahl C, et al. Operation for infective endocarditis: Results after implantation of mechanical valves. *Ann Thorac Surg* 1998;65: 359–364.
13. McGiffin DC, Galbraith AJ, McLachlan GJ, et al. Risk factors for death and recurrent endocarditis after aortic valve replacement. *J Thorac Cardiovasc Surg* 1992;104:511–520.
14. Haydock D, Barratt-Boyes B, Macedo T, et al. Aortic valve replacement for active infectious endocarditis in 108 patients: A comparison of freehand allograft valves with mechanical prostheses and bioprostheses. *J Thorac Cardiovasc Surg* 1992;103:130–139.
15. Dossche KM, Defauw JJ, Ernst SM, et al. Allograft aortic root replacement in

prosthetic aortic valve endocarditis: A review of 32 patients. *Ann Thorac Surg* 1997;63:1644–1649.

16. David TE, Kuo J, Armstrong S. Aortic and mitral valve replacement with reconstruction of the intervalvular fibrous body. *J Thorac Cardiovasc Surg* 1997; 114:766–772.

17. Zwischenberger JB, Shalaby TZ, Conti VR. Viable cryopreserved aortic homograft for aortic valve endocarditis and annular abscesses. *Ann Thorac Surg* 1989;48:365–370.

18. Nataf P, Vaissier DE, Bors V, et al. Extra-annular procedures in the surgical management of prosthetic valve endocarditis. *Eur Heart J* 1995;16 (suppl B): 99–102.

19. Kirklin JK, Kirklin JW, Pacifico AD. Aortic valve endocarditis with aortic root abscess cavity: Surgical treatment with aortic valve homograft. *Ann Thorac Surg* 1988;45:674–677.

20. David TE, Feindel CM, Armstrong S, et al. Reconstruction of the mitral annulus: A ten year experience. *J Thorac Cardiovasc Surg* 1995;110:1323–1332.

21. Tuna IC, Orszulak TA, Schaff HV, et al. Results of homograft aortic valve replacement for active endocarditis. *Ann Thorac Surg* 1990;49:619–624.

IV

Special Considerations

Chapter 13

Surgical Therapy of Infective Endocarditis in Children

Ralph S. Mosca, M.D.
Edward L. Bove, M.D.

Introduction

Infective endocarditis (IE) continues to pose significant morbidity and mortality in the pediatric population despite major advances in clinical diagnostics and therapeutics. Once nearly 100% fatal, the advent of antibiotics and aggressive medical care has improved this ominous prognosis.[1] Current reviews of IE in children report an overall mortality rate of approximately 25%.[2] Ironically, the same advances in medical care that have lowered the mortality rate are contributing to a rise in its incidence. Historically, infective endocarditis in children was a complication of congenital or rheumatic heart disease. At present, rheumatic heart disease has been all but eradicated in the United States. Concurrently there has been a rapid rise in the incidence of neonates with infective endocarditis in the absence of congenital heart disease.[3] This appears to correlate with more invasive procedures and the use of indwelling vascular catheters. Also, the mean age of children suffering from endocarditis is increasing, principally due to increasing patient longevity following surgical repair or palliation.[4]

Although any congenital heart defect may predispose a child to develop infective endocarditis, lesions that precipitate turbulent blood flow and result in endothelial damage predominate. (These include ventricular septal defect, aortic and mitral valve disease, stenotic valved conduits and patent ductus arteriosus.[5]) The presence of cyanotic congenital heart

From: Vlessis AA, Bolling S (eds): *Endocarditis: A Multidisciplinary Approach to Modern Treatment.* © Futura Publishing Co., Armonk, NY, 1999.

disease is an independent risk factor for IE as well.[6] Endothelial damage promotes platelet and fibrin deposition, which results in the formation of a nonbacterial thrombotic vegetation (NBTV) believed to be essential in the pathogenesis of IE. The NBTV then becomes infected as a result of intravascular bacteremia. Once inoculated, the vegetation may "protect" the bacteria between a zone of necrotic endocardium and an exterior coat of leukocytes and fibrin.[7] These boundaries make penetration by antibiotics difficult. Often, surgical therapy is necessary to remove infected prosthetic material and debride walled-off abscesses.

Medical Therapy

Streptococcal species continue to be the most frequently encountered microorganisms, followed closely by staphylococci, an occasional gram-negative organism and fungi. In most cases microorganisms gain entry into the blood via dental procedures, cutaneous penetration, or as a result of cardiac surgery. A minimum course of 4 to 6 weeks of intravenous bactericidal antibiotics is necessary to sterilize vegetations and prevent relapse. Currently, empirical therapy includes penicillin G and an aminoglycoside. Patients suspected of harboring *Staphylococcus aureus* should receive a penicillinase-resistant penicillin, and in those cases where *Staphylococcus epidermidis* is likely, they should be treated with intravenous vancomycin. The culture results then allow for the proper tailoring of the antibiotic regimen.

Approximately 70% of patients with native valve endocarditis (NVE) can be cured by appropriate antibiotic therapy. However, up to 60% of these patients will eventually require an operation to replace the damaged cardiac valve.[8] Extrapolating from the adult literature, prosthetic valve endocarditis is a much more virulent process and carries approximately a 10% to 50% overall mortality depending upon the time of presentation after surgery, as well as the causative organism.[9,10] In prosthetic valve endocarditis, eradication of the infection often involves early operative intervention.

Echocardiography

Echocardiography has become an important tool in the diagnosis and treatment of infective endocarditis. It should be performed in all patients in whom infective endocarditis is suspected.[11] Many patients can be adequately imaged using transthoracic echocardiography (TTE); however, biplane transesophageal echocardiography (TEE) with color flow Doppler has greatly improved diagnostic accuracy. In patients with proven IE the sensitivity of TEE has been shown to be between 90% and 100% with relatively infrequent false positive results.[12]

Although echocardiography cannot determine causality, it can provide valuable anatomic and physiologic information. The presence, location, size and mobility of vegetations can be evaluated, as can changes in these parameters that relate to the patient's clinical course. Valvar dysfunction as a result of deformation or destruction of tissue and obstructing vegetations can be evaluated with Doppler. Documentation of the anatomic substrate causing valvar insufficiency or stenosis in the beating, working heart can aid significantly in planning the operative strategy. For example, mitral insufficiency related to a perforated posterior mitral valve leaflet, with associated shortened and fibrotic chordae, and mitral annular dilatation may be treated by chordal lengthening, removal of the infected portion of the mitral valve leaflet, replacement of this lost tissue with pericardium and mitral valve annuloplasty. Intraoperative TEE provides immediate information concerning the adequacy of the repair.

Echocardiography can also be helpful in defining extension of infection beyond the valve itself. Myocardial abscesses, aneurysms of the sinus of Valsalva, intracardiac fistulae, involvement of the interventricular septum and pericarditis can all be demonstrated prior to operative intervention.

Surgical Therapy

The mainstay of treatment for infective endocarditis continues to be intravenous antibiotics. In the hemodynamically stable patient, a complete course of antibiotic therapy is given, followed by the evaluation of cardiac function and observation for signs of recurrent infection. Surgery is reserved for the treatment of the complications of IE such as congestive heart failure secondary to valvar dysfunction or recurrent septal defects, uncontrolled infection including myocardial abscesses, recurrent systemic emboli, and prosthetic valve dysfunction. In addition, some believe that the presence of aggressive microorganisms (for example S. aureus) or organisms known to be difficult to eradicate such as gram-negative or fungal infections warrants early surgical intervention.

The first report of successful surgical therapy for endocarditis complicating congenital heart disease was in 1940 when Touroff and Vessel described ligation of a patent ductus arteriosus and eradication of the infection.[13] In 1965, Wallace and colleagues showed the possibility and efficacy of operative intervention and valve replacement in the face of active endocarditis.[14] Subsequently, other authors described the successful treatment

Table 1
Pediatric Valve Prostheses

	Size Match	Durability	Thromboembolic Complications	Availability	Calcification
Mechanical	poor	excellent	poor	excellent	excellent
Heterograft	poor	poor	good	excellent	poor
Allograft	good	good	excellent	poor	fair
Autograft	excellent	excellent	excellent	excellent	excellent

of endocarditis following removal of infected foreign material and wide excision of infected or necrotic cardiac structures. Schollin et al outlined guidelines for surgical therapy in children with endocarditis.[15] Two more recent series described the results of children operated on for infective endocarditis at a single institution.[16,17]

An aggressive combined medical and surgical therapy for infective endocarditis has resulted in improved survival in adults.[10] A similar approach is likely warranted in children. However, a variety of additional factors must be considered. Pediatric patients are undergoing continual somatic growth and thus may quickly outgrow prosthetic valves. Currently available metallic and bioprosthetic valves may not fit into their respective cardiac positions in smaller children and neonates due to the relatively large circumferences and high profiles of these devices. Bioprosthetic (xenograft) valves tend to be become quickly calcified and obstructive to flow when used in children. Females of childbearing age are best served by a valve which avoids anticoagulation. Lastly, the risks of anticoagulation may be somewhat higher in this accident-prone pediatric age group and certainly will accumulate over the patient's lifetime.

All of these factors must be considered when determining the most appropriate type of valve replacement and timing of surgery. The optimal pediatric valve would be viable, capable of unlimited growth, easily implantable at a low operative risk and would not require anticoagulation. Unfortunately, such a valve is not currently available. (See Table 1 for a comparison of the intrinsic qualities of available valve substitutes in the pediatric population. Depicted are appropriate size valves, durability, freedom from thromboembolic complications, availability, and freedom from dystrophic calcification.)

Preoperative Evaluation

The evaluation of a child with endocarditis prior to surgery should include an assessment of the patient's major organ systems function as well as specific studies focused upon the clinical situation and known complications of bacterial endocarditis. Once suspected by history and physical examination, the pathology can be confirmed by echocardiography and often by positive blood cultures. Other pertinent investigations should be directed towards the known sequelae of endocarditis and include determination of hematologic disorders, renal or hepatic dysfunction, cerebral embolization, distal septic foci, and dental consultation as guided by the patient's clinical exam.

Right-sided Endocarditis

Tricuspid and pulmonary valve endocarditis account for approximately 10% to 15% of all cases of infective endocarditis in children. Right-sided endocarditis is commonly associated with intravenous drug users in the adult population, but most cases in children are associated with a ventricular septal defect (VSD), congenitally abnormal valves (pulmonic stenosis, or Ebstein's anomaly), the placement of prosthetic materials (VSD closure and right ventricle to pulmonary artery conduits), or intravascular catheter use.[18]

Tricuspid Valve

The tricuspid valve appears to be at increased risk for infective endocarditis when it is adjacent to a VSD, is dysplastic and regurgitant as in Ebstein's anomaly, when it is adjacent to an indwelling central venous cathether, or following VSD closure.[19] In otherwise normally structured hearts, tricuspid valve endocarditis should be treated by removal of any associated central venous catheters, and intravenous antibiotic therapy. Surgical therapy is recommended for cases of persistent sepsis, recurrent clinically significant pulmonary emboli, and severe, poorly tolerated tricuspid regurgitation.[20] Severe tricuspid regurgitation will often lead to right-sided heart failure, central venous congestion, hepatomegaly and ascites. When feasible, surgical treatment should include tricuspid valve repair even if a mild to moderate degree of regurgitation persists, given the inherent problems of valve replacement in the pediatric population.

If valve repair is not possible or unsatisfactory, valve replacement may be necessary. Although some authors have recommended valvectomy in adult patients with tricuspid valve endocarditis, it is often poorly tolerated in the pediatric population, especially in neonates and infants.[21] The use of metallic prosthetic valves in the pulmonary circulation of children has been marked by an alarmingly high incidence of thrombosis and embolization, and therefore a xenograft valve should be employed. Currently, the smallest such valves are 19 mm in size, relatively high profile, and thus are not feasible for use in patients less than 2 to 3 years of age in the absence of a markedly dilated tricuspid valve annulus.

Pulmonary Valve

Endocarditis involving the native pulmonary valve is relatively rare. In the majority of cases the pulmonary valve will become regurgitant, which is well tolerated by the normal right ventricle. Thus, no surgical intervention may be necessary if the valve has been sterilized. In those cases of pulmonary valve endocarditis associated with pulmonic stenosis, pulmonary hypertension or elevated pulmonary vascular resistance, a replacement valve may be necessary. Under these circumstances either a pulmonary valve allograft or heterograft may be utilized. Each has inherent advantages and disadvantages. The pulmonary allograft valve is pliable, easy to implant and tends to promote hemostasis. However, it will have a greater tendency towards regurgitation in the early postoperative period, it may be in short supply, and it will ultimately fail by regurgitation in approximately 7 to 12 years. The heterograft valves are readily available in a variety of sizes and confer a maximal degree of competency in the early postoperative period. These valves, however, may be more technically difficult to implant in infants and neonates, will tend to become obstructive relatively rapidly due to dystrophic calcification, and may have a somewhat higher incidence of early reinfection due to the large amount of prosthetic material.

Left-sided Endocarditis

Most series dealing with pediatric endocarditis have shown that the aortic and mitral valves are affected approximately 2 to 3 times as frequently as the tricuspid and pulmonary valves.[5,15,22] This may be related to numerous factors, among them the mean pressure to which the valve is exposed, the density of the inoculant, the ability of the valve to self-sterilize, and perhaps the impact of different oxygen tensions.

Mitral Valve

The normal mitral valve may become infected as the result of an unsuspected bacteremia. This risk increases when the valve is structurally abnormal resulting in turbulent flow (mitral stenosis or insufficiency) or following surgical exposure and/or repair. If the infection can not be eradicated by antibiotic therapy alone, or if valve destruction results in congestive heart failure, surgical therapy may be necessary.

Exposure of the mitral valve in pediatric patients, particularly infants and neonates, may be quite difficult, especially when associated with a normal sized left atrium. A variety of techniques may be helpful in improving visualization of the valve. In the case of postoperative left atrioventricular valve endocarditis following repair of an AV septal defect, the "mitral valve" can usually be adequately exposed by elevating or removing the atrial portion of the septal patch. Approaching the mitral valve in an otherwise normal heart may be improved by utilizing a transseptal incision. If an approach through the intra-atrial groove is used, adequate exposure may require extensive mobilization of the intra-atrial groove and extension of the incision well behind the superior vena cava toward the left atrial appendage. Transsection of the superior vena cava allows the right atrium to be rotated to the patient's left and maximal exposure achieved through the dome of the left atrium.

Emphasis should be on the repair of the mitral valve whenever feasible.[23] Tissue loss as occurs in perforated leaflets or destruction of the base of the leaflet can be repaired using tanned autogenous or xenograft pericardium. Gore-Tex sutures can be used as substitutes for damaged chordae, and annular enlargement due to insufficiency can be alleviated through the use of annuloplasty techniques with or without a supporting ring.

If mitral valve replacement is necessary, the current readily available choices include xenograft or mechanical prostheses. Given the relatively high profile and early failure of the xenograft valve in the pediatric population, a mechanical valve should be used. Although a mechanical valve will necessitate anticoagulation, the risk of reinfection appears to be no higher than with a bioprosthetic valve. Homograft replacement of the mitral valve has been reported in adults and may someday extend the surgical options for mitral valve replacement in children.[24]

Aortic Valve

The aortic valve is the valve most often involved in infective endocarditis in the pediatric population.[17] (Figure 1) Although the majority (75% to 80%) of infections can be cured by intravenous antibiotic therapy alone, approximately 15% will require surgical therapy in the acute phase of the disease. Of those patients in whom early surgery is avoided for control of the infection, 60% will require aortic valve repair or replacement due to structural damage of the valve impairing its function.[8]

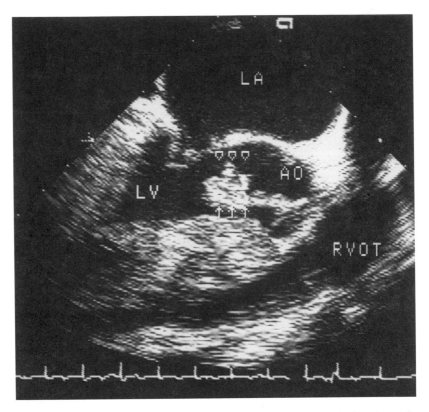

Figure 1. Transesophageal echocardiogram (longitudinal view) showing a large mobile vegetation attached to the aortic valve.

Although repair of the aortic valve is possible, extensive distortion of the valve leaflets, deformation of the aortic root, spread of the infection beyond the valve itself, and associated LV outflow tract anomalies all may necessitate aortic valve replacement. Current replacement options in the pediatric population include metallic and xenograft prostheses, aortic homografts and pulmonary autografts.[25]

Mechanical devices are the most durable, but have the highest risk of embolic events, require systemic anticoagulation, and may not be available in the appropriate sizes. Xenograft bioprostheses have a lower rate of thromboembolic events and usually do not require anticoagulation but are limited in smaller patients by size availability, and fail relatively quickly in children secondary to calcification producing aortic stenosis.

When the aortic valve must be replaced in the presence of active infection there is some evidence that the use of homografts or autografts confers a somewhat lower risk of early reinfection. The use of an aortic homograft with its attached mitral valve leaflet can be useful in situations of extensive infection in which debridement of the interventricular septum or aortic root is necessary. Late follow-up in a series of adolescents and young adults has shown that 85% of patients are free of reoperation at 10 years when an aortic homograft is used.[26] The use of aortic homografts for aortic valve replacement in infants and children has a less favorable prognosis. Pulmonary autograft replacement of the aortic valve is a double valve procedure for single valve disease. As such, it requires a more extensive operation, is embarked upon at a slightly higher risk, and involves opening additional tissue planes, which may be counterproductive in cases of acute infection. The advantages of the pulmonary autograft over the aortic homograft may be its availability, growth potential and longevity.[25,27,28] In addition, the native pulmonary valve and artery, by virtue of their location, have been treated with the same systemic antibiotics prior to repair. Among those patients treated with autografts in the treatment of aortic valve disease, 85% are free of reoperation at 20 years.[26] Therefore, in children, the choice of the optimal aortic valve substitute is dependent upon many factors: patient age and size, severity and extent of infection, clinical status, availability of materials, the status of the native pulmonary valve, the need for additional operations on the left ventricular outflow tract and subjective factors of patient preference and reliability. After all these factors are considered, an aortic homograft is probably the best choice to replace an aortic valve operated upon to control sepsis, or in the face of extensive tissue destruction beyond the aortic valve itself. The pulmonary autograft may be best reserved for those patients requiring operation for a sterilized, but deformed aortic valve producing increasing aortic insufficiency.

Prosthetic Material

The current practice of pediatric cardiac surgery involves the frequent use of prosthetic material in a variety of cardiac locations. Aside from the occasional use of prosthetic valves and angioplasty rings, prosthetic patch material is used to close cardiac septal defects, partition and channel intracardiac blood flow (hemi-Fontan and Fontan procedures), and septate the great vessels (repair of aortopulmonary window). It is also used in a variety of procedures on the right ventricular outflow tract. Although infective endocarditis after cardiac surgery for congenital heart disease is relatively rare, historically a high mortality rate has been reported for infective endocarditis involving prosthetic material.[29] Furthermore, the appearance of aggressive antibiotic-resistant organisms has been associated with a worse prognosis: only a few successful surgical outcomes have been reported.[30]

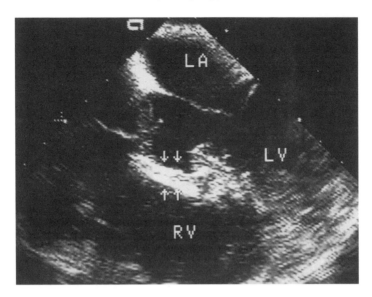

Figure 2. Transesophageal echocardiogram (longitudinal view). Infective endocarditis involving a ventricular septal defect patch. Note how bright and irregular the patch appears.

The diagnosis of active patch-related endocarditis may be difficult. Echocardiography can be helpful in delineating residual intracardiac shunts, visualizing abnormal masses attached to the patch, and noting an echobright appearance of the patch or an irregularity in the outline of the patch.[11,31] (Figure 2.) However, it is by no means definitive. Changes in the appearance of these findings can be documented during treatment and can help establish indications for surgery and optimal timing.

The selection of replacement material is also controversial. The choices include additional foreign material, autogenous pericardial tissue, allograft patches, or xenograft tissue (bovine pericardium). Although autogenous tissue appears to be more resistant to reinfection, some authors have reported the late development of patch dilatation or aneurysms.[32] On the other hand, others have reported successfully replacing prosthetic patch material with the same material. Lastly, bovine pericardium, which is thicker, may tend to resist aneurysmal dilatation more effectively than the thinner human pericardium. The final decision should center upon the severity and extent of the infection and the pressure gradient to which the tissue will be exposed.

Summary

Infective endocarditis in children is a relatively rare, yet complex, heterogeneous disease that despite the advent of potent antimicrobial therapy still portends a significant morbidity and mortality. Approximately 1 in 1500 admissions to major children's hospitals are for the treatment of endocarditis. The mean age of children with infective endocarditis appears to be rising, likely due to increasing longevity following surgery for the treatment of congenital heart defects. Concurrently, there has been a rapid rise in the incidence of neonates with infective endocarditis associated with advances in neonatal intensive care, invasive procedures, and indwelling venous catheters.

Any congenital heart lesion may predispose a child to developing infective endocarditis. However, the most common sites in order of decreasing frequency remain ventricular septal defect, VSD in association with tetralogy of Fallot, aortic valve, mitral valve, followed by tricuspid valve and pulmonary valve. Many studies have shown that the presence of cyanosis further increases the risk of developing infective endocarditis.

Viridans streptococci account for approximately 40% of cases of infective endocarditis in childhood. Staphylococcal species cause 25% to 30% of cases, most of which are due to coagulase-positive staphylococci. However, coagulase-negative and methicillin-resistant staphylococci are causing an increasing number of infections following cardiac surgery. The remainder of infections are caused by gram-negative organisms, fungi and parasites.

Bactericidal antimicrobial therapy is the treatment of choice. Surgical intervention is reserved for the treatment of complications associated with infective endocarditis. Accepted indications for surgery include:

1. Congestive heart failure secondary to valvar dysfunction
2. Persistent infection despite appropriate antimicrobial therapy
3. Extension of the infection beyond the valve despite appropriate antimicrobial therapy (including involvement of the conduction system)
4. Multiple systemic emboli

Optimal timing of surgery in the pediatric patient must take into account the patient's clinical condition, patient size, available surgical options and durability of the proposed surgical therapy. In those in whom the infection persists, surgery should be performed before the infection extends beyond the valve leaflets and annulus. In cases of extravalvar infection, extensive debridement of the infected tissue is essential. The subpopulation of patients with progressive congestive heart failure should be treated prior to cardiac decompensation. Patients with aortic or prosthetic endocarditis benefit greatly from early surgical intervention. A combined treatment plan incorporating initial medical therapy and carefully applied surgical therapy will result in improved survival.

References

1. Kaplan EL. Infective endocarditis in the pediatric age group: An overview. In: Kaplan EL, Taronta AV (eds.) *Infective Endocarditis: An American Heart Association Symposium*. Dallas, TX. American Heart Association, 1977. pp 51–54.

2. Thekekara AG, Denham B, Duff DF. Eleven year review of infective endocarditis. *Ir Med J* 1994;87;(3):80–82.

3. Rastogi A, Luken JA, Pildes RS, et al. Endocarditis in neonatal intensive care unit. *Pediatr Cardiol* 1993;14:183–186.

4. Karl T, Wensky D, Stark J, et al. Infective endocarditis in children with congenital heart disease: Comparison of selected features in patients with surgical correction or palliation and those without. *Br Heart J* 1987;58;57–62.

5. Robard S. Blood velocity and endocarditis. *Circulation* 1963;27:18–?

6. Saiman L, Prince A, Gersony WM. Pediatric infective endocarditis in the modern era. *J Pediatr* 1993;122:847–853.

7. Fantin B, Leclercq R, Ottaviani M, et al. In vivo activities and penetration of the two components of the streptogramin RP 59500 in cardiac vegetations of experimental endocarditis. *Antimicrob Agents Chemother* 1994;38:432–437.

8. Arbulu A, Asfaw I. Management of infective endocarditis: Seventeen years' experience. *Ann Thorac Surg* 1987;43:144–149.

9. Petrov M, Wong K, Albertucci M, et al. Evaluation of unstented aortic homografts for the treatment of prosthetic aortic valve endocarditis. *Circulation* 1994:90 (5 pt2):II 198–204.

10. Vlessis AA, Hovaguimian H, Jaggers J, et al. Infective endocarditis: Ten year review of medical and surgical therapy. *Ann Thorac Surg* 1996;61:1217–1222.

11. Jessurun C, Mesa A, Wilansky S. Utility of transesophageal echocardiography in infective endocarditis: A review. *Tex Heart Inst J* 1996;23(2):98–107.

12. Mügge A. Echocardiographic detection of cardiac valve vegetations and prognostic implications. *Infect Dis Clin North Am* 1993;7:877–898.

13. Touroff ASW, Vessel H. Subacute *Streptococcus viridans* endarteritis complicating patent ductus arteriosus. *JAMA* 1940;115:1270–1272.

14. Wallace AG, Young WG Jr, Osterhout S. Treatment of acute bacterial endocarditis by valve excision and replacement. *Circulation* 1965;31:450–453.

15. Schollin J, Bjarke B, Wesstrom G. Infective endocarditis in Swedish children II. Location, major complications, laboratory findings, delay of treatment, treatment and outcome. *Acta Paediatr Scand* 1986;75:999–1004.

16. Citak M, Rees A, Mauroudis C. Surgical management of infective endocarditis in children. *Ann Thorac Surg* 1992;54(4):755–760.

17. Tolan RW Jr, Kleinman MB, Frank M, et al. Operative intervention in active endocarditis in children: Report of a series of cases and review. *Clin Infect Dis* 1992;14(4):852–862.

18. Awadallah SM, Kavey REW, Byrum CJ, et al. The changing pattern of infective endocarditis in childhood. *Am J Cardiol* 1991;63:90–94.

19. Hofstetter R, Toussaint R, Quintenz R, et al. Echocardiographic detection of endocarditis vegetations of the tricuspid valve in two children with ventricular septal defect. *Klin Paediatr* 1984;196(5):5277–5280.

20. Ribeiro PJ, Evora PR, Brasil JC, et al. Surgical approach in bacterial endocarditis at the tricuspid valve in children: Report of two cases. *Arq Bras Cardiol* 1989;52(2):153–157.

21. Arbulu A, Holmes RJ, Asfaw I. Surgical treatment of intractable right-sided infective endocarditis in drug addicts: 25 years experience. *J Heart Valve Dis* 1993;2(2):129–139.

22. Normand J, Bozio A, Etienne J, et al. Changing patterns and prognosis of infective endocarditis in childhood. *Eur Heart J* 1995;16 (Suppl B):28–31.

23. Muehicke DD, Cosgrove DM III, Lytle BW, et al. Is there an advantage to repairing infected mitral valves? *Ann Thorac Surg* 1997;63(6):1718–1724.

24. Acar C, Tolan M, Berrebi A, et al. Homograft replacement of the mitral valve, graft selection, technique of implantation, and results in 43 patients. *J Thorac Cardiovasc Surg* 1996;111(2):367–380.

25. Kovchovkos NT, Pavila-Roman VG, Spray TL, et al. Replacement of the aortic root with a pulmonary autograft in children and young adults with aortic valve disease. *N Engl J Med* 1994;330:1–6.

26. Doty D. Aortic valve replacement with homograft and autograft. *Semin Thorac Cardiovasc Surg* 1996;8(3):249–258.

27. Joyce F, Tingleff J, Pettersson G. The Ross operation: Results of early experience including treatment for endocarditis. *Eur J Cardiothorac Surg* 1995;9: 384–392.

28. Elkins RC, Knott-Craig CJ, Ward KE, et al. Pulmonary autograft in children: Realized growth potential. *Ann Thorac Surg* 1994;57:1387–1394.

29. Amoury RA, Bowman FO Jr, Malm JR. Endocarditis associated with intracardiac prostheses. *J Thorac Cardiovasc Surg* 1966;51:36–48.

30. Imoto Y, Sese A, Veno Y, et al. Methicillin-resistant *Staphylococcus aureus* endocarditis following patch closure of a ventricular septal defect. *J Jpn Assoc Thorac Surg* 1992;40:294–298.

31. Shrivastava S, Radhakrishnan S. Infective endocarditis following patch closure of a ventricular septal defect: A cross sectional Doppler echocardiographic study. *Int J Cardiol* 1989;25:27–32.

32. Kawashima Y, Nakano S, Kato M. Fate of pericardium utilized for the closure of ventricular septal defect: Postoperative ventricular septal aneurysm. *J Thorac Cardiovasc Surg* 1974;68:209–218.

Chapter 14

Prosthetic Valve Endocarditis

Bruce W. Lytle, M.D.

Introduction

Prosthetic valve endocarditis (PVE) is the most serious complication of cardiac valve replacement. Advances in diagnostic techniques and in the medical and surgical treatment of PVE have changed PVE from the death sentence that it represented in the early years of cardiac surgery to the status of a serious complication that most patients will survive today. However, it still remains a problem that challenges the clinician and adversely affects the patient's long-term outcome.

Assessing the existing data regarding the occurrence, diagnosis and treatment of PVE is difficult for a variety of reasons. First, different subspecialties such as internal medicine, cardiology, infectious disease and cardiac surgery have an impact upon the care of patients with suspected or real PVE. These different subspecialties interact with different patient subsets, and studies concerning PVE are scattered in different regions of the medical literature. Second, few single institutions have treated large numbers of patients with PVE, making statistical analyses difficult. Third, the criteria for the diagnosis of PVE have been drastically changed by the advent of echocardiography. Fourth, the organisms causing PVE and the antibiotics used to treat those organisms have evolved and continue to evolve. Fifth, the safety and effectiveness of the surgical treatment of PVE have improved dramatically. Sixth, the population of patients undergoing valve replacement—and who are, therefore, subject to PVE—has evolved in the direction of older patients with more complex cardiac and noncardiac disease. For today's clinician, it is important to realize that because

From: Vlessis AA, Bolling S (eds): *Endocarditis: A Multidisciplinary Approach to Modern Treatment.* © Futura Publishing Co., Armonk, NY, 1999.

of changing diagnostic and therapeutic techniques, past studies of PVE can provide only limited guidance for today's clinical decisions.

The goal of this chapter is to assess the current issues involved with the diagnosis and treatment of PVE. For some of the reasons listed above, data from the past have limited applicability to the current situation and principles of treatment must at times be based on logic as much as on historical data.

Incidence and Bacteriology of PVE

Early PVE

Studies of patients undergoing valve replacement have documented an increased "early phase" incidence of PVE that appears to extend for 2 to 6 months after operation, then decreases to a lower rate (late phase risk) that appears to extend indefinitely (Figure 1).[1] In studies of operations

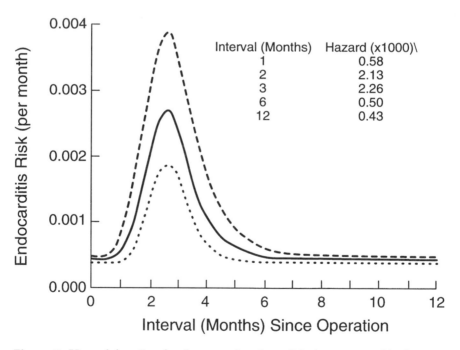

Figure 1. Hazard function for the rate of endocarditis (events/month) after primary aortic valve replacement, follow-up of 2443 patients. The early peaking phase gives way to a constant phase at about 5.5 months after operation. (From Agnihotri AK, McGiffin DC, Galbraith AJ, et al. The prevalence of infective endocarditis after aortic valve replacement. *J Thorac Cardiovasc Surg* 1995;110:1708–1724. Reprinted by permission.)

during which standard mechanical or xenograft prostheses were implanted, the magnitude of the early phase risk has appeared to be approximately 3%. Blackstone and Kirklin studied patients undergoing primary valve surgery from 1975 through 1979 and documented a 3% incidence of PVE by the end of the first postoperative year,[2] and Calderwood et al examined 2608 patients surviving valve replacement during a similar time period (1975–1982) and noted 3.1% incidence during the first postoperative year.[3] Grover et al authored the Veterans Affairs Cooperative Study (VA study) of valvular heart disease and reported a 1.5% incidence of PVE within 2 months after operation.[4] Gordon et al have reviewed our recent (1992–1997) experience with 7043 patients undergoing valve replacement or repair and with prospective surveillance identified 74 cases of PVE (1%) within the first postoperative year.[5] For patients with valve repair and prosthetic rings the incidence was 4 of 1992 (0.2%), versus 28 of 1731 (1%) for mechanical and 38 of 3320 (1%) for bioprostheses (P<0.001).

In a recent study of patients undergoing aortic valve replacement (AVR), some of whom received aortic valve homografts, Agnihotri et al documented an overall risk of endocarditis of approximately 1% during the first postoperative year.[1] This risk was increased for patients undergoing AVR for the treatment of native valve endocarditis; patients suffering from native valve endocarditis due to *Staphylococcus aureus* were at particularly high risk.[1] In addition, patients undergoing aortic root replacement with a synthetic graft were at increased risk, as were those who suffered a postoperative wound infection. Patients who received homograft valves did not experience an increased early risk of PVE. The VA cooperative study also noted that active native valve infection was a predictor of early phase risk and documented an increased risk of PVE associated with multivalve operations.[4]

In patients undergoing valve replacement for the treatment of active native valve endocarditis, early phase PVE usually results from persistent infection, but in other patients, early PVE generally represents nosocomial infection and is related to either a microbial contamination of the prosthesis at operation or the occurrence of a postoperative bacteremia in a patient where the prosthesis is not yet endothelialized and thus is more susceptible to infection. Keys studied patients undergoing valve replacement between 1986 and 1990 and identified 68 patients who were documented to have a bacteremia or fungemia in the early postoperative period.[6] He noted that 16 patients (24%) were eventually found to have documented or probable PVE. Fang et al reported on a similar group of patients in a multicenter study and found that of 115 patients who were not considered to have PVE at the time of a bacteremia, 18 subsequently developed endocarditis.[7] In both of these studies the most common portals of entry were intravascular catheters and skin infections. Urinary tract and gastrointestinal sources were uncommon. Despite the documented relationship between postoperative bacteremia and early PVE, most cases of PVE do not occur subsequent to a documented bacteremia, and logic would dictate that surgical contamination must play a role in many of those cases. Early onset PVE appears to be equally as common for patients receiving mechanical valves and standard bioprostheses (porcine or bovine heterografts) but much less common for patients receiving aortic valve homografts or pulmonic valve to aortic valve autotransplantation (Ross operation). Newer xenograft designs ("stent-less" valves) have smaller cloth stents than those on older models but whether or not that characteristic will decrease the incidence of PVE is as yet unknown. PVE is also extremely uncommon after mitral valve reparative procedures even in situations where prosthetic rings are used in association with mitral valve repair. Thus, the likelihood of early PVE becoming established appears to be a function of the interaction of the rate of bacteremia or bacterial contamination, the effectiveness of antibiotic prophylaxis and the prosthesis.

The microbiology of early phase PVE is indicative of a nosocomial origin of these infections. In the study by Calderwood, PVE within the first postoperative year was usually associated with coagulase-negative Staphylococcus, gram-negative organisms and fungi, all indicative of hospital-acquired infections.[3] Most other authors have documented similar findings. The majority of cases of early PVE are caused by gram-positive organisms, and despite the fact that gram-negative infection is more common in early PVE than in late PVE, gram-negative bacteria still cause only a small proportion of early PVE. Table 1 shows the distribution of causative organisms in our study (1975–1992) of surgically treated cases of PVE.[8] A report from Dusseldorf, Germany, noted a similar distribution

Table 1
Causative Organisms: 146 Surgical Cases of PVE

	Early (46 patients)	Late (100 patients)
S. Epidermidis	20	17
S. Aureus	11	20
Streptococcus	5	22
Enterococcus	1	10
Gram-negative	9	9
Fungus	3	5
Culture-negative	2	23
Multiple organisms	11*	

* Refers to number of patients with multiple organisms both early and late.

of organisms in the European setting.[9] Gordon's more recent review (1992–1997) of PVE occurring in patients undergoing valve surgery at the Cleveland Clinic Foundation noted that 54% of patients with early PVE had coagulase-negative Staphylococcus, 15% had fungi, and only 11% S. aureus. These changes may represent more effective prophylaxis against S. aureus and changes in hospital pathogens.[5]

The definition of "early" versus "late" PVE has varied among authors. In our studies we have defined "early" PVE as a situation in which infection becomes manifest within one year after operation.[8] Although that is a longer time period than many other authors have chosen, we have done so because the pathology and the microbiology of our surgical cases was consistent within the first postoperative year. Although relatively few cases of PVE occur between 6 months and a year after original surgery, those that do occur during that time period tend to have characteristics of early PVE. It is our opinion that they represent nosocomial infections in which the clinical manifestations of PVE have been delayed by perioperative antibiotic treatment and indolent organisms.

Late PVE

The time-related likelihood of acquiring late PVE is much less than that during the early phase but appears to be present indefinitely. Documentation of the incidence of late PVE requires careful long-term follow-up. Grover et al found an overall incidence of PVE of 0.8% per year and did not detect a difference in the incidence of late PVE between bioprosthetic and mechanical prostheses.[4] Over an 11-year follow-up, Hammermeister et al noted an incidence of PVE ranging from 7% for mechanical aortic valve prostheses to 17% for mitral valve bioprostheses,[10] but the differences in incidence between prosthesis type and valve position were not statistically significant. In a study examining the long-term outcomes of patients after primary isolated AVR, we found that the linearized incidence of endocarditis was 0.91% per patient-year for patients with bioprostheses versus 0.42% per patient-year for those with mechanical valves.[11] The aortic valve study by Agnihotri et al also found that the late phase risk of PVE was lower for patients with bileaflet mechanical valves compared to those with porcine or allograft valves.[1] In their study the constant phase risk was increased for all patients with previous endocarditis whether it was active or not at the time of operation, and that risk was particularly high for patients with previous S. aureus-related endocarditis. Other factors increasing the late phase risks were renal dysfunction and young age. In the VA study, late endocarditis was also related to superficial wound infection at the time of operation.[4] To sum up, the late phase incidence of PVE appears to be between 0.5% and 1% per year, and that risk is probably slightly increased for patients with bioprostheses relative to those with mechanical valves.

It is important to realize that during the last 20 years, there were virtually no nosocomial organisms that were resistant to all antibiotics. The emergence of resistant organisms could dramatically change the incidence and profile of PVE.

When cases of early versus late PVE are compared, it can be seen that the distribution of microbial agents differs, although there is substantial overlap (Table 1).[8] Those differences may become smaller as organisms previously considered to be "hospital-acquired" become more common in the general population. In both early and late PVE the causative agents are usually gram-positive. We have also found that culture-negative PVE is much more common in the late phase than in the early phase, probably because out-of-hospital febrile illnesses are more likely to be treated with oral antibiotics without blood cultures being obtained.

Pathology of Prosthetic Valve Endocarditis

The pathology of PVE is influenced by the type of the prosthesis, the route of the infection, the microbial organism, the time of occurrence of the infection and the length of time the infection is present. In our surgical series, we classified the pathological findings into infections involving the prosthesis alone, infections involving the junction of the prosthesis and the native valve annulus (annular infection), and infections that cause tissue destruction beyond the native valve annulus (extensive infection).[8] These subgroups can be helpful because they have been predictive of outcome, and the extent of infection may be detectable with echocardiography. Early PVE almost always involves at least the junction of the prosthesis and the native valve annulus, and it is rarely limited to the prosthesis alone. Early PVE is often associated with periprosthetic leak, and depending upon the length of time the infection has been present without effective treatment, the extension of the infection may create extensive tissue destruction including fistulae into cardiac chambers and abscess formation. In our surgical series, 83% of the patients with early PVE had involvement of at least the annulus and 39% had evidence of tissue destruction beyond the annulus. In addition, the infection will often produce vegetations that can create the danger of embolization.

Patients with late PVE are much more likely to have involvement of the prosthesis alone, particularly if the infection involves a bioprosthesis or a homograft. In our surgical series, 100 patients had late PVE and of those 58 had involvement of the prosthesis alone: 49 of those cases involved a bioprosthesis, 3 a homograft, and only 6 a mechanical prosthesis.[8] Therefore, there is a specific late pathological entity, infection of the prosthesis alone for patients with a bioprosthesis, that represented about half of the cases of late endocarditis in our surgical series, a type of infection uncommon in early PVE.

Another important pathological distinction in assessing the diagnosis and treatment of PVE is "active" versus "healed" endocarditis. We have felt that the definition of "active" endocarditis must include the demonstration of organisms either preoperatively or intraoperatively. Therefore, in order to classify a case of PVE as "active" we have required positive blood cultures prior to operation, or positive culture of the explanted valve, or organisms identified by microscopic examination of the explanted valve. Cases not exhibiting any of those characteristics have been classed as "healed" PVE.

Clinical Syndromes and Diagnosis of PVE

The accuracy of the diagnosis of PVE is important. In the case of an individual patient, failure to make the diagnosis jeopardizes outcome. The false positive diagnosis of PVE also creates problems because the treatments for PVE are expensive and may entail some patient risk. Furthermore, "soft" diagnoses of PVE may lead to an erroneously optimistic view of the efficacy of treatment for PVE. The advent of echocardiography has dramatically changed the diagnostic criteria for PVE. Previous clinical criteria proposed by von Reyn et al for diagnostic categories of "definite," "probable" and "possible" endocarditis are helpful in establishing the need for further investigation,[12] but often do not provide enough information to determine therapy or lack of it for patients with PVE. Durack et al have added echocardiographic criteria to aid in the evaluation of patients with possible PVE[13] and it is likely that in the future other imaging modalities such as magnetic resonance imaging will also be helpful.

For patients with suspected PVE the issues that are critical to determining therapy are whether or not there is evidence of systemic infection, whether or not there is a documented bacteremia or fungemia, and whether or not there is anatomic evidence that localizes an infection to the prosthetic valve. The diagnostic tests that provide the answers to these questions in the overwhelming majority of cases are blood cultures and echocardiography.

The documentation of a bacteremia or a fungemia is a very important issue for patients with a prosthetic heart valve as is the decision to begin any type of antibiotic therapy. Any patient with a prosthetic heart valve should have blood cultures drawn before antibiotic therapy is instituted for any reason other than prophylaxis. Patients who are inadequately treated with oral antibiotics started as empirical therapy for symptoms thought to be minor run the risk of suffering progressive and extensive PVE during a time when their oral antibiotic therapy may prevent identification of the presence of PVE and of the organism causing it. Even for patients who do not have established PVE, documentation of bacteremia is important and directs therapy. In a multicenter study by Fang et al, 16% of patients with a documented bacteremia who did not have evidence of PVE at the time of that bacteremia eventually developed clear-cut PVE.[7] The extent to which antibiotic therapy will prevent the development of PVE in patients who present with a bacteremia is not known, but logic dictates that documentation of a gram-positive bacteremia in a patient with a prosthetic heart valve is an indication for 6 weeks of intravenous antibiotic therapy. For patients with a gram-negative bacteremia but without evidence of PVE, decision- making in regard to the length of antibiotic therapy is more difficult. However, in a patient with a prosthetic heart valve it is a sound general principle that documentation of any blood stream infection is an indication for relatively long-term intravenous treatment with the appropriate antimicrobial agent, regardless of whether that infection can be localized to the valve.

To clearly establish the diagnosis of PVE with a degree of confidence that will justify reoperation requires documentation of a new anatomic abnormality involving a prosthetic heart valve. The most reliable way to accomplish this is transesophageal echocardiography.[13–15] Echocardiographic characteristics of PVE include the presence of vegetations, periprosthetic leak, intracardiac fistulae and abscess cavities. A negative echocardiogram does not exclude the diagnosis of PVE. In particular, patients with early PVE may have extensive infection of the annulus without presence of a periprosthetic leak or valvular vegetations that can be seen on TEE. In some of these uncommon situations magnetic resonance imaging (MRI) can highlight differences in tissue consistency and may provide evidence of infection before abnormalities of blood flow, detectable by echo, are present.

The most common scenarios that physicians are called upon to evaluate in reference to the diagnosis of PVE and institution of appropriate treatment are a) fever; b) fever and documented bacteremia; c) new periprosthetic leak with or without fever; d) embolization with or without fever; and e) clear-cut PVE with a combination of positive blood cultures and anatomic abnormality of the prosthetic valve. Persistent fever, new periprosthetic leak and evidence of embolization occurring in a patient with a prosthetic heart valve all represent indications for blood cultures and transesophageal echocardiography, and the results of these studies will determine the initial approach to therapy.

Patients with a clinical scenario that is suggestive of PVE but who do not have either positive blood cultures or a diagnostic valve lesion seen on echocardiography represent difficult diagnostic problems. It is usually a good idea to avoid starting antibiotics blindly in this situation and to continue drawing blood cultures unless the patient is clinically very unstable. To achieve a cure of PVE it is a tremendous advantage to have identified a specific organism.

For patients with a documented blood stream infection, appropriate intravenous antibiotics should be started regardless of the echocardiographic findings. If patients have positive blood cultures but no anatomic abnormality via echocardiography or small valvular vegetations, it is possible that they either do not have PVE or that they have early PVE that may be treatable with antibiotics alone. However, patients with positive blood cultures and anatomic abnormalities involving the valve annulus are highly likely to need combined medical and surgical treatment and management should point in that direction. Most patients with clear PVE will eventually need operation. The issues involved in their management include a) evidence of metastatic infection; b) coronary anatomy; c) end organ function; d) evidence of control of infection; and e) duration of preoperative antibiotic therapy.

Complications of metastatic infections can be a significant source of morbidity and mortality for patients with PVE. Although CT scanning prior to surgery for PVE is not absolutely routine, abdominal symptoms are an indication for abdominal CT scanning to investigate the possibility of a hepatic or splenic abscess. The identification of hepatic or splenic abscesses is not a contraindication to valve re-replacement, nor is it necessarily an indication for splenectomy or hepatic abscess drainage either at the time of cardiac surgery or prior to cardiac surgery. However, once these visceral abscesses have been documented, their failure to improve with antibiotics may indicate subsequent surgery.

Stroke has been documented in 10% to 25% of patients with PVE. In a study by Davenport and Hart of 61 patients with PVE,[16] 18% suffered embolic strokes and 10% experienced brain hemorrhage. In 2 patients hemorrhage occurred following an embolic stroke. Most of the strokes occurred soon after the diagnosis was made and the initiation of antibiotic therapy appeared to decrease the subsequent risk of stroke. Occurrence of a stroke for a patient with PVE (or for a patient without known PVE but with a prosthetic heart valve) is an indication for echocardiography and cerebral CT scanning. The presence of residual vegetations (particularly those greater than 1 cm in diameter) on a prosthetic heart valve is a relative indication for operation. Also, the presence of a CT-documented embolic stroke is not a contraindication to valve replacement surgery. Fears that heparinization and cardiopulmonary bypass will convert embolic strokes into intracranial hemorrhage have rarely been borne out. However, for a patient who presents with PVE and intracranial hemorrhage, decision-making is often difficult and the risk of immediate surgery must be weighed against the risks of a worsening infection. While it has been our experience that valve replacement surgery did not often worsen the existing neurological deficit, it has also been true that patients with a clearly documented focal stroke on CT scan did not commonly exhibit improvement in the neurological deficit after operation.

The need to investigate the coronary anatomy of patients with PVE is also a complex issue. In the past coronary angiography has not been routinely carried out for patients with PVE, both because of the possible risk of producing embolization of vegetations and because most patients did not have coronary artery disease. However, many patients undergoing valve replacement are at an age when they may also have coronary artery disease and, in fact, may have had previous bypass surgery. Most patients with PVE who have had previous bypass surgery should undergo coronary angiography that is extensive enough to define their bypass graft anatomy. It is important for the surgeon to understand the bypass graft anatomy and to know whether or not atherosclerotic vein grafts are present, both from the standpoint of achieving good intraoperative myocardial protection and to know what grafts may need to be replaced in case of an intraoperative graft injury or a need to replace the aortic root and/or the ascending aorta. For patients with mitral valve PVE, coronary angiography is unlikely to be a high-risk procedure. For patients with aortic valve endocarditis and vegetations there is some risk of embolization associated with coronary angiography, and judgement must be used in recommending these studies.

Prior to operation, patients with PVE will often exhibit organ system failure. Although there are few absolute contraindications to operation, an understanding of the end-organ failure that has already occurred is important. Renal and hepatic function particularly need to be assessed. In addition, hemostatic mechanisms are important to evaluate in patients with PVE. Many have been anticoagulated because of a mechanical prosthetic heart valve, and both preoperative and postoperative coagulopathies are common. Both the surgeon and the blood bank should be prepared for this eventuality.

The choice of medical therapy versus combined medical-surgical therapy for PVE will be addressed more completely in the Results section of this chapter, but even in patients who seem destined for operation, the question often arises of how long to continue preoperative antibiotic therapy. At issue is the possible benefit of preoperative antibiotic therapy in the control of systemic and local sepsis versus the risk of progressive infection worsening the patient's clinical or anatomic status. In terms of preventing reinfection after operation, 2 principles of treatment are that some antibiotics are better than no antibiotics, and if a bacteriologic cure is possible with antibiotics prior to surgery, the risk of reinfection is less. However, it is also true that our ability to surgically manage active infection has improved greatly; thus it is not wise to allow the patient to undergo local anatomic extension of the infection or systemic organ failure while unsuccessfully trying to achieve a bacteriologic cure. Most patients with evidence of an annular or invasive infection will not be curable with antibiotics alone; waiting for that to happen risks making a bad situation worse. Therefore, once antibiotics have been started, continued delay of surgery requires that clinical improvement be prompt and sustained. Any worsening of the situation (judged by persistent or recurrent fever, new signs of peripheral embolization, or worsening anatomy as identified by serial echocardiography) is an indication to proceed with operation.

Surgery for Prosthetic Valve Endocarditis

There has been substantial improvement in the combined medical-surgical therapy of PVE within the last decade in terms of perioperative survival, long-term survival, freedom from reinfection and freedom from reoperation. The factors that have been involved in producing these improved outcomes are multiple and include 1) effective myocardial protection;[17] 2) improved capability of blood banks to provide component therapy for treatment of coagulopathies; 3) the use of intraoperative transesophageal echo; 4) the use of aortic valve homografts;[17-20] 5) the use of biological tissue such as autologous pericardium and glutaraldehyde-treated bovine pericardium for intracardiac reconstruction;[21-24] 6) improved antibiotics; 7) surgical approaches that include aggressive debridement of infected tissue and foreign material;[21-24] and 8) the increased experience of surgeons. However, operations for PVE have not become simpler but rather have become longer, larger, and more effective. These are operations that may involve multiple cardiac chambers, long cross-clamp times, extensive intracardiac reconstructions, and coronary bypass grafting. Because of the complexity of these procedures and their demands on resources, they are best performed in at least semi-elective settings if possible. Wise preoperative assessment of these patients will usually permit avoidance of emergency operations.

Most operations for PVE are best carried out through a median sternotomy. Regardless of the preoperative echo findings, the surgeon never can be sure of doing a "limited" operation for a "limited" infection and should be prepared for anything during an operation for PVE. For example, mitral valve reoperations can be accomplished through a right or left thoracotomy, and multiple routes for "minimally" invasive valve surgery are available, but when PVE is thought to be present, involvement of all valves as well as the fibrous trigone of the heart is possible, and these situations are difficult to remedy except through a median sternotomy. The repeat median sternotomy is carried out with the use of an oscillating saw. The sternal wires from the previous sternotomy are divided anteriorly but left in place posteriorly, allowing the surgeon to tell when the posterior table of the sternum has been divided. Situations that create an increased risk of complications associated with repeat sternotomy include right ventricular enlargement, aortic false aneurysm, previous aortic graft, multiple coronary bypass grafts, a right internal thoracic artery graft crossing the midline and multiple atherosclerotic vein grafts. In these situations it may be helpful to perform a small right anterior thoracotomy before making the sternotomy. This allows the surgeon to place a hand beneath the sternum to assess the danger and, if needed, dissection through this right thoracotomy may allow separation of the sternum from underlying structures.

An alternative approach is peripheral arterial and venous cannulation, establishing cardiopulmonary bypass, and reopening the sternotomy either with the heart beating and decompressed, or after systemic deep hypothermia has produced circulatory arrest. We do not use this approach routinely because of the disadvantages of prolonged heparinization and cardiopulmonary bypass. However, in the presence of an aortic false aneurysm beneath the sternum, the circulatory arrest strategy may be useful. For patients with prolonged heparinization, the use of aprotinin combined with monitoring of heparin levels may help control potential coagulopathies.

Once the sternum is divided, the pleural cavities are entered as soon as possible. This maneuver allows the cardiac structures to fall posteriorly and helps achieve some separation of the sternum from those cardiac structures. In addition, this allows a hand to be placed into the left chest to accomplish cardiac decompression if cardiac arrest should occur. The right-sided cardiac structures are then exposed along with the aorta. It is usually not necessary to completely expose the left side of the heart unless coronary bypass grafting will be needed or a patent left ITA graft must be controlled. During the dissection, segments of autologous pericardium should be preserved if possible for use during reconstructive procedures.

Once the aorta, right atrium, and caval structures are exposed, cannulation is undertaken. Cannulation usually involves separate cannulation of the superior (SVC) and inferior vena cava, and it is helpful to cannulate the SVC directly so that it can be divided if necessary to enhance the exposure of the left atrium, aortic root and fibrous trigone of the heart. Aortic pathology can make SVC exposure difficult, and if that is the case a small venous cannula can be placed in the innominate vein for drainage. The inferior vena cava can be cannulated through the right atrium or the femoral vein. With the use of relatively small (22–28 fr) long femoral venous cannulae and vacuum-assisted drainage for cardiopulmonary bypass, excellent drainage and flows can be obtained via the femoral route, limiting the cannulae that transverse the operative field. A self-inflating coronary sinus retrograde cardioplegia cannulae is placed transatrially.

Since operations for PVE will often be extensive, myocardial protection is critical. We use systemic hypothermia to 32°C and a combination of antegrade and retrograde substrate-enhanced cold blood cardioplegia as described by Buckberg.[17] Maintenance cardioplegia is given every 15 to 20 minutes for intervals of approximately 2 minutes. If retrograde cardioplegia delivery is effective, most maintenance regimens are via that route, particularly for patients with coronary atherosclerosis and previous bypass surgery. Many different strategies for cardioplegia can be effective. However, for today's population of patients with prosthetic valve endocarditis, some adjustment to the presence of patent and/or stenotic bypass grafts and the presence of severe coronary artery disease must often be made. Retrograde cardioplegia is often the best solution in these situations.

Once cannulation is undertaken and cardiopulmonary bypass is possible, the operation is carried out. The general principles of operations for PVE are 1) remove the prosthetic valve and debride away infected tissue and foreign material; 2) close the holes in the heart; 3) replace the valves; and 4) use biologic tissue as much as possible.

Aortic Valve PVE

For patients with aortic valve PVE it is our intention to replace the infected prosthesis with an aortic valved homograft, usually implanted as an aortic root replacement. After aortic cross- clamping and cardioplegia delivery, the aortic valve is exposed through an oblique aortotomy extending toward the annulus through the noncoronary cusp. The aortic prosthesis is removed and infected tissue is debrided along with any residual suture material and Teflon felt pledgets. If it is clear that a homograft is to be used, the aortic tissue around the coronary artery orifices is debrided as well and the coronary orifices are prepared as buttons for reanastomosis

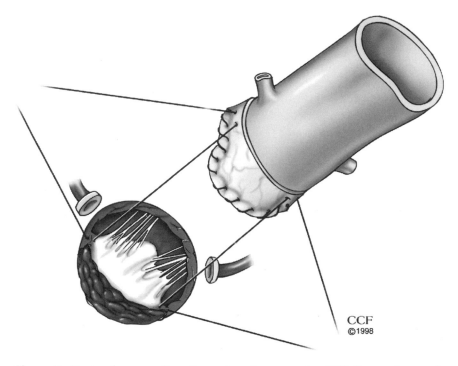

Figure 2. During homograft aortic root replacement for PVE the aortic root is extensively debrided and coronary buttons are created. Spacing the homograft by matching its mitral valve to the native mitral valve is a reliable way to orient the homograft in a distorted aortic root. The most common location for an annular abscess is in the area of the anterior leaflet of the mitral valve.

to the homograft (Figure 2). In the reoperative aortic root it is often necessary to dissect along the length of the coronary arteries for up to 1 cm in order to obtain mobility. If communications between the aortic outflow tract and the right ventricle or right and left atrium existed prior to operation or have been created by the debridement, those holes are closed with large pericardial patches sewn into place with 4-0 Prolene suture material. Autologous pericardium is our first choice of material to close holes and reconstruct annular structures, but in situations of multiple previous operations, autologous pericardium is sometimes not available. Under these circumstances, we used glutaraldehyde-treated bovine pericardium.

Once the aortic valve has been removed, the mitral valve is inspected. If continuous active infection appears to extend directly to the mitral valve from the prosthetic aortic valve and the mitral valve is insufficient, then it is probable that the mitral valve and probably the fibrous trigone of the heart will need to be replaced along with the aortic prosthesis. However,

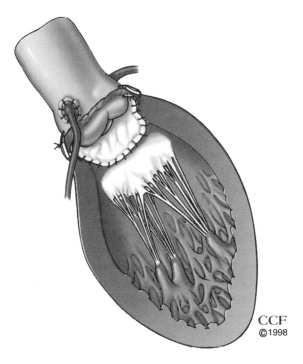

CCF
©1998

Figure 3. One strategy for management of an abscess cavity as seen in Figure 2 is to use the homograft mitral valve as an extension, sewing it to the superior rim of the native mitral valve. This allows the homograft to bridge the gap created by the abscess cavity and usually positions the homograft correctly for the coronary artery anastomoses.

that situation is not common. It is more common for isolated mitral valve perforations (drop lesions) to be created by a jet of aortic insufficiency. If those perforations are discrete and separated from the infected annulus of the aortic valve prosthesis, they are usually not an indication for mitral valve replacement and can usually be closed by freshening the edges of the perforation and closing it with a pericardial patch.

The most common location for extension of infection from the aortic annulus is the creation of an abscess cavity extending posteriorly in the location of the fibrous trigone and the anterior leaflet of the mitral valve (Figure 2). As long as the active infection can be debrided and the anterior leaflet of the mitral valve is not unstable, these situations can usually be managed without removal of the fibrous trigone of the heart. If an aortic valve homograft will be used for valve replacement it is not usually necessary to close these cavities separately. The inferior rim of the defect is the superior aspect of the native mitral valve and the continuity of the aortic

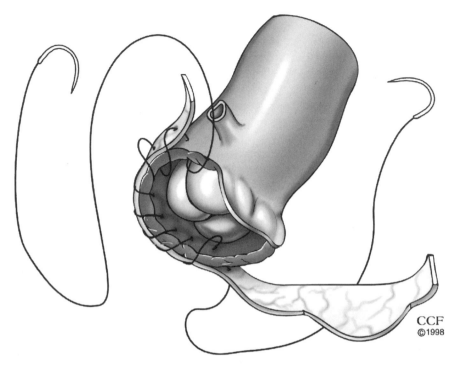

Figure 4. The sewing of a pericardial "skirt" around the base of the homograft with 5-0 Prolene suture material is helpful during homograft aortic root replacement. This strategy "bulks up" the homograft, establishing a better size match if the annulus is enlarged. In addition, when the anastomotic sutures pass through the homograft and pericardium, hemostasis is very secure.

outflow tract can be constructed by sewing the mitral valve anterior leaflet of the homograft to the superior rim of the native mitral valve anterior leaflet (Figure 3). If a standard valve prosthesis is used, then that cavity will need to be closed separately with a biological patch in order to provide an annulus to support the new valve.

    Placement of an aortic valve homograft for PVE has some aspects that may not be present when replacing a noninfected native valve. First, if tissue destruction in the aortic root has been extensive, there may be a large size discrepancy between the smaller homograft and the larger remnant of the aortic annulus. Aortic valve annular "shrinking" techniques that have been described to aid in the use of smaller homografts in elective operations for aortic root replacement have usually involved some sort of commissural plication. However, these annular "shrinking" techniques are difficult in the setting of infection because the periannular tissue is usually quite rigid and fixed in position. When faced with a large size discrepancy, it helps to not debride any of the muscular tissue from the homograft itself and also to leave the homograft mitral valve as long as possible. In addition, a pericardial "skirt" may be sewn circumferentially to the inferior portion of the homograft with continuous 5-0 Prolene suture (Figure 4). This technique bulks up the homograft. In addition, during construction of the proximal homograft to annulus anastomosis, the sutures pass through the homograft musculature and also through the pericardial skirt, essentially creating a pericardial "sewing ring" for the homograft. This helps in securing hemostasis.

The second problem common to situations with infection is that extensive tissue destruction may make orientation of the homograft and spacing of the sutures difficult. If the patient still has a native mitral valve, the best orientation strategy is to ignore the location of the aortic valve commissures and orient the mitral valve of the homograft to the patient's mitral valve (Figure 3). Each edge of the 2 mitral valves then establishes 2 points of fixation that encompass approximately one third of the annulus. Bisecting the remainder of the homograft and the remainder of the native annulus then allows a reasonable spacing of sutures around the homograft. In addition, since the left coronary orifice of the homograft is usually just medial to the lateral edge of the anterior leaflet of the mitral valve, positioning the homograft in this way helps in the orientation of the native and homograft left coronary orifices despite what may be a distorted aortic root.

For construction of the homograft-aortic root anastomosis we use 4-0 Prolene suture material, usually in an interrupted fashion, employing somewhere between 32 and 38 sutures around the circumference of the aortic root. The homograft is held just above the aortic root while the sutures are placed in the annulus, septum, and superior rim of the mitral valve (whatever is left after debridement), then through the homograft. Once all the sutures have been placed, the homograft is parachuted into position and all sutures are tied. In situations where extensive annular destruction has occurred, the proximal end of the homograft will be placed on the ventricular side of the former annulus and the homograft will transverse the destroyed annulus. Thus, the sutures are commonly placed through ventricular muscle rather than the annulus. In extensive infections, heart block is common. Following construction of the proximal anastomosis, the coronary artery buttons are anastomosed in an anatomic fashion to the left and right coronary sinuses, usually into orifices created by removal of the homograft coronary arteries (Figure 3). Since the coronary arteries are usually not aneurysmal, large buttons can be used. Either 4-0 or 5-0 Prolene suture material is used for these anastomoses. The left coronary artery is constructed first and is followed with the right coronary artery. At this point the homograft and coronary anastomoses are tested for competency by running cardioplegia solution into the homograft itself. The host aorta is then divided distally and an end-to-end anastomosis is constructed between the homograft and native aorta.

Early in our homograft experience we performed some free hand or "mini-root" homograft operations for PVE, but we now usually perform a total root replacement for the treatment of PVE. With this strategy, debridement of infected or foreign material is more complete, exposure and reconstruction are actually simpler, and in the often distorted aortic root anatomy of patients with PVE, total root replacement helps minimize homograft distortion and early aortic insufficiency.

Although homograft aortic valve replacement is our first choice of procedures for the treatment of isolated aortic valve PVE, if a surgeon is not familiar with homograft techniques, then initiating a homograft experience with a difficult reoperation on a critically ill patient is probably not a good idea. In addition, our previous experience has shown that with radical debridement of infected tissue and foreign material, valve replacement with standard prostheses can also result in good outcomes.[8] When placing standard prostheses, the aortic root is reconstructed with pericardium before the prosthesis is placed. In this setting, placing sutures from the prosthesis sewing ring through the aorta and tying those sutures down outside the aorta is often an effective way to seat the prosthesis (Figure 5). In the area of the noncoronary cusp or right coronary cusp the surgeon may be able to tie sutures outside the aorta. Opening the right atrium, pulmonary artery or right ventricle will allow sutures to be tied inside those structures. There does not appear to be a fundamental advantage of mechanical versus heterograft valves in terms of the likelihood of reinfection when operating for PVE. Our choice is usually to use a bioprosthesis because of its more forgiving sewing ring, the avoidance of impingement of subvalvular structures on opening and closing of the valve, and the ability to avoid anticoagulants postoperatively.

A variant form of aortic root endocarditis that creates special considerations is infection of a composite aortic valve and ascending aorta and/or aortic arch graft (Bentall operation). (Figure 6) For patients with previous Bentall operations, PVE usually involves the prosthesis/native aortic valve annulus junction. The diagnosis of PVE in this circumstance may be difficult because the one piece aortic valve/ascending aortic graft makes a perivalvular leak impossible, and an anatomic abnormality of the graft may be difficult to recognize by echocardiogram until a large perivalvular and perigraft abscess cavity is created. Secondarily the infection may extend along the length of the graft. Periannular false aneurysms rarely create danger in terms of sternal reopening, but if infection of the coronary buttons has occurred, right coronary artery false aneurysms can be dangerous during the repeat sternotomy.

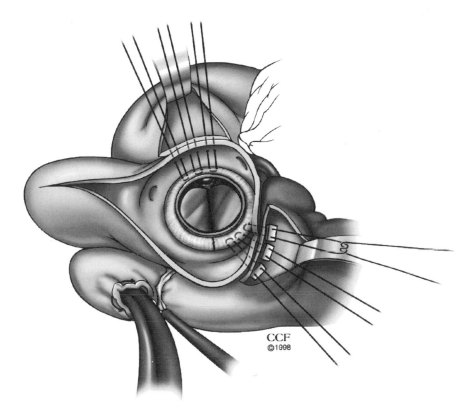

Figure 5. When placing a standard prosthesis into an infected aortic root after debridement, it may help to open the pulmonary artery and right atrium, allowing suture placement through the prosthesis and the residual wall of the annulus and aorta, and finally into these structures.

For patients with PVE and composite grafts, our goal is to remove all the prosthetic material and to replace everything with homografts. Circulatory arrest is usually required for construction of the distal homograft to aortic arch anastomosis and in this situation we employ axillary artery cannulation, deep hypothermia, circulatory arrest and retrograde superior vena cava cerebral perfusion for cerebral protection. Once systemic hypothermia has been achieved, the systemic circulation is arrested and we first approach the distal graft to aorta anastomosis, removing all the prosthetic material. For patients who have had ascending aortic grafts a single homograft is usually not long enough to reach all the way from the aortic root to the aortic arch, and so we usually need to use 2 homografts. The first homograft can be reversed to take advantage of the larger aortic root size for anastomosis to the aortic arch (after the aortic leaflets

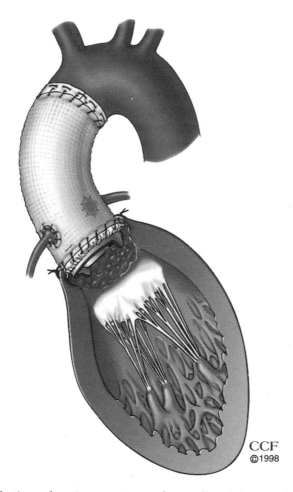

CCF
©1998

Figure 6. Infections of aortic composite grafts usually originate at the valve-native annulus interface.

are removed), and that homograft is sewn into place in the aortic arch with continuous 4-0 Prolene suture material. We then restart the systemic circulation and clamp the homograft with an atraumatic clamp (Figure 7). Systemic rewarming is then possible while the aortic root situation is addressed. If the patient has a residual aortic arch dilatation, it may not be wise to anastomose the homograft directly to the dilated arch because tension on the smaller homograft may cause suture line bleeding. On a few occasions we have used a small cuff of prosthetic graft beveled at one end to match the aortic arch size, then constructed an end-to-end anastomosis of the nonbeveled end of the graft with the homograft at its

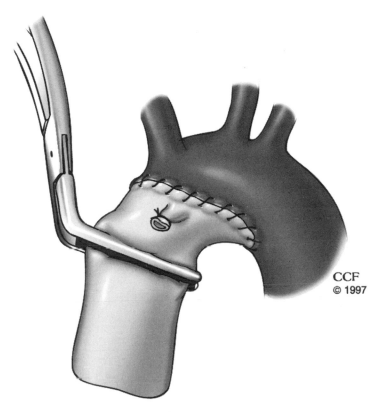

Figure 7. For the treatment of an infected composite graft, the distal anastomosis is approached first. It sometimes helps to reverse a homograft and excise the valve leaflets, allowing the larger end of the homograft to be anastomosed to the aortic arch. Once that is completed the homograft is clamped allowing systemic perfusion to be restarted and systemic rewarming to begin.

distal end to help make the size transition. Although we do not think it ideal to leave any prosthetic material in place, the focus of the infection is usually around the aortic valve annulus, and so this strategy is a compromise that may be acceptable. In the 2 cases in which we have used this approach, late reinfection has not occurred. A second homograft is used to replace the aortic root, as described above, and when that is completed the 2 homografts are sewn together (Figure 8).

Mitral Valve PVE

For patients thought to have isolated mitral valve endocarditis, the mitral valve is exposed by a left atriotomy anterior to the right superior pulmo-

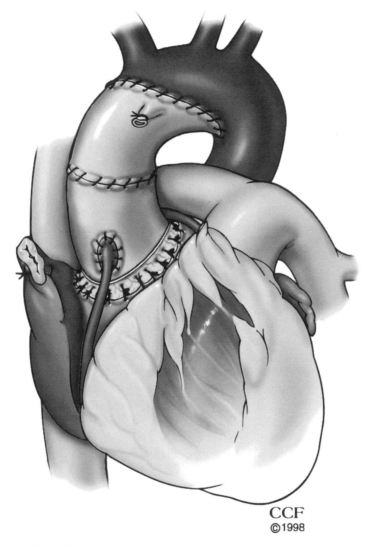

CCF
©1998

Figure 8. Once the aortic root replacement is completed, the 2 homografts are sewn together to complete the replacement of the composite graft.

nary vein. If necessary, exposure can be improved by dividing the superior vena cava and extending the left atrial incision toward the fibrous trigone of the heart and the aortic root (see Figure 12).

Once exposed, the prosthetic mitral valve is then removed with all infected tissue. It is relatively common for annular infections to burrow within the mitral valve annulus, essentially creating atrial ventricular dis-

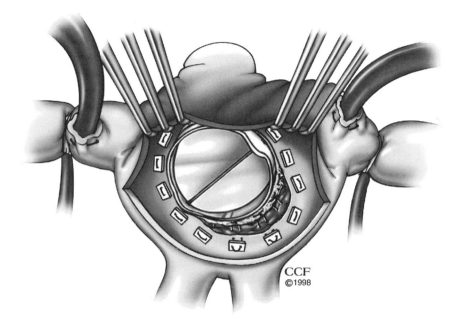

Figure 9. Infection of the posterior mitral valve annulus often creates an abscess cavity that essentially produces atrioventricular dissociation.

sociation, particularly posteriorly (Figure 9). Once the infected tissue has been radically debrided it is often necessary to reconstruct that annulus with pericardium. The atrioventricular discontinuity is repaired by sewing one edge of the patch to noninfected ventricular muscle and continuing the suture line across the annulus to the atrial edge of the defect (Figure 10). A standard prosthesis of either the mechanical or heterograft type is then placed in the normal position using the pericardial patch as the annulus (Figure 11). Thus, the abscess cavity is not pulled together and closed but is covered with pericardium. In the setting of PVE these abscess cavities are usually fixed with friable tissue surrounding them, and trying to close the cavity with sutures that are then used as valve sutures will often fail as the sutures tear through. Adding the pericardial tissue to bridge the gap created by the abscess allows closure without tension.

Mitral valve homografts have been used for the treatment of PVE although experience with this strategy has not been extensive. It is possible that they will provide advantages in the treatment of infection as aortic valve homografts have done, but for the present time the most common strategy is the placement of standard prostheses. With radical debride-

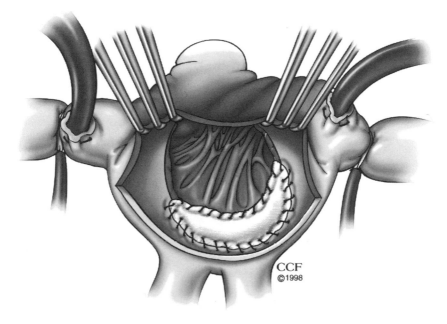

Figure 10. Once the valve, prosthetic material, and infected tissue are debrided, the abscess cavity is closed with pericardium before the valve is replaced.

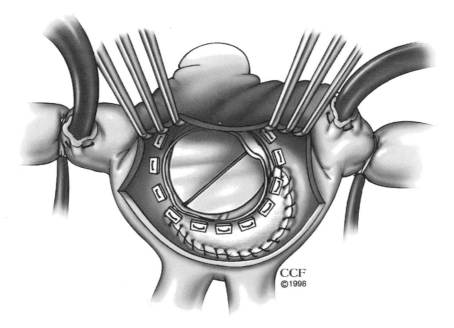

Figure 11. The mitral valve is replaced using the pericardium as part of the annulus. The valve sutures are not used to attempt to close the cavity.

ment of infected tissue and postoperative antibiotics, the outcomes with the use of standard prostheses have been good. My own preference is to use porcine heterografts in the mitral position because of the favorable sewing ring on a porcine valve and because it is often an advantage not to be forced to anticoagulate a patient with severe PVE.

PVE with Fibrous Trigone Infection

In patients with previous mitral valve replacement, aortic valve replacement, or both, it is possible for infection of either prosthesis to extend directly into the fibrous trigone of the heart in the area between the aortic and mitral valve. In this situation, the only real possibility of removing infection is to remove the entire fibrous trigone of the heart, along with the aortic and the mitral valve. To gain exposure to this area it is helpful to divide the superior vena cava (Figure 12). A left atrial incision can then be extended up through the fibrous trigone of the heart and on to the aorta, exposing both the aortic and the mitral valve. Both valves are then excised and the infected tissue debrided, producing at that point a continuous chamber encompassing the left atrium, left ventricle, and aorta (Fig-

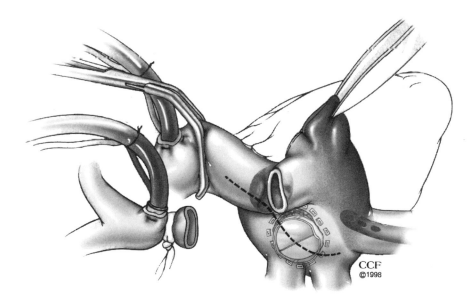

Figure 12. Division of the superior vena cava provides good exposure of the aortic root, mitral valve and fibrous trigone.

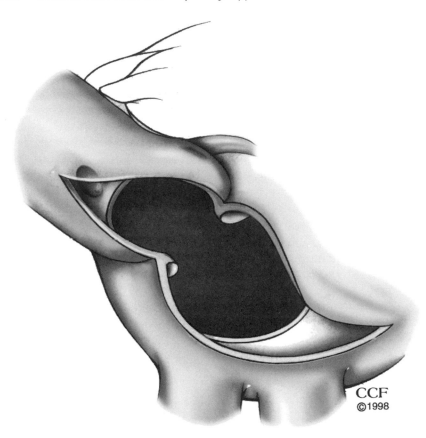

Figure 13. Debridement of the aortic and mitral valves and fibrous trigone leaves a continuous chamber.

ure 13). The reconstruction is accomplished by first placing the posterior, medial and lateral aspects of the mitral prosthesis in the remaining area of the mitral valve annulus. Once that prosthesis is tied into place, the superior portion of the mitral valve annulus can be reconstructed with a segment of autologous or bovine pericardium. Mattress sutures are then placed through the pericardium which then forms the superior aspect of the mitral valve annulus (Figure 14). An aortic valve prosthesis is then placed around two thirds to three quarters of its circumference and the pericardium is used to create the medial aspect of the aortic valve annulus (Figure 15). The closure of the left atrium and the aorta are then completed using the pericardial patch (Figure 16) and the superior vena cava is reattached. Thus, the fibrous trigone of the heart, the aortic valve and the mitral valve are replaced by this reconstruction. Despite the extensive

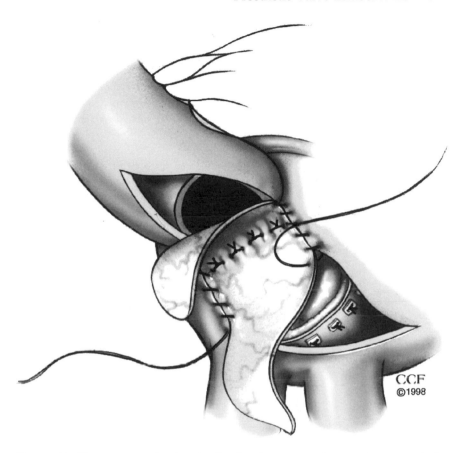

Figure 14. The new prosthetic mitral valve is sewn to the annulus posteriorly, medially and laterally, but the superior portion of the mitral valve annulus is created by an elongated pericardial patch that replaces the fibrous trigone.

nature of this type of repair, effective myocardial protection allows this approach to invasive infection.

Results of the Treatment of PVE

The treatment options for patients with PVE are long-term intravenous antibiotic treatment alone (medical treatment) or long-term intravenous antibiotic treatment combined with reoperation for valve re-replacement (medical-surgical treatment). No randomized studies exist comparing these 2 strategies and, in fact, they are complementary. An initial decision to begin antibiotic treatment does not by itself preclude the possibility of

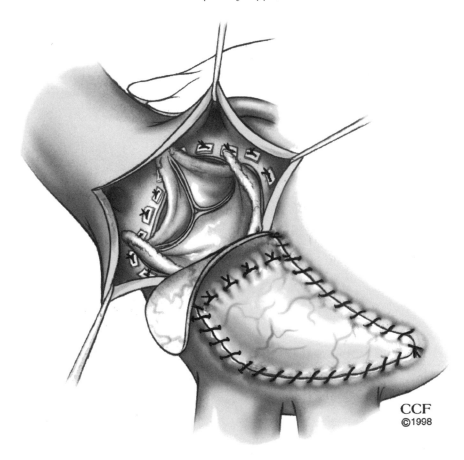

Figure 15. Once the mitral valve is in place, the aortic valve is secured throughout most of the annulus, and the pericardial patch recreates the medial part of the aortic valve annulus.

performing surgery. However, the downside of prolonged medical management can be that delaying surgery in the hope of achieving a cure with antibiotics alone may jeopardize the outcome once the decision for surgery is made because of the worsening of the patient's local or systemic infection. In assessing older studies of the medical treatment of endocarditis, it is important to remember that prior to the echocardiographic era the diagnosis of PVE for patients treated without surgery was often imprecise. Therefore, it is probable that some patients in older "medically treated" groups did not, in fact, have PVE. Despite the advent of echocardiography, this is still a danger in comparing the results of medical and medical-surgical treatment.

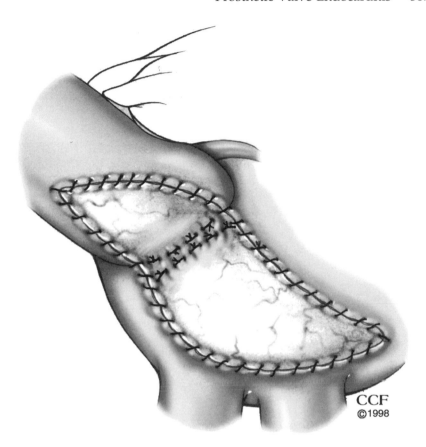

Figure 16. Once the valve replacements are completed the pericardial patch is extended to close the aorta and the left atrium.

Despite imprecision in the diagnosis of PVE for patients who do not come to surgery or autopsy, it is still clear that patients thought to have PVE who are treated with antibiotics alone usually do not have good outcomes. Ivert noted a mortality rate of 70%.[25] Calderwood et al divided patients into "uncomplicated" and "complicated" PVE groups.[26] "Complicated" PVE was defined as 1) a new or worsening murmur of valve dysfunction; 2) congestive heart failure; 3) ECG conduction abnormalities; and 4) an intracardiac abscess. Of patients in their "complicated" group, only 21% survived the hospital stay and did not need further therapy. More recent studies have not shown improved outcomes for medical treatment alone. In a multicenter study, Yu et al noted a mortality rate of 56% with medical therapy alone over a one-year follow-up, compared to a 23%

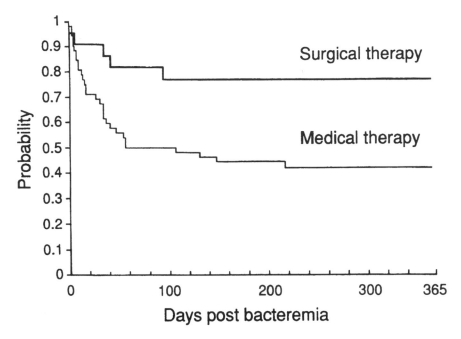

Figure 17. Comparison of Kaplan-Meier curves demonstrating improved survival with surgical therapy compared to medical therapy for patients with early prosthetic valve endocarditis. (From Yu et al. Prosthetic valve endocarditis: Superiority of surgical valve replacement versus medical therapy only. *Ann Thorac Surg* 1994; 58:1073–1077. Reprinted by permission.)

mortality rate for medical-surgical treatment (Figure 17).[27] A recent study by John et al of patients with *S. aureus* PVE noted that 22 of 33 (67%) presented with cardiac complications (as previously defined by Calderwood et al).[26] Of the medically treated patients, 10 of 12 (83%) with cardiac complications died within 90 days (versus 2 of 10 with surgery) and 2 of 7 (29%) without cardiac complications died within 90 days (versus 0 of 4 with surgery).[28] It is also important to note that 90-day outcome is a very short follow-up for patients with PVE, and one cannot assume that a cure has been effected for at least a few years after treatment.

Many of the cases in these series were patients with early PVE. Most patients with early endocarditis will need surgery to be cured of PVE. What is not yet clear is whether or not there are patients who fulfill the criteria for early PVE but with a relatively benign course who can be predictably treated with antibiotics alone.

There are some patients with late PVE who fall into categories wherein it appears they can be reasonably safely treated with antibiotics alone, at least to the point of achieving a bacteriologic cure. Specifically, patients with bioprostheses who present with a late infection not involving *S. aureus* or fungi and without evidence of annular or more extensive involvement can often be successfully treated with antibiotics. However, it has been apparent to us that even those patients successfully treated with antibiotics appeared to have an accelerated failure rate of bioprostheses and often come to reoperation within a few years. The advantage of treating those patients medically, however, is that they may come to operation at a point where they do not have active endocarditis. Anecdotal reports have shown that patients with annular involvement will on occasion be successfully treated with antibiotics alone, but that is not a predictable outcome.[29,30]

One reason that the medical treatment of PVE has been prevalent is that in the past the in-hospital risk of combined medical-surgical treatment of patients with PVE has been substantial, even at centers known for their experience with PVE. Reported in-hospital mortality rates for patients with PVE included 23% in 1982 by Baumgartner and colleagues from Stanford University,[31] 23% in 1986 by Calderwood et al from the Massachusetts General Hospital[26] and 20% in our own pre-1984 series at the Cleveland Clinic Foundation.[8]

Fortunately, things have changed for the better despite a higher-risk group of patients who are now presenting for treatment of PVE. To evaluate the changing results on our own surgical series, we divided the 1975–1992 time frame into 2 parts: 1975–1984 (44 patients) and 1985–1992 (102 patients). The in-hospital mortality rate between those time periods decreased from 20% to 10% in the later surgical period. Furthermore, higher-risk categories of patients experienced substantial improvement in mortality rate. The mortality for patients with active endocarditis dropped from 24% to 13% and for patients with annular or more extensive infection it decreased from 36% to 9%.[8] More recently, a study of the specific subgroup of our patients undergoing homograft aortic root replacement for aortic valve endocarditis documented a 6% risk.[20] Other groups have reported a similar experience. David et al documented a 4.8% in-hospital risk for 62 patients with active PVE and Dossche et al reported a risk of 9.4% for 32 patients undergoing allograft root replacement for PVE.[21,32]

Active infection and end-organ failure (e.g. renal failure, stroke, shock) are still factors that increase the risk of operations for PVE although their influence is not as dramatic as it has been in the past.

The long-term outcome after reoperation for PVE is not equivalent to that for patients undergoing routine valve surgery. In our own surgical series the 5-year and 10-year survival of patients surviving the operation and hospitalization was 82% and 40% respectively, and survival free from

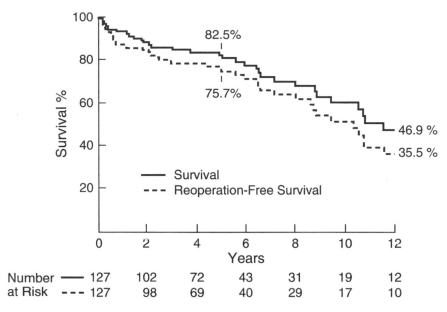

Figure 18. Late survival and reoperation-free survival for the in-hospital survivors undergoing surgery for prosthetic valve endocarditis. (From Lytle BW, Priest BP, Taylor PC, et al. Surgical treatment of prosthetic valve endocarditis. *J Thorac Cardiovasc Surg* 1996;111:198–210. Reprinted by permission.)

reoperation was 76% and 36%, respectively (Figure 18). In assessing adverse events during the follow-up of patients treated for PVE, it is important to focus on reoperation rather than reinfection. For patients who have received long-term antibiotic treatment, the recurrence of active infection is often difficult to document despite the need for reoperation, perhaps because extensive antibiotic treatment makes cultures relatively unproductive. David et al noted a 67% 5-year survival for their patients who underwent surgery for active PVE. In our series, the time (early versus late), activity and extent of the infection did not appear to influence long-term outcomes. We have interpreted this observation to mean that with aggressive surgical and antibiotic treatment, the activity and extent of the infection can be neutralized.

An interesting observation from our series is the fact that of the 127 in-hospital survivors, 19 underwent a subsequent reoperation and active infection could be documented in only 5. Furthermore, the 5-year survival of the patients who underwent a second valve re-replacement was 61%, not ideal but not futile either. In other words, an apparently successful operation for PVE does not necessarily mean that all the patient's troubles are over, but if valve insufficiency does recur it is worthwhile to operate again.

Reports by Haydock et al[33] and McGiffin et al[18] have provided substantial evidence that the use of aortic valve homografts for the treatment of aortic valve infection produces better long-term outcomes when compared to the use of standard mechanical or bioprosthetic valves (Figure 19). Joyce et al have carried this concept one step further and advocate the use of pulmonary autotransplantation (Ross operation) to treat aortic root infection.[34] While they have shown that this concept is feasible for the treatment of PVE and so far have demonstrated good short-term and long-term outcomes, it is too early to know whether pulmonary autotransplantation has incremental advantage over the use of an aortic valve homograft.

Intensive postoperative treatment with intravenous antibiotics is an important part of preventing recurrent endocarditis even when operation with homografts or autografts is possible. It is our preference to treat all patients with any evidence of active endocarditis for at least 6 weeks with intravenous antibiotics after the date of the operation. All patients receive early postoperative transesophageal echo studies and are followed care-

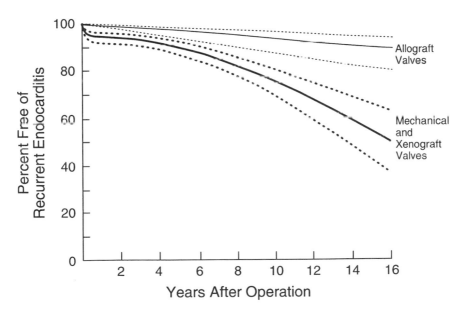

Figure 19. Parametric estimate of freedom from recurrent endocarditis for patients with mechanical and xenograft valves versus allograft aortic valves with 70% confidence limits (dotted lines). (From McGiffin DC, Galbraith AJ, McLachlan GJ, et al. Aortic valve infection: Risk factors for death and recurrent endocarditis after aortic valve replacement. *J Thorac Cardiovasc Surg* 1992;104:511–520. Reprinted by permission.)

fully during their postoperative antibiotic treatment for any evidence of anatomic change or systemic symptoms.

A special subgroup that highlights the combined medical-surgical treatment of prosthetic valve endocarditis is that of patients with fungal prosthetic valve endocarditis. Our early experience included a patient who underwent successful treatment for *Candida* endocarditis and was placed postoperatively on oral ketoconazole. After being well for approximately 2 years, the patient unilaterally discontinued her antifungal treatment and 6 months later had recurrent *Candida* endocarditis. After another replacement with a heterograft combined with perioperative treatment with amphotericin and long-term oral suppressive treatment, she has remained well.

Therefore, our approach to the treatment of fungal prosthetic valve endocarditis is valve replacement with perioperative amphotericin treatment, and lifelong oral antifungal therapy. This strategy has resulted in a survival of 8 of 12 patients for more than 48 months after treatment. Furthermore, of 8 patients treated with aortic valve homografts plus this regimen, only one recurrence has been noted and that was related to an organism that was resistant to all antifungal agents.

Indications for Surgery

Based on the considerations listed above, our current indications for surgery for PVE are as follows. Surgery clearly offers the best outcome for patients whose early PVE is marked by annular involvement, periprosthetic leak, congestive heart failure or vegetations greater than 1 cm. We prefer some intravenous antibiotic therapy prior to operation but do not expect to achieve a bacteriologic cure. It is important to perform these operations at a time of our choosing prior to hemodynamic deterioration, and we may proceed with operation after only a few days of antibiotics. Obviously, patients with shock or significant hemodynamic deterioration at the time of presentation will need to be operated on emergently. For clinically stable patients with early PVE who do not have annular involvement by echo and who have only small vegetations, decision-making is more difficult. However, the fact remains that most patients with early PVE will end up having surgery despite the disease's initially benign course. In this setting we would begin intravenous antibiotic therapy and perform frequent serial echocardiograms. If there is any evidence of anatomic progression we recommend operation even in the absence of clinical deterioration; any sign of clinical deterioration is an indication for immediate operation. It is important to remember that in some situations where echocardiac abnormalities are mild, the patient may not have PVE. If that is the case, serial echocardiography is the best way to arrive at the correct diagnosis.

In patients with late PVE, we persist with medical treatment for those who show no echocardiographic evidence of annular involvement and who are clinically well. Again, once there is clear evidence of annular involvement, surgery is likely to be necessary, and we usually proceed with operation at a time of our choosing once severe deterioration has occurred. Patients with infections that involve only the leaflets of bio-prostheses who exhibit rapid clinical improvement once antibiotic therapy has been started may be treatable with antibiotics alone, at least over the short term.

Despite new generations of antibiotics, treatment with intravenous antibiotics alone for prosthetic valve endocarditis has plateaued in terms of achieving favorable outcomes. The concepts of surgical treatment and means of support to achieve complicated operations have improved greatly and are still improving. Further improvement in the treatment of PVE is likely to be achieved through the combined medical-surgical approach.

References

1. Agnihotri AK, McGiffin DC, Galbraith AJ, et al. The prevalence of infective endocarditis after aortic valve replacement. *J Thorac Cardiovasc Surg* 1995;110: 1708–1724.
2. Blackstone EH, Kirklin JW. Death and other time-related events after valve replacement. *Circulation* 1985;72:753–767.
3. Calderwood SB, Swinski LA, Waternaux CM, et al. Risk factors for the development of prosthetic valve endocarditis. *Circulation* 1985;72:31–37.
4. Grover FL, Cohen DJ, Oprian C, et al. Determinants of the occurrence of and survival from prosthetic valve endocarditis: Experience of the Veterans Affairs Cooperative Study on valvular heart disease. *J Thorac Cardiovasc Surg* 1994; 108:207–214.
5. Gordon S, Serkey J, Longworth D, et al. Early-onset prosthetic valve endocarditis (EO-PVE) at The Cleveland Clinic Foundation, 1992–1997. Abstracts of the IDSA 36th Annual Meeting. Nov. 12–15, 1998.
6. Keys TF. Early onset prosthetic valve endocarditis. *Cleve Clin J Med* 1993;60: 455–459.
7. Fang G, Keys TF, Gentry LO, et al. Prosthetic valve endocarditis resulting from nosocomial bacteremia: A prospective, multicenter study. *Ann Int Med* 1993;119:560–567.
8. Lytle BW, Priest, BP, Taylor PC, et al. Surgical treatment of prosthetic valve endocarditis. *J Thorac Cardiovasc Surg* 1996;111:198–210.
9. Horstkotte D, Piper C, Niehues R, et al. Late prosthetic valve endocarditis. *Eur Heart J* 1995;16 (Supp B):39–47.
10. Hammermeister KE, Sethi GK, Henderson WG, et al. A comparison of out-

comes in men 11 years after heart-valve replacement with a mechanical valve or bioprosthesis. *N Engl J Med* 1993;328:1289–1296.

11. Lytle BW, Cosgrove DM, Taylor PC, et al. Primary isolated aortic valve replacement: Early and late results. *J Thorac Cardiovasc Surg* 1989;97:675–694.

12. von Reyn CF, Levy BS, Arbeit RD, et al. Infective endocarditis: An analysis based on strict case definitions. *Ann Intern Med* 1981;94:505–518.

13. Durack DT, Lukes AS, Bright DK. New criteria for diagnosis of infective endocarditis: Utilization of specific echocardiographic findings. *Am J Med* 1994;96: 200–209.

14. Stewart WJ, Shan K. The diagnosis of prosthetic valve endocarditis by echocardiography. *Semin Thorac Cardiovasc Surg* 1995;7:7–12.

15. Daniel WG, Mügge A, Grote J, et al. Comparison of transthoracic and transesophageal echocardiography for detection of abnormalities of prosthetic and bioprosthetic valves in the mitral and aortic positions. *Am J Cardiol* 1993;71: 210–215.

16. Davenport J, Hart RG. Prosthetic valve endocarditis 1976–1987: Antibiotics, anticoagulopathy and stroke. *Stroke* 1990,21:993–999.

17. Buckberg GD. Studies of controlled reperfusion after ischemia: A series of experimental and clinical observations from the Division of Thoracic and Cardiovascular Surgery, UCLA School of Medicine. *J Thorac Cardiovasc Surg* 1986; 92:483.

18. McGiffin DC, Galbraith AJ, McLachlan GJ, et al. Aortic valve infection: Risk factors for death and recurrent endocarditis after aortic valve replacement. *J Thorac Cardiovasc Surg* 1992;104:511–520.

19. McGiffin DC, Kirklin JK. The impact of aortic valve homografts on the treatment of aortic prosthetic valve endocarditis. *Semin Thorac Cardiovasc Surg* 1995; 7:25–31.

20. Camacho MT, Cosgrove DM. Homografts in the treatment of prosthetic valve endocarditis. *Semin Thorac Cardiovasc Surg* 1995;7:32–37.

21. David TE, Bos J, Christakis GT, et al. Heart valve operations in patients with active infective endocarditis. *Ann Thorac Surg* 1990;49:701–705.

22. Lytle BW. Surgical treatment of prosthetic valve endocarditis. *Semin Thorac Cardiovasc Surg* 1995;7:13–19.

23. Ergin MA. Surgical techniques in prosthetic valve endocarditis. *Semin Thorac Cardiovasc Surg* 1995;7:54–60.

24. Ergin MA, Raissi S, Follis F, et al. Annular destruction in acute bacterial endocarditis: Surgical techniques to meet the challenge. *J Thorac Cardiovasc Surg* 1989;97:755–763.

25. Ivert TS, Dismukes WE, Cobbs CG, Blackstone EH, et al. Prosthetic valve endocarditis. *Circulation* 1984;69:223–232.

26. Calderwood SB, Swinski LA, Karchmer AW, et al. Prosthetic valve endocarditis: Analysis of factors affecting outcome of therapy. *J Thorac Cardiovasc Surg* 1986;92:776–783.

27. Yu VL, Fang GD, Keys TF, et al. Prosthetic valve endocarditis: Superiority of surgical valve replacement versus medical therapy only. *Ann Thorac Surg* 1994; 58:1073–1077.

28. John MD, Hibberd PL, Karchmer AW, et al. *Staphylococcus aureus* prosthetic valve endocarditis: Optimal management and risk factors for death. *Clin Infect Dis* 1998;26:1302–1309.

29. Kanawaty DS, Stalker MJ, Munt PW. Nonsurgical treatment of Histoplasma endocarditis involving a bioprosthetic valve. *Chest* 1991;99:253–256.

30. Tucker KJ, Johnson JA, Ong T, et al. Medical management of prosthetic aortic valve endocarditis and aortic root abscess. *Am Heart J* 1993;125:1195–1197.

31. Baumgartner WA, Miller DC, Reitz BA, et al. Surgical treatment of prosthetic valve endocarditis. *Ann Thorac Surg* 1983;35:87–104.

32. Dossche KM, DeFauw JJ, Ernst SM, et al. Allograft aortic root replacement in prosthetic aortic valve endocarditis: A review of 32 patients. *Ann Thorac Surg* 1997;63:1644–1649.

33. Haydock D, Barratt-Boyes B, Macedo T, et al. Aortic valve replacement for active infectious endocarditis in 108 patients: A comparison of freehand allograft valves with mechanical prostheses and bioprostheses. *J Thorac Cardiovasc Surg* 1992;103:130–139.

34. Joyce F, Tingleff J, Pettersson G. The Ross operation in the treatment of prosthetic aortic valve endocarditis. *Semin Thorac Cardiovasc Surg* 1995;7:38–46.

Chapter 15
Fungal Endocarditis

John Blizzard, M.D.

God grant me the serenity
To accept the things I cannot change,
The courage to change the things I can,
And the wisdom to know the difference.
The Serenity Prayer

Introduction

Treatment of fungal endocarditis requires expert management with meticulous attention to detail. Timely diagnosis and intervention are paramount to an optimal outcome. The overall care of the patient involves the primary physician, the cardiologist, the infectious disease specialist, the cardiac surgeon and the nursing staff as well as the patient and family. Despite the best of management, the outcome may still be dismal due to the severity of this disease process and the usual host in which it becomes manifest.

History

The yeast *Candida albicans* was first described in 1841 by Bergin.[1] The first description of fungal endocarditis followed nearly 100 years later.[2] Through 1998, more than 1000 cases have been cited in the literature. Undoubtedly, many more cases have gone unreported and undetected.

From: Vlessis AA, Bolling S (eds): *Endocarditis: A Multidisciplinary Approach to Modern Treatment.* © Futura Publishing Co., Armonk, NY, 1999.

Pathogens

Candida

C. albicans is by far the most prevalent causative organism in both native and prosthetic valve fungal endocarditis. This yeast usually exists in symbiosis with humans, becoming invasive only when host defense mechanisms have been lowered. Microscopically, *C. albicans* appears as a thin-walled, oval, budding yeast with or without brachial elements (Figure 1). *C. albicans* is easily cultured on blood agar or Sabouraud dextrose agar in 24 to 48 hours. Positive germ tube test can yield a presumptive diagnosis in 2 to 3 hours. Definite species identification, by visual identification, requires an additional 2 to 10 days. Antibody detection techniques are not recommended due to the high rate of false positive results.[3]

  C. tropicalis, a less commonly identified pathogen, is the most virulent of the candidal species.[4,5] Neutropenic patients are predisposed to this yeast. Diagnosis relies on positive cultures, and definitive identification is made via rapid yeast identification panel or grown cultures examined histologically.

  C. krusei, C. parapsilosis,[6–22] *C. lusitaniae*,[23] *C. stellatoidea*,[24] *C. zeylanoides*,[25] and *Torulopsis (Candida) glabrata*[26–30] are all reported pathogens

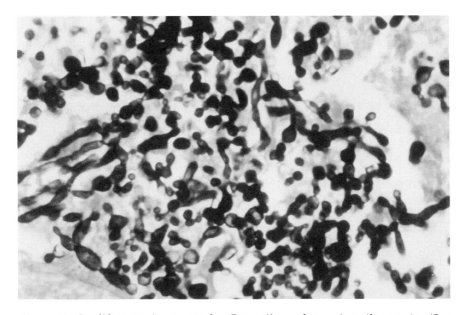

Figure 1. *Candida* organisms seen by Gomori's methenamine silver stain. (See color appendix.)

of native and prosthetic valve fungal endocarditis. Typical histological appearance and cultures are used to differentiate species.

Aspergillus

Aspergillus species are the next most common organisms after *Candida* species that cause native or prosthetic valve fungal endocarditis. They represent approximately one sixth of the reported cases. Although there are over 200 reported species of this saprophytic mold, the most common are *A. fumigatus* and *A. flavus*.[31–71] Other less commonly reported pathogens of this genus are *A. clavatus*,[72] *A. niger*,[73,74] *A. terreus*,[75,76] and *A. ustus*.[77] These ubiquitous molds are easily aerosolized, and airborne transmission is the presumed mode in cases after open heart surgery. Microscopically, *Aspergillus* shows coarse filamented, branching septate hyphae in clusters (Figure 2). Evidence of clinical and pathological invasiveness is necessary to rule out specimen contamination. Blood cultures are rarely positive (less than 10%).

Blastomyces dermatitidis

Another dimorphous fungus, *Blastomyces dermatitidis*, has been reported predominantly in severely immunocompromised hosts, most commonly

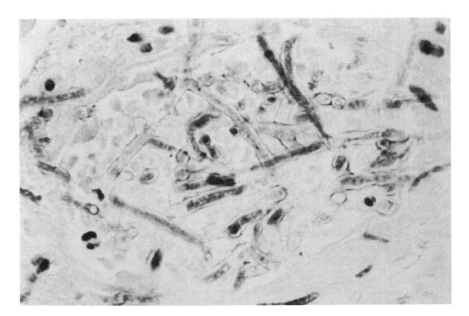

Figure 2. *Aspergillus* organisms seen by hematoxylin and eosin stain. (See color appendix.)

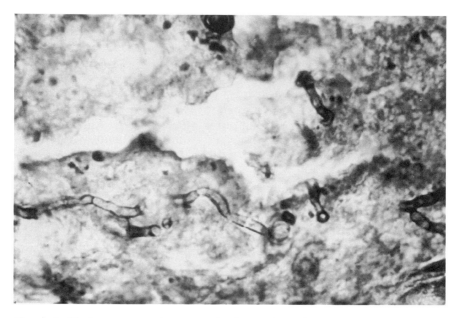

Figure 3. *Blastomyces* organisms seen by Gomori's methenamine silver stain. (See color appendix.)

those with autoimmune deficiency syndrome.[78] Microscopically they have a refractive, thick cell wall with multiple nuclei and reproduce via a broad-based bud. (Figure 3). Identification is by typical histologic appearance or DNA probe directed to *Blastomyces dermatitidis*.

Histoplasma capsulatum

Histoplasma capsulatum is the causative organism in the most common systemic fungal infection in the United States. It rarely produces endocarditis, representing only 5% to 7% of reported cases of fungal endocarditis.[78–102] When identified as the etiologic agent in endocarditis, it is usually in immune compromised patients. *H. capsulatum* is also dimorphous and, as with other infectious yeasts, biopsied tissues should be both cultured and stained. Intracellular organisms are identified with periodic acid-Schiff or Gomori's methenamine silver. A commercially marketed DNA probe is currently the diagnostic tool of choice. A urine screen is also available.

Cryptococcus

Cryptococcus neoformans more commonly produces meningitis and encephalitis in the immunocompromised host. There are reported cases of cryptococcal native and prosthetic valve endocarditis.[103] Diagnosis of the encapsulated yeast is by direct identification after staining with India ink or Wright's stain.

Coccidioides immitis

Coccidioides immitis, the causative agent of San Joaquin fever, has also been reported as a cause of endocarditis.[104–106] This is exceedingly rare and usually confined to the immunocompromised host or to patients with disseminated malignancies. Detection is by either complement fixation or culture of the organism. Additional confirmation is now available with a DNA probe.

Sporothrix

Sporothrix schenckii was first described by Link in 1809. Cutaneous pathogenicity was discovered in 1898 by Schenck. It has rarely been reported as a causative agent in endocarditis. Histopathological identification of the cigar-shaped organisms is unusual. Cultures are very difficult to grow and blood cultures are frequently negative. A definitive diagnosis is very difficult to obtain.

Miscellaneous Fungi

Over the last 30 years, 26 other fungi have been reported in the world literature as causative agents of endocarditis. These include *Acremonium kiliense*,[107,108] *Arnium leporinum*,[109] *Blastoschizomyces capitatus*,[110] *Conidiobolus coronatus*,[111] *Curvularia lunata*,[112,113] *Drechslera longirostrata*[114] and *D. specifera*,[115] *Exophiala dermatitidis*[116,117] and *E. jeanselmei*,[118] *Fusarium solani*,[119] *Paecilomyces javanicus*[120,121] and *P. varioti*,[122,123] *Penicilliosis marneffei*,[124] *Phacoacremonium parasiticum*,[125] *Phialophora dermatitidis*[126] and *P. richardsiae*,[127] *Pseudallescheria boydii*,[128–131] *Pseudoonas*,[132] *Rhodotorula pilimanae*,[133,134] *Saccharomyces* species,[135] *Scedosporium*[136,137] *apiospermum*[64,65] and *S. inflatum*,[138] *Scopulariopsis brevicaulis*,[139,140] *Thermomyces lanuginosus*,[141] *Trichosporon beigelii*[142–147] and *T. cutanean*,[148] and *Wangiella dermatitidis*.[149]

Epidemiology

Fungal endocarditis generally manifests as a native valve or a prosthetic valve infection. However, numerous cases of fungal endocarditis have been reported from permanent pacemaker wires or automatic implantable cardiac defibrillator leads.[107,131,150,151] Fungal endocarditis has also been reported after placement of peritoneal-venous shunt for intractable ascites,[152] and after percutaneous transluminal coronary angioplasty.[153]

Risk factors for developing fungal and fungal prosthetic valve endocarditis include autoimmune deficiency syndrome,[154] solid organ transplantation, bone marrow transplantation, indwelling catheters, intravenous drug use, heart valve prostheses, and severe burns.

The incidence of developing fungal endocarditis after prosthetic valve implantation is small, less than 0.1% per year;[155] however, with over 100,000 valve replacements per year in the United States alone, fungal endocarditis is a serious clinical reality that cannot be overlooked. Fungal infections represent approximately 5% of cases of prosthetic valve infection.[156,157]

Fungemia in the presence of a prosthetic valve carries a significant (10%) risk of subsequent valve infection. Of patients who present with fungemia, 10% to 15% actually have endocarditis at the time of positive blood cultures. Therefore, fungemia is associated with a 20% to 25% early and late risk of fungal prosthetic valve infection.[158–160]

Clinical Signs and Symptoms

Most patients with fungal endocarditis, like their counterparts with bacterial endocarditis, will present with fever, chills, night sweats, anorexia, weight loss, fatigue and dyspnea.[161,162] Clinical signs point to one of 3 underlying causes. First, the local destruction of valvular tissue can cause signs and symptoms of left and/or right-sided heart failure accompanied by a murmur of valvular insufficiency. Second, vegetations, often quite large, may lead to acute valvular obstruction or massive embolization of systemic organs with stroke or organ failure. Lastly, signs of microembolization, such as Roth's spots (retinal embolism), petechiae (usually with pale center), splinter hemorrhages (linear emboli of the nail beds), Osler's nodes (hemorrhagic emboli to the pulp of the fingers), and Janeway's lesions (painful, irregular, bordered, blanching lesions of the palms and soles) may be evident on physical examination.

Diagnosis

The diagnosis of fungal endocarditis is aided by the work of Fang et al[162] and the classification systems of von Reyn[161] and Durack.[163] (See preceding chapters for a detailed discussion of their clinical utility.)

The clinical history should elucidate immunosuppressive states and other risk factors for endocarditis. The physical exam looks for the clinical signs and symptoms described above. Necessary tests include an electrocardiogram, blood cultures, complete blood count with differential, C-reactive protein and a chest roentgenogram. Cardiac catheterization may be necessary to determine if there is concomitant coronary disease. Echocardiography assesses valvular function and the paravalvular tissues. Right heart catheterization may be of use in selected cases, especially with tricuspid involvement associated with multiple pulmonary emboli. Newer modalities such as helical computed tomography and magnetic resonance imaging are of little value at this time.

Chemotherapy

The choice of antifungal chemotherapeutic agents is not a simple matter. Organism susceptability and drug side effects must be weighed into the drug choice.[164]

Amphotericin B

The mainstay of therapy remains amphotericin B. Amphotericin B was first isolated in 1956 by Vandeputte from *Streptomyces nodosus*.[165] The mechanism of action depends on the ability to bind primarily to ergosterol to form pores in the fungal cell wall. These pores allow egress of fluids, solutes and small molecules from the fungi, thus facilitating their demise. Synergism of amphotericin B with flucytosine,[166] rifampin and minocycline[167] has been documented. Antagonism with ketoconazole has also reported.[168] Adverse side effects include fever, chills, nausea, vomiting, nephrotoxicity, thrombophlebitis, anemia and electrolyte imbalance.

Abelcet is a formulation of amphotericin B with dimyristoyl phosphatidylcholine and dimyristoyl phosphatidylglycerol. This combination alters the pharmacokinetics by increasing the volume of distribution, lengthening the half-life and lowering the blood levels. This lowers the side effect profile and allows once-a-day dosing.

Flucytosine

Flucytosine (Ancobon, Roche Laboratories, Nutley, NJ), a fluorinated pyrimidine, is converted to 5-fluorouracil in fungal cells.[169] The fluorinated pyrimidine becomes incorporated into DNA and RNA in place of thymidine, thereby blocking cellular replication and synthetic processes. It is administered orally and is most effective in treating cryptococcus and candidal infection. Adverse side effects include bone marrow suppression, nausea, vomiting, rise in serum hepatic enzymes, diarrhea and rash.

Ketoconazole

Ketoconazole (Nizoral, Janssen Pharmaceutica, Titusville, NJ) blocks the synthesis of ergosterol, the primary sterol of susceptible fungi. The mechanism is via inhibition of lanosterol demethylase, the last enzyme in the production of ergosterol. Lack of ergosterol alters fungal membrane permeability and slows fungal growth. The effect is fungistatic, not fungicidal. Synergism is noted with flucytosine and antagonism with amphotericin B.[167] After oral administration, an acidic gastric environment is necessary for absorption. It is highly protein- bound and therefore numerous drug-drug interactions exist. Metabolism is hepatic with inactive metabolites excreted via the urine. Adverse side effects include dysmenorrhea, impotence and decreased libido, alopecia, gastrointestinal upset, rash, pruritus and hepatotoxicity.

Fluconazole

Fluconazole (Diflucan, Pfizer Inc., New York, NY) was released in 1990 and, like ketoconazole, is fungistatic by virtue of its ability to inhibit ergosterol synthesis. Intravenous and oral forms are available, with oral bioavailability exceeding 90%. Dosing must be modified in patients with hepatic or renal insufficiency. Adverse side effects include gastrointestinal upset, rash, headache and transient elevation of serum hepatic enzymes.

Itraconazole

Itraconazole (Sporanox, Janssen Pharmaceutica, Titusville, NJ) is an oral agent with a 64- hour half-life. It was released in 1992 for treatment of histoplasmosis and blastomycosis, but has a broad spectrum of activity and is now approved for use with infections due to *Aspergillus, Candida, Cryptococcus* and *Sporothrix*. The fungistatic properties are related to similar mechanisms seen with ketoconazole and fluconazole, ergosterol synthesis inhibition. Absorption is greatly enhanced by administration with food. Itraconazole has a better side effect profile than ketoconazole and is similar to fluconazole. No dosage adjustments are necessary in patients with renal insufficiency, but drug monitoring is recommended in patients with hepatic insufficiency or failure.

Surgical Treatment

Although there are numerous case reports of medical therapy alone in the treatment of fungal endocarditis, a combination of chemotherapy and surgical intervention is associated with the best outcomes in suitable patients. Isolated medical therapy is usually reserved only for patients whose circumstances preclude major surgery. Although details of exact surgical procedures appear elsewhere in this book, the goal of surgical treatment can be summarized as the removal of all affected tissues and functional reconstruction of the heart and valvular structures. This usually requires thorough debridement and complex reconstruction. Homografts have demonstrated tremendous utility when reconstructing the right and left ventricular outflow tracts. Elsewhere, others have used the Ross procedure successfully.[170] In prosthetic valve fungal endocarditis, there are only 10 case reports of successful outcomes without surgical intervention.[8,9,11,27,102,112,171–174]

Indications for surgical treatment must be tailored to the individual patient.[175] In the patient with fungal endocarditis, surgery is almost always indicated unless other medical circumstances preclude it, profound neurological devastation being the usual reason for delaying or not proceeding with surgery. Indications for surgical treatment include congestive heart failure, major embolic or continued microembolic events, persistent infection on medical treatment and evidence of extension of infection beyond the valve.

Right heart fungal endocarditis seems to be better tolerated than left heart fungal endocarditis, and the timing of surgery becomes more liberal, because the embolic and valvular disruption consequences are less profound. The main indications for surgical treatment include complications of right-sided heart failure, extra-valvular extension of disease, presence of right to left heart defects and failure of infection to respond to medical therapy alone.

Results of Treatment

In the past, outcomes of fungal endocarditis have been abysmal. Until 1969, no one survived prosthetic fungal endocarditis. Today, species of fungi remain that have not yet been successfully treated. For candidal prosthetic infections, a recent report has yielded a 67% survival with a 52- month follow-up in a small number of patients.[175] A large portion of the problem is obtaining a timely and accurate diagnosis. Fortunately, newer techniques of molecular typing have improved both speed and accuracy in identifying fungal species.[176]

Conclusions

Native or prosthetic fungal endocarditis is a challenging therapeutic problem. Due to the increased prevalence of immunosuppressive states and a resurgence in intravenous drug use, the incidence of fungal endocarditis is increasing. A combined multidisciplinary approach is necessary for timely diagnosis and treatment and, ultimately, for optimal patient outcome. Surgery remains the mainstay of treatment. The successful management of this serious condition falls to the experience and interest of the treating physicians coupled with patient compliance and family devotion.

References

1. Baue AE. *Glenn's Thoracic and Cardiovascular Surgery*, 6th ed. Stamford, CT. Appleton & Lange, 1996. p 315.
2. Joachin H, Polayes SH. Subacute endocarditis and systemic mycosis. *JAMA* 1940;115:205–208.
3. Hallum JL, Williams TW. Candida endocarditis. In Body GP (ed.) *Candidiasis Pathogenesis: Diagnosis and Treatment*. New York, NY. Raven Press, 1993. pp 357–369.
4. Mansur AJ, Safi J Jr, Markus MR et al. Late failure of surgical treatment for prosthetic valve endocarditis due to *Candida tropicalis*. *Clin Infect Dis* 1996; 22(2):380–381.
5. Malouf J, Nasrallah A, Daghir I, et al. *Candida tropicalis* endocarditis in idiopathic hypertrophic subaortic stenosis [letter]. *Chest* 1984;86(3):508.
6. Inoue Y, Yozu R, Ueda T, et al. Case report of *Candida parapsilosis* endocarditis. *J Heart Valve Dis* 1998;7(2):240–242.
7. Diekema DJ, Messer SA, Hollis RJ, et al. An outbreak of *Candida parapsilosis* prosthetic valve endocarditis. *Diagn Microbiol Infect Dis* 1997;29(3):147–153.
8. Lejko-Zupanc T, Kozelj M. A case of recurrent *Candida parapsilosis* prosthetic valve endocarditis: Cure by medical treatment alone. *J Infect* 1997;35(1):81–82.
9. Baddour LM. Long-term suppressive therapy for *Candida parapsilosis*-induced prosthetic valve endocarditis. *Mayo Clin Proc* 1995;70(8):773–775.
10. Cancelas JA, Lopez J, Cabezudo E, et al. Native valve endocarditis due to *Candida parapsilosis*: A late complication after bone marrow transplantation-related fungemia. *Bone Marrow Transplant* 1994;13(3):333–334.
11. Zahid MA, Klotz SA, Hinthorn DR, et al. Medical treatment of recurrent candidemia in a patient with *Candida parapsilosis* prosthetic valve endocarditis. *Chest* 1994;105(5):1597–1598.
12. Weems JJ Jr. *Candida parapsilosis*: Epidemiology, pathogenicity, clinical manifestations and antimicrobial susceptibility. *Clin Infect Dis* 1992;14(3):756–766.
13. Blinkhorn RJ Jr, Eckhauser ML, Snow N, et al. Saddle embolism complicating *Candida parapsilosis* aortic valve endocarditis. *J Vasc Surg* 1992;16(1):128–129.
14. Faix RG, Feick HJ, Frommelt P, et al. Successful medical treatment of *Candida parapsilosis* endocarditis in a premature infant. *Am J Perinat* 1990;7(3):272–275.
15. Severo LC, Alves AM, Bassanesi MC, et al. Endocarditis in biological prosthesis by *Candida parapsilosis*. *Rev Inst Med Trop Sao Paulo* 1987;29(1):43–46.

16. Romero Vivas J, Sanchez Sousa A, Rodriguez Creixems M, et al. *Candida parapsilosis* endocarditis. *Med Clin (Barc)*1985;84(15):618–619.

17. Marrie TJ, Cooper JH, Costerton JW, et al. Ultrastructure of *Candida parapsilosis* endocarditis. *Infect Immun* 1984;45(2):390–398.

18. Herling IM, Kotler MN, Segal BL, et al. *Candida parapsilosis* endocarditis without predisposing cause. *Int J Cardiol* 1984;5(6):753–756.

19. Auger PR, Pelletier LC, Dyrda I, et al. Endocarditis caused by *Candida parapsilosis*. *Arch Mal Coeur Vaiss* 1983;76(10):1231–1234.

20. Samelson LE, Lerner SA, Resnekov L, et al. Relapse of *Candida parapsilosis* endocarditis after long-term suppression with flucytosine. *Ann Intern Med* 1980;93(6):838–839.

21. Mayrer AR, Brown A, Weintraub RA, et al. Successful medical therapy for endocarditis due to *Candida parapsilosis*. *Chest* 1978;73(4):546–549.

22. Chevy S, Yu L. *Candida parapsilosis* endocarditis following heart surgery: Case report. *Hawaii Med J* 1970;29(8):637–640.

23. Wendt B, Haglund L, Razavi A, et al. *Candida lusitaniae:* An uncommon cause of prosthetic valve endocarditis. *Clin Infect Dis* 1998;26(3):769–770.

24. Marsten JH, Greenberg JJ, Piccini JC, et al. Aortitis due to *Candida stellatoidea* developing in a supravalvular suture line. *Ann Thorac Surg* 1969;7(2):134–138.

25. Whitby S, Madu EC, Bronze MS, et al. Case report: *Candida zeylanoides* infective endocarditis complicating infection with the human immunodeficiency virus. *Am J Med Sci* 1986;312(3):138–139.

26. Rubinstein E, Lang R. Fungal endocarditis. *Eur Heart J* 1995;16 (Suppl B): 84–89.

27. Nishida T, Mayumi H, Kawachi Y, et al. The efficacy of fluconazole in treating prosthetic valve endocarditis caused by *Candida glabrata*: Report of a case. *Surg Today* 1994;24(7):651–654.

28. Alaya M, Ouerghemmi D, Blin D, et al. *Torulopsis glabrata* endocarditis after cardiac surgery for heart valve replacement. *Presse Med* 1988;17(19):962–963.

29. Heffner DR, Franklin WA. Endocarditis caused by *Torulopsis glabrata*. *Am J Clin Path* 1978;70(3):420–423.

30. Sharp DN. *Torulopsis glabrata* endocarditis complicating aortic homograft valve treated with 5-fluorocytosine. *N Z Med J* 1975;81(536):294–298.

31. Ellis M. Fungal endocarditis. *J Infect* 1997;35(2):99–103.

32. Sergi C, Weitz, J, Hofmann WJ, et al. Aspergillus endocarditis, myocarditis and pericarditis complicating necrotizing fasciitis: Case report and subject review. *Virchows Archiv* 1996;429(2–3):177–180.

33. Casson DH, Riordan FA, Ladusens EJ. Aspergillus endocarditis in chronic granulomatous disease. *Acta Paediatr* 1996;85(6):758–759.

34. Keating MR, Guerrero MA, Daly RC, et al. Transmission of invasive aspergillosis from a subclinically infected donor to three different organ transplant recipients. *Chest* 1996;109(4):1119–1124.

35. Hosking MC, MacDonald NE, Cornel G. Liposomal amphotericin B for postoperative *Aspergillus fumigatus* endocarditis. *Ann Thorac Surg* 1995;59(4): 1015–1017.

36. Stavridis GT, Shabbo FP. Aspergillus prosthetic valve endocarditis. *Eur J Cardiothorac Surg* 1993;7(1):50–51.

37. Roux JP, Koussa A, Cajot MA, et al. Primary Aspergillus endocarditis: Apropos of a case and review of the international literature. *Ann Chir* 1992;46(2): 110–115.

38. Kuijer PM, Kuijper EJ, van den Tweel JG, et al. *Aspergillus fumigatus*, a rare cause of fatal coronary artery occlusion. *Infection* 1992;20(1):45–47.

39. Light JT Jr, Hendrickson M, Sholes WM, et al. Acute aortic occlusion secondary to Aspergillus endocarditis in an intravenous drug abuser. *Ann Vasc Surg* 1991;5(3):271–275.

40. Rahman M, Rahman M, Kundi A, et al. *Aspergillus fumigatus* endocarditis. *JPMA* 1990;40(4):95–96.

41. Bogner JR, Lufti S, Middeke M, et al. Successful drug therapy in Aspergillus endocarditis. *Dtsch Med Wochenschr* 1990;115(48):1833–1837.

42. Corrigan C, Horner SM. Aspergillus endocarditis in association with a false aortic aneurysm. *Clin Card* 1988;11(6):430–432.

43. Galed I, Alvarez A, Garcia J, et al. Endocarditis caused by *Aspergillus fumigatus*. *Med Clin* 1987;89(7):305.

44. Wagner DK, Werner PH, Bonchek LI, et al. Successful treatment of postmitral valve annuloplasty *Aspergillus flavus* endocarditis. *Am J Med* 1985;79(6): 777–780.

45. McFadden PM, Gonzalez-Lavin L, Remington JS. Limited reliability of the "negative" two- dimensional echocardiogram in the evaluation of infectious vegetative endocarditis: Diagnostic and surgical implications. *J Card Surg* 1985;26(1):59–63.

46. Rinaldi MG. Invasive aspergillosis. *Rev Infect Dis* 1983;5(6):1061–1077.

47. Vishniavsky N, Sagar KB, Markowitz SM. *Aspergillus fumigatus* endocarditis on a normal heart valve. *South Med J* 1983;76(4):605–608.

48. Vo NM, Russell JC, Becker DR. Mycotic emboli of the peripheral vessels: Analysis of forty- four cases. *Surgery* 1981;90(3):541–545.

49. Garcia Gomez R, Valdespino Estrada A, Lopez Ortiz R. Aspergillus endocarditis: Report of a case treated surgically with success. *Arch Inst Cardiol Mex* 1981;51(6):549–553.

50. Barst RJ, Prince AS, Neu HC. Aspergillus endocarditis in children: Case report and review of the literature. *Pediatrics* 1981;68(1):73–78.

51. Wilson WR, Nichols DR, Thompson RL, et al. Infective endocarditis: Therapeutic considerations. *Am Heart J* 1980;100(5):689–704.

52. Walsh TJ, Hutchins GM, Bulkley BH, et al. Fungal infections of the heart: Analysis of 51 autopsy cases. *Am J Card* 1980;45(2):357–366.

53. Stinson EB. Surgical treatment of infective endocarditis. *Prog Cardiovasc Dis* 1979;22(3):145–168.

54. Otto T, Halweg H, Pietraszek A, et al. Aspergillus endocarditis following aortic valve replacement. *Kardiologia Polska* 1979;22(2):221–226.

55. Puig LB, Verginelli G, Kawabe L, et al. Four years' experience with dura mater cardiac valves. *J Card Surg* 1977;18(3):247–255.

56. Brandt G, Tulusan AH. Scanning electron microscope observations of tissue invasion by opportunistic mycoses. *Mykoses* 1976;19(9):337–343.

57. Petheram IS, Seal RM. Aspergillus prosthetic valve endocarditis. *Thorax* 1976; 31(4):380–390.

58. Case records of the Massachusetts General Hospital. Weekly clinicopathological exercises. Case 39-1976. *N Engl J Med* 1976;295(13):718–724.

59. Kammer RB, Utz JP. Aspergillus species endocarditis: The new face of a not so rare disease. *Am J Med* 1974;56(4):506–521.

60. Tuazon CU, Hill R, Sheagren JN. Microbiologic study of street heroin and injection paraphernalia. *J Infect Dis* 1974;129(3):327–329.

61. Lerner PI. Infective endocarditis: A review of selected topics. *Med Clin North Am* 1974;58(3):605–622.
62. Harford CG. Postoperative fungal endocarditis: Fungemia, embolism and therapy. *Arch Intern Med* 1974;134(91):116–120.
63. Friedman AH, Chishti MI, Henkind P. Endogenous ocular aspergillosis. *Ophthalmologica* 1974;168(3):197–205.
64. Meyer RD, Fox ML. Aspergillus endocarditis: Therapeutic failure of amphotericin B. *Arch Intern Med* 1973;132(1):102–106.
65. Case records of the Massachusetts General Hospital. Weekly clinicopathological exercises. Case 24-1973. *N Engl J Med* 1973;288(24):1290–1296.
66. Lonyai T, Feher C, Timar K. Aspergillus endocarditis following aortic valve replacement. *Acta Chir Hung* 1973;14(1):43–51.
67. Roberts WC, Buchbinder NA. Right-sided valvular infective endocarditis: A clinicopathologic study of twelve necropsy patients. *Am J Med* 1972;53(1):7–19.
68. Grabowski H, Holak L, Musiatowicz B. Case of Aspergillus endocarditis in a patient following surgery for Fallot's tetralogy. *Pol Tygodnik Lek* 1971;26(14):520–521.
69. Cohen DM, Goggans EA. Sclerosing mediastinitis and terminal valvular endocarditis caused by fungus suggestive of Aspergillus species. *Am J Clin Pathol* 1971;56(1):91–96.
70. Hairston P, Lee WH Jr. Mycotic (fungal) endocarditis after cardiovascular surgery. *Am Surg* 1969;35(2):135–143.
71. Doughten RM, Pearson HA. Disseminated intravascular coagulation associated with Aspergillus endocarditis: Fatal outcome following heparin therapy. *J Pediatr* 1968;73(4):576–582.
72. Opul SM, Reller LB, Harrington G, et al. *Aspergillus clavatus* endocarditis involving a normal aortic valve following coronary artery surgery. *Rev Infect Dis* 1986;8(5):781–785.
73. Moore RS, Hasleton PS, Lawson RA, et al. *Aspergillus niger* endocarditis complicating aortic tissue valve replacement. *Thorax* 1984;39(1):76–77.
74. Malivi TA, Webb HM, Dixon CD, et al. Systemic aspergillosis caused by *Aspergillus niger* after open-heart surgery. *JAMA* 1968;203(7):520–522.
75. Laham MN, Carpenter JL. *Aspergillus terreus*, a pathogen capable of causing infective endocarditis. *Am Rev Resp Dis* 1982;125(6):769–772.
76. Drexler L, Rytel M, Keelan M, et al. *Aspergillus terreus* infective endocarditis on a porcine heterograft valve. *J Thorac Cardiovasc Surg* 1980;79(2):269–274.
77. Carrizosa J, Levison ME, Lawrence T, et al. Cure of *Aspergillus ustus* endocarditis on a prosthetic valve. *Arch Intern Med* 1974;133(3):486–490.
78. Stiver HG, Telford GO, Mossey JM, et al. Intravenous antibiotic therapy at home. *Ann Intern Med* 1978;89 (5 Part 1):690–693.
79. Case records of the Massachusetts General Hospital. Weekly clinicopathological exercises. *N Engl J Med* 1975;293(5):247–253.
80. Smith JW, Utz JP. Progressive disseminated histoplasmosis: A prospective study of 26 patients. *Ann Intern Med* 1972;76(4):557–565.
81. Reimann HA. Infectious diseases: Annual review of significant publications. *Postgrad Med J* 1971;47(548):332–353.
82. Stefani DV. Human immunoglobulins and their role in infectious pathology. *Zhurnam Mikrobiologii, Epidemiologii I Immunobiologii* 1971;48(6):126–131.

83. Cherry JD, Lloyd CA, Quilty JF, et al. Amphotericin B therapy in children: A review of the literature and a case report. *J Pediatr* 1969;75(6):1063–1069.
84. Segal C, Wheeler CG, Tompsett R. Histoplasma endocarditis cured with amphotericin. *N Engl J Med* 1969;280(4):206–207.
85. Weaver DK, Batsakis JG, Nishiyama RH. Histoplasma endocarditis. *Arch Surg* 1968;96(1):158–162.
86. Hartley RA, Remsberg JR, Sinaly NP. Histoplasma endocarditis: Case report and review of the literature. *Arch Intern Med* 1967;119(5):527–531.
87. Gerber HJ, Schoonmaker FW, Vazquez MD. Chronic meningitis associated with Histoplasma endocarditis. *N Engl J Med* 1966;275(2):74–76.
88. Korns ME. Coincidence of mycotic (*Histoplasma capsulatum*) vegetative endocarditis of the mitral valve and the Lutembacher syndrome: Report of a case. *Circulation* 1965;32(4):589–592.
89. Blair T, Raymond L. *Histoplasma capsulatum* endocarditis. *Chest* 1981;79(6): 620.
90. Raymond LW, Donaldson JC, Elliott RC, et al. Scars without wounds: Spectrum of delayed manifestations of histoplasmosis outside of the endemic area. *Clin Rev Diagn Imaging* 1980;14(1):37–72.
91. Bradsher RW, Wickre CG, Savage AM, et al. *Histoplasma capsulatum* endocarditis cured by amphotericin B combined with surgery. *Chest* 1980;78(5): 791–795.
92. Blair TP, Waugh RA, Pollack M, et al. *Histoplasma capsulatum* endocarditis. *Am Heart J* 1980;99(6):783–788.
93. Waterhouse G, Burney DP, Prager RL. *Histoplasma capsulatum* endocarditis requiring aortic valve replacement for aortic insufficiency. *South Med J* 1980; 73(5):683–684.
94. Goodwin RA Jr, Shapiro JL, Thurman GH, et al. Disseminated histoplasmosis: Clinical and pathologic correlations. *Medicine* 1980;59(1):1–33.
95. Alexander WJ, Mowry RW, Cobbs CG, et al. Prosthetic valve endocarditis caused by *Histoplasma capsulatum*. *JAMA* 1979;242(13):1399–1400.
96. Olive T, Lagier A, Dumas D, et al. Generalized histoplasmosis with laryngeal localization and endocarditis. *Nouvelle Presse Med* 1978;7(30):2662.
97. Rogers EW, Weyman AE, Noble RJ, et al. Left atrial myxoma infected with *Histoplasma capsulatum*. *Am J Med* 1978;64(4):683–690.
98. Pankey GA. Infective endocarditis: Changing concepts. *Hosp Prac(Off Ed)* 1986;21(3):103–110.
99. Hutton JP, Durham JB, Miller DP, et al. Hyphal forms of *Histoplasma capsulatum*: A common manifestation of intravascular infections. *Arch Path Lab Med* 1985;109(4):330–332.
100. Svirbely JR, Ayers LW, Buesching WJ. Filamentous *Histoplasma capsulatum* endocarditis involving mitral and aortic valve porcine bioprostheses. *Arch Pathol Lab Med* 1985;109(3):273–276.
101. Wilmshurst PT, Venn GE, Eykyn SJ. Histoplasma endocarditis on a stenosed aortic valve presenting as dysphagia and weight loss. *Br Heart J* 1993;70(6): 565–567.
102. Kanawaty DS, Stalker MJ, Munt PW. Nonsurgical treatment of Histoplasma endocarditis involving a bioprosthetic valve. *Chest* 1991;99(1):253–256.
103. Banerjee U, Gupta K, Venugopal P. A case of prosthetic valve endocarditis caused by *Cryptococcus neoformans var. neoformans*. *J Med Vet Mycol* 1997;35(2): 139–141.

104. Reimann HA. Infectious diseases: Annual review of significant publications. *Postgrad Med J* 1971;47(548):332–353.
105. Olavarria R, Fajardo LF. Ophthalmic coccidioidomycosis: Case report and review. *Arch Pathol* 1971;92(3):191–195.
106. Cherry JD, Lloyd CA, Quilty JF, et al. Amphotericin B therapy in children: A review of the literature and a case report. *J Pediatr* 1969;75(6):1063–1069.
107. Heitman L, Cometta A, Hurni M, et al. Right-sided pacemaker endocarditis due to Acremonium species. *Clin Infect Dis* 1997;25(1):158–160.
108. Lucuz C da S, Porto E, Carnciro JJ, et al. Endocarditis in dura mater prosthesis caused by *Acremonium killiense*. *Rev Inst Med Trop Sao Paulo* 1981;23(6): 274–279.
109. Restrepo A, McGinnis MR, Malloch D, et al. Fungal endocarditis caused by *Arnium leporinum* following cardiac surgery. *Sabourandin* 1984;22(3):225–234.
110. Polacheck I, Salkin IF, Kitzes-Cohen N, et al. Endocarditis caused by *Blastoschizomyces capitatus* and taxonomic review of the genus. *J Clin Microbiol* 1992;30(9):2318–2322.
111. Jaffey PB, Hague AK, el-Zaatari M, et al. Disseminated Conidiobolus infection with endocarditis in a cocaine abuser. *Arch Pathol Lab Med* 1990;114(12): 1276–1278.
112. Bryan CS, Smith CW, Berg DE, et al. *Curvularia lunata* endocarditis treated with terbinafine: Case report. *Clin Infect Dis* 1993;16(1):30–32.
113. Kaufman SM. *Curvularia* endocarditis following cardiac surgery. *Am J Clin Pathol* 1971;56(4):466–470.
114. Drouhet E, Guilmet D, Kouvalchouk JF, et al. First human case of *Drechslera longirostrata* mycosis. *Nouvelle Press Medicale* 1982;11(19):3631–3635.
115. Rolston KV, Hopfer RL, Larson DL. Infections caused by *Drechslera* species: Case report and review of the literature. *Rev Infect Dis* 1985;7(4):525–529.
116. Gold WL, Vellend H, Sulit IE, et al. Successful treatment of systemic and local infections due to *Exophiala* species. *Clin Infect Dis* 1994;19(2):339–341
117. Ventia M, Ramirez C, Garau J. *Exophiala dermatitidis* le Hoog from a valvular prosthesis. *Mycopathologia* 1987;99(1):45–46.
118. Roncoroni AJ, Smayevsky J. Arthritis and endocarditis from *Exophiala jeanselmei* infection. *Ann Intern Med* 1988;108(5):773.
119. Guinvarc'h A, Guilbert L, Marmorat-Khuong A, et al. Disseminated *Fusarium solari* infection with endocarditis in a lung transplant patient. *Mycoses* 1998; 41(1–2):59–61.
120. Ho RL, Allevato PA, King P, et al. Cerebral *Paecilomyces javanicus* infection: An ultrastructural study. *Acta Neuropathol* 1986;72(2):134–141.
121. Allevato PA, Ohorodnik JM, Mezger E, et al. *Paecilomyces javanicus* endocarditis of native and prosthetic aortic valve. *Am J Clin Pathol* 1984;82(2):247–252.
122. Kalish SB, Goldschmidt R, Li C, et al. Infective endocarditis caused by *Paecilomyces varioti*. *Am J Clin Pathol* 1982;78(2):249–252.
123. Haldane EV, MacDonald JL, Gittens W, et al. Prosthetic valvular endocarditis due to the fungus *Paecilomyces*. *Can Med Assoc J* 1974;111(9):963–965, 968.
124. DelRossi AJ, Morse D, Spagna PM, et al. Successful management of *Penicillium* endocarditis. *J Thorac Cardiovasc Surg* 1980;80(6):945–947.
125. Heath C, Lendrum JL, Wetherall BL, et al. *Phaeoacremonium parasiticum* infective endocarditis following liver transplantation. *Clin Infect Dis* 1997;25(5): 1251–1252.

126. Engleman RM, Chase RM, Spencer FC, et al. Mycotic infections on prosthetic and homograft heart valves: Report of first case of endocarditis caused by *Hormodendrum dermatitidis. Ann Surg* 1971;173(3):455–461.

127. Juma A. *Phialophora richardsiae* endocarditis of aortic and mitral valves in a diabetic man with a porcine mitral valve. *J Infect* 1993;27(2):173–175.

128. Welty FK, McLeod GX, Ezratty C, et al. *Pseudallescheria boydii* endocarditis of the pulmonic valve in a liver transplant recipient. *Clin Infect Dis* 1992; 15(5):858–860.

129. Raffanti SP, Fyfe B, Carreiro S, et al. Native valve endocarditis due to *Pseudallescheria boydii* in a patient with AIDS. *Rev Infect Dis* 1990;12(6):993–996.

130. Gordon G, Axelrod JL. Case report: Prosthetic valve endocarditis caused by *Pseudallescheria boydii* and *Clostridium limosum. Mycopathologia* 1985;89(3): 129–134.

131. Davis WA, Isner JM, Bracey AW, et al. Disseminated *Pseudallescheria boydii* and pacemaker endocarditis. *Am J Med* 1980;69(6):929–932.

132. Ellenberger C Jr, Sturgill BC. Endogenous *Pseudomonas panophthalmitis. Am J Ophthalmol* 1968;65(4):607–611.

133. Naveh Y, Friedman A, Merzbach D, et al. Endocarditis caused by *Rhodotorula* successfully treated with 5-fluorocytosine. *Br Heart J* 1975;37(1):101–104.

134. Leeber DA, Scher I. *Rhodotorula fungemia* presenting as "endotoxic" shock. *Arch Intern Med* 1969;123(1):78–81.

135. Stein PD, Folkens AT, Hruska KA. *Saccharomyces fungemia. Chest* 1970;58(2): 173–175.

136. Ogihara A, Chino M, Yoshiro H, et al. A case of prosthetic valve endocarditis due to *Scedosporium apiospermum. J Jpn Soc Int Med* 1989;78(3):432–433.

137. Bloom SM, Warner RR, Weitzman I. Maxillary sinusitis: Isolation of *Scedosporium apiospermum*, anamorph of *Petriellidium boydii. Mt Sinai J Med* 1982;49(6): 492–494.

138. Toy EC, Rinaldi MG, Savitch CB, et al. Endocarditis and hip arthritis associated with *Scedosporium inflatum. South Med J* 1990;83(8):957–960.

139. Migrino RQ, Hall GS, Longworth DL. Deep tissue infections caused by *Scopulariopsis brevicollis*: Report of a case of prosthetic valve endocarditis and review. *Clin Infect Dis* 1995;21(3):672–674.

140. Gentry LO, Nasser MM, Kielhofner M. *Scopulariopsis* endocarditis associated with Duran ring valvuloplasty. *Tex Heart Inst J* 1995;22(1):81–85.

141. Lesco-Bornet M, Gueho E, Barbier-Boehm G, et al. Prosthetic valve endocarditis due to *Thermomyces lanuginous* Tsiklinsky: First case report. *J Med Vet Mycol* 1991;29(3):205–209.

142. Nesher N, Erez A, Nezer D, et al. Acute fungal endocarditis due to *Trichosporon beigelii. Harefuah* 1997;132(6):396–398, 447–448.

143. Miralles A, Quiroga J, Farinola T, et al. Recurrent *Trichosporon beigelii* endocarditis after aortic valve replacement. *Cardiovasc Surg* 1994;2(1):119–123.

144. Sidarous MG, O'Reilly MV, Cherubin CE. A case of *Trichosporon beigelii* endocarditis eight years after aortic valve replacement. *Clin Cardiol* 1994;17(4): 215–219.

145. Martinez-Lacasa J, Mana J, Niubo R, et al. Long-term survival of a patient with prosthetic valve endocarditis due to *Trichosporon beigelii. Eur J Clin Microbiol Infect Dis* 1991;10(9):756–758.

146. Keay S, Denning DW, Stevens DA. Endocarditis due to *Trichosporon beigelii*: In vitro susceptibility of isolates and review. *Rev Infect Dis* 1991;13(3):383–386.

147. Reinhart HH, Urbanski DM, Harrington SD, et al. Prosthetic valve endocarditis caused by *Trichosporon beigelii*. *Am J Med* 1988;84(2):355–358.

148. Marier R, Zakhireh B, Downs J, et al. *Trichosporon cutaneum* endocarditis. *Scand J Infect Dis* 1978;10(3):225–226.

149. Vartian CV, Shaes DM, Padhye AA, et al. *Wangiella dermatitidis* endocarditis in an intravenous drug user. *Am J Med* 1985;78(4):703–707.

150. Joly V, Belmatoug N, Leperre A, et al. Pacemaker endocarditis due to *Candida albicans*: Case report and review. *Clin Infect Dis* 1997;25(6):1359–1362.

151. Shmuely H, Kremer I, Sagie A, et al. *Candida tropicalis* multifocal endophthalmitis as the only initial manifestation of pacemaker endocarditis. *Am J Ophthalmol* 1997;123(4):559–560.

152. Reyes CV, Stanley MM, Rippon JW. *Trichosporon beigelii* endocarditis as a complication of peritoneovenous shunt. *Hum Pathol* 1985;16(8):857–859.

153. Wang JH, Liu YC, Lee SS. Candida endocarditis following percutaneous transluminal coronary angioplasty. *Clin Infect Dis* 1998;26(1):205–206.

154. Mertens TE, Low-Beer D. HIV and AIDS: Where is the epidemic going? *Bull World Health Organ* 1996;74(2):121–129.

155. Ramsey ES, Lytle BW. Repair of fungal aortic prosthetic valve endocarditis associated with periannular abscess. *J Heart Valve Dis* 1998;7(2):255–259.

156. Invert T, Dismukes W, Cobb C, et al. Prosthetic valve endocarditis. *Circulation* 1984;69:223–232.

157. Arnett E, Robert W. Prosthetic valve endocarditis. *Am J Cardiol* 1979;38:281–292.

158. Gordon S, Keys T. Bloodstream infections in patients with prosthetic cardiac valves. *Semin Thorac Cardiovasc Surg* 1995;7:2–6.

159. Nasser RM, Melgar GR, Longworth DL, et al. Incidence and risk of developing fungal prosthetic valve endocarditis after nosocomial candidemia. *Am J Med* 1997;103:25–32.

160. Nguyen MH, Nguyen ML, Yu VL, et al. Candida prosthetic valve endocarditis: Prospective study of six cases and review of the literature. *Clin Infect Dis* 1996;22:262–267.

161. Von Reyn CF, Levy BS, Arbeit RD, et al. Infective endocarditis: An analysis based on strict case definitions. *Ann Intern Med* 1981;94(4):505–518.

162. Fang G, et al. Prosthetic valve endocarditis resulting from nosocomial bacteremia. *Ann Intern Med* 1993;119(7):560–567.

163. Durack DT, Lukes AS, Bright DK. New criteria for diagnosis of infective endocarditis: Utilization of specific echocardiographic findings. *Am J Med* 1994;96:200–209.

164. Terrell CL, Hughes CE. Antifungal agents used for deep-seated mycotic infections. *Mayo Clin Proc* 1992;67(1):69–91.

165. Vandeputte J, Wachtel JL, Stiller ET. Amphotericins A & B, antifungal antibiotics produced by a streptomyces. *Antibiotic Annual 1955–1956*. New York, NY. Medical Encyclopedia, Inc. pp 587–591.

166. Medoff G, Dismukes WE, Meade RH III, et al. A new therapeutic approach to Candida infections. *Arch Intern Med* 1972,130:241–245.

167. Odds FC. Interactions among amphotericin B, 5-fluorocytosine, ketoconazole and miconazole against pathogenic fungi in vitro antimicrobial agents. *Chemotherapy* 1982;22:63–70.

168. Iwen PC, Miller NG, McFadden HW Jr. Treatment of murine pulmonary

cryptococcosis with ketoconazole and amphotericin B. *J Infect Dis* 1984;149: 650.

169. Hardman JG, Limbird LE (eds.) *Goodman & Gilman's The Pharmacological Basis of Therapeutics.* 9th ed. New York, NY. McGraw-Hill, 1995.

170. Joyce FS, Tingleff J, Pettersson G. The Ross operation in the treatment of prosthetic aortic valve endocarditis. *Semin Thorac Cardiovasc Surg* 1995;7: 38–46.

171. Roel JD, Gamba A, Curone M, et al. Successful medical treatment of *Candida tropicalis* in prosthetic valve endocarditis. *Medicina B Aires* 1998;58(3):301–302.

172. Thakur RK, Skelcy KM, Kahn RN, et al. Successful treatment of Candida prosthetic valve endocarditis with a combination of fluconazole and amphotericin B. *Crit Care Med* 1994;22(4):712–714.

173. Czwerwiec FS, Bilsker MS, Kamerman ML, et al. Long-term survival after fluconazole therapy of candidal prosthetic valve endocarditis. *Am J Med* 1993; 94(5):545–546.

174. Dupont B, Drouhet E, Lapresle C. First medical cure of Candida endocarditis on a valve prosthesis. *Ann Med Int* 1977;128(8–9):699–703.

175. Muehrcke DD, Lytle BW, Cosgrove DM III. Surgical and long-term antifungal therapy for fungal prosthetic valve endocarditis. *Ann Thorac Surg* 1995;60(3): 538–543.

176. Pfaller MA. Epidemiology of fungal infections: The promise of molecular typing. *Clin Infect Dis* 1995;20:1535–1539.

Index

Color Appendix

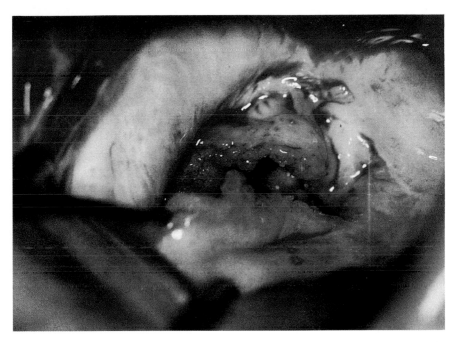

Chapter 2, Figure 1. Mitral valve endocarditis intraoperative view involving both the anterior and posterior leaflets, a "kissing" lesion. Reproduced with permission: Antunes, MJ. *Mitral Valve Repair*. Starnberg, Germany, Verlag RS Schulz, 1989. p 49.

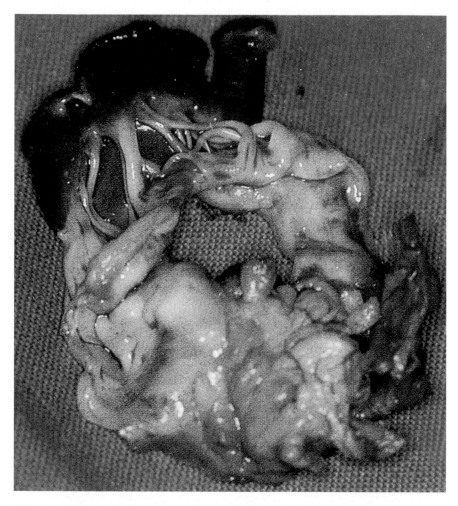

Chapter 2, Figure 2. Fungal mitral valve endocarditis with extensive destruction of the anterior leaflet. Note the large size. Reproduced with permission: Antunes MJ. *Mitral Valve Repair*. Starnberg, Germany, Verlag RS Schulz, 1989. p 49.

Chapter 2, Figure 4. Normal atrioventricular valve. The thin endothelial layer is represented with the occasional hyperchromatic oblong nucleus covering the valve surface. The endothelium is commonly abraded during process and may not be seen on routine examination. The layering of valve material is vaguely discernible with hematoxylin and eosin stain. Trichrome stain highlights collagen bundles with a deep blue hue. The fibrosa contains densely packed collagen bundles. Elastic von Giesen delineates the elastic fibers of the ventricularis with silver, resulting in a black appearance.

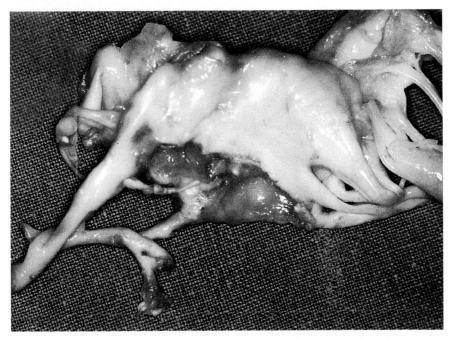

Chapter 2, Figure 3. Ruptured chordae tendineae of mitral valve endocarditis. This patient had been operated on for extensive infective endocarditis of the aortic valve and mitral valve vegetations were found incidentally. Reproduced with permission: Antunes MJ. *Mitral Valve Repair*. Starnberg, Germany, Verlag RS Schulz, 1989. p 51.

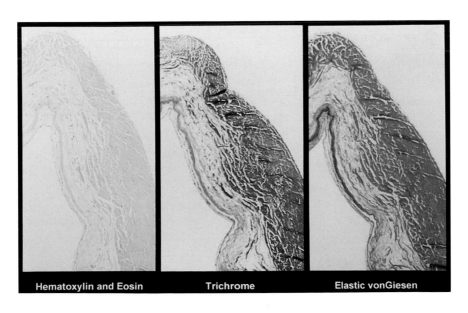

Hematoxylin and Eosin   Trichrome   Elastic vonGiesen

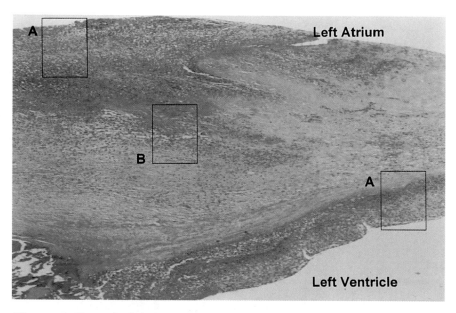

Chapter 2, Figure 6. Infective endocarditis vegetation. A gradient of inflammatory cells present in the vegetation is apparent, with fewer inflammatory cells over the atrial and ventricular surfaces (A) and numerous inflammatory cells at the vegetation and supporting connective tissue junction (B). The vegetation is composed primarily of fibrin, platelets, inflammatory cells and microorganisms.

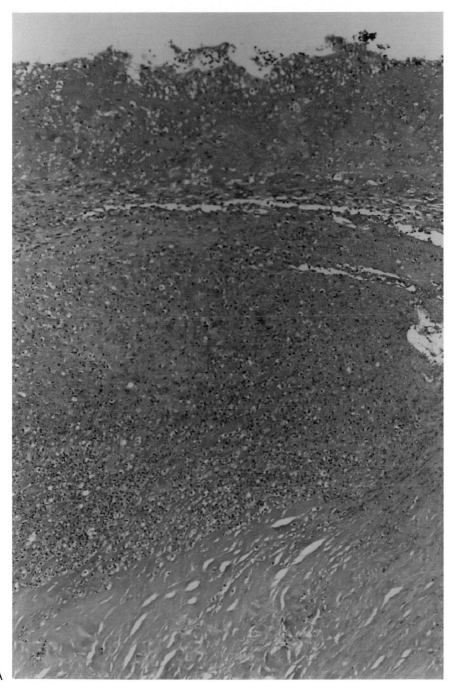

A

Chapter 2, Figure 7. Higher magnification corresponding to Figure 6, area delimited in (A). Note the paucity of inflammatory cells within the dense eosinophilic fibrin matrix at the vegetation surface.

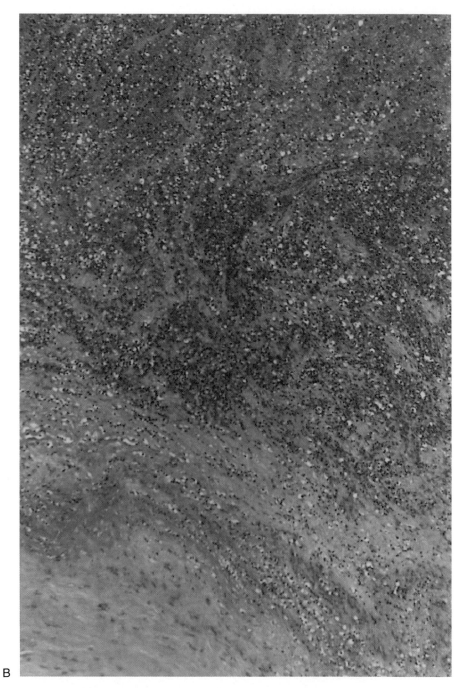

B

Chapter 2, Figure 7. *(continued)* (B) The inflammatory cells are seen in dense collections within the valve tissue.

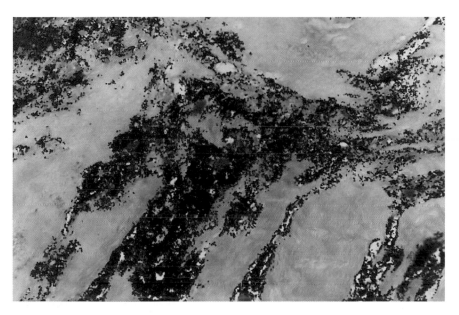

Chapter 2, Figure 8. Tissue Gram's stain highlights the dense collections of cocci deep within the vegetation. The area depicted corresponds to Figure 6, area delimited in (B).

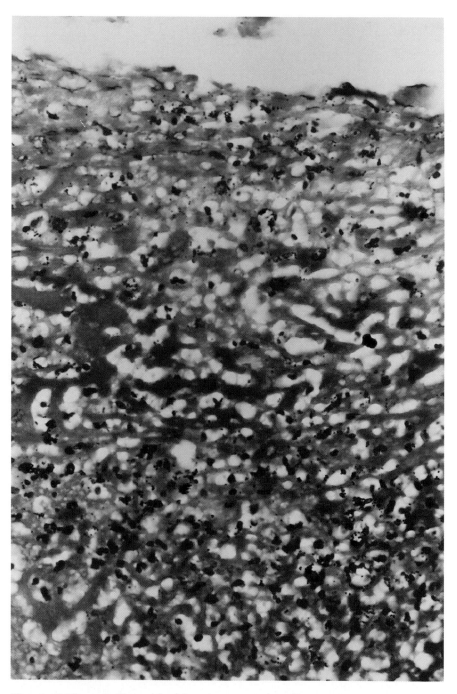

Chapter 2, Figure 9. Exosaccharide polymers produced by some bacteria along with fibrin polymers create a seal over the vegetation (a "biofilm") which may inhibit the diffusion of antimicrobial drugs into the deeper layers within the vegetation.

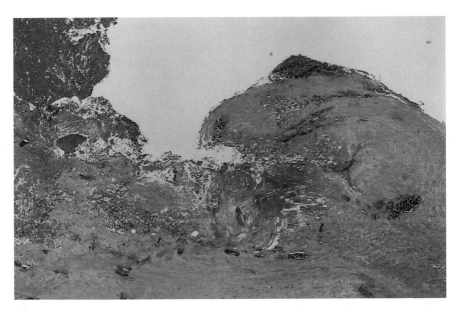

Chapter 2, Figure 10. Virulent microorganisms may produce colonies that are visible on routine hematoxylin and eosin microscopic preparations. The organism in this case was *Staphylococcus aureus*.

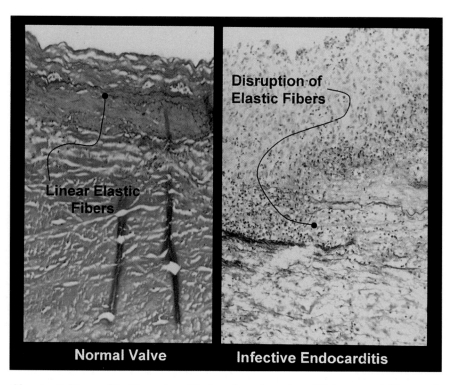

Chapter 2, Figure 11. Normal and infected aortic valve with intact and disrupted elastic layers, respectively, stained with elastic von Giesen. Neutrophils are evident in the background of the infected specimen.

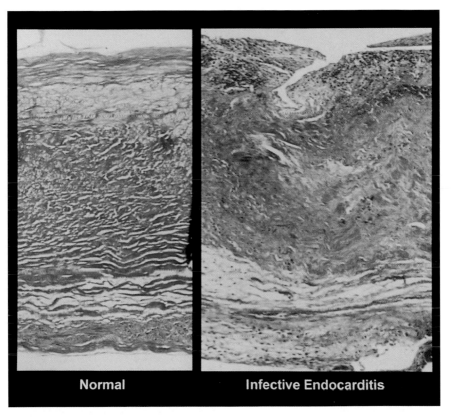

Normal **Infective Endocarditis**

Chapter 2, Figure 12. Normal and infected aortic valve stained with trichrome, highlighting the collagen bundles of the fibrosa blue. The fulminant inflammatory process destroys the fibrillar organization and integrity of the valve.

A11

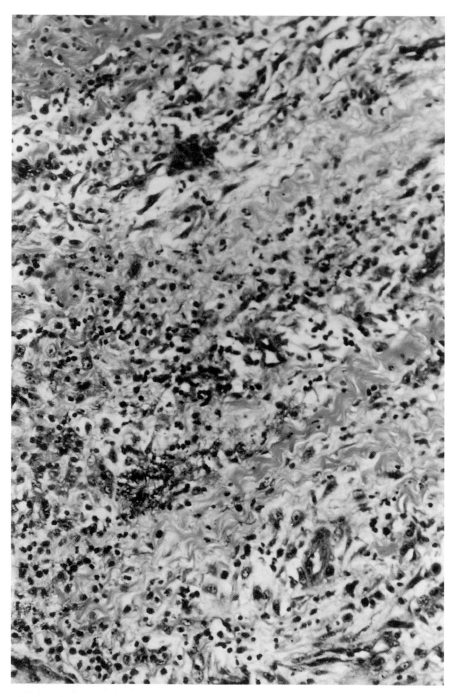

Chapter 2, Figure 13. Trichrome stain of infected aortic valve. Neutrophils, extravasated red blood cells and edema separate the fibrosa collagen bundles. (Magnification 400X.)

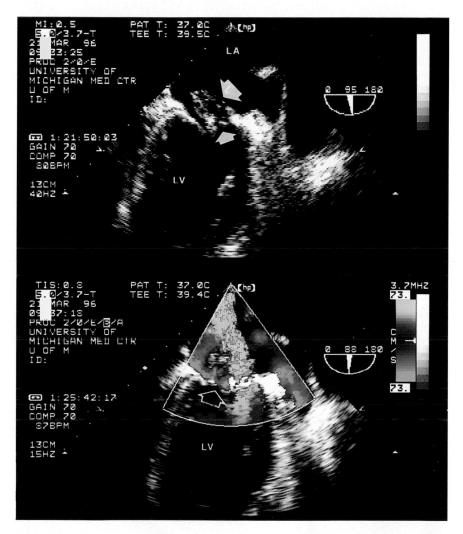

Chapter 6, Figure 10. Top panel: Large anterior mitral leaflet vegetation (large arrow) with accompanying perforation (small arrow). Bottom panel: Color flow Doppler demonstrates large regurgitant jet through perforation. Note site of jet origin distinct from point of leaflet coaptation with posterior mitral leaflet (open arrow). LA = left atrium; LV = left ventricle.

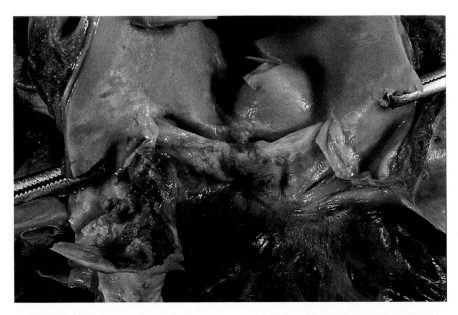

Chapter 9, Figure 2. Photo of an aortic native valve demonstrating the vegetations that typically occur at the line of valve closure on the ventricular side.

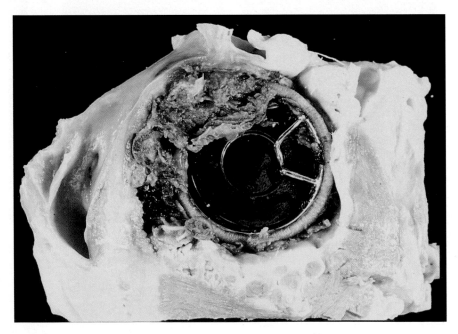

Chapter 9, Figure 3. Vegetations on a prosthetic valve in the aortic position. The vegetations in PVE commonly occur along the sewing ring, which can lead to periprosthetic leaks.

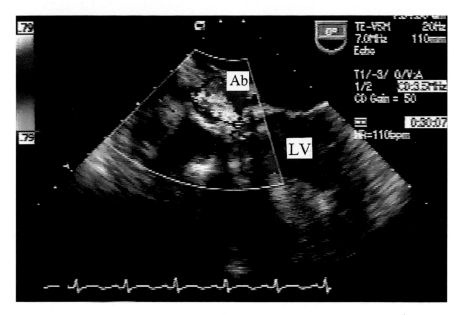

Chapter 12, Figure 6. Color doppler demonstrates flow into the abscess cavity (Ab) from the left ventricle (LV) during systole. The left atrium is seen in the upper portion of the figure in close proximity to the abscess cavity.

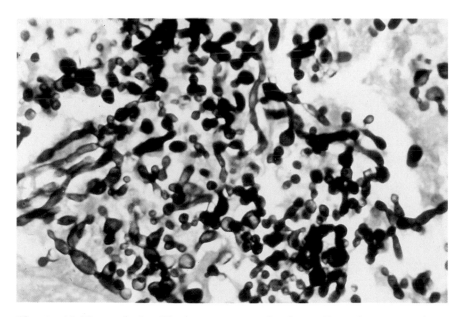

Chapter 15, Figure 1. *Candida* organisms seen by Gomori's methenamine silver stain.

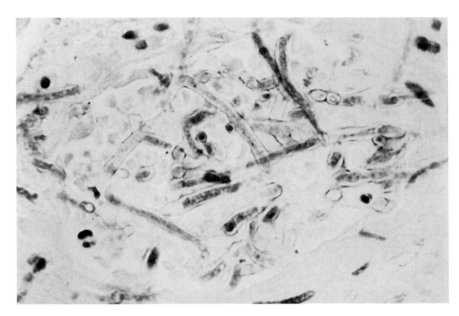

Chapter 15, Figure 2. *Aspergillus* organisms seen by hematoxylin and eosin stain.

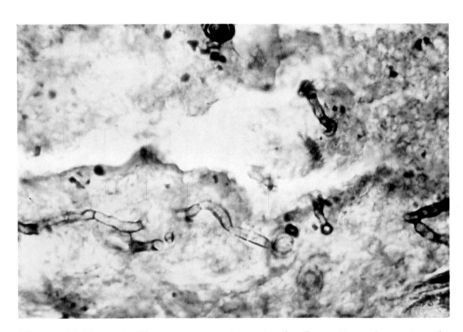

Chapter 15, Figure 3. *Blastomyces* organisms seen by Gomori's methenamine silver stain.